Challenging Concepts in Neurosurgery

Titles in the Challenging Concepts in series

Anaesthesia (Edited by Dr Phoebe Syme, Dr Robert Jackson, and Professor Tim Cook)

Cardiovascular Medicine (Edited by Dr Aung Myat, Dr Shouvik Haldar, and Professor Simon Redwood)

Emergency Medicine (Edited by Dr Sam Thenabadu, Dr Fleur Cantle, and Dr Chris Lacy)

Infectious Diseases and Clinical Microbiology (Edited by Dr Amber Arnold and Professor George E. Griffin)

Interventional Radiology (Edited by Dr Irfan Ahmed, Dr Miltiadis Krokidis, and Dr Tarun Sabharwal)

Neurology (Edited by Dr Krishna Chinthapalli, Dr Nadia Magdalinou, and Professor Nicholas Wood)

Obstetrics and Gynaecology (Edited by Dr Natasha Hezelgrave, Dr Danielle Abbott, and Professor Andrew H. Shennan)

Oncology (Edited by Dr Madhumita Bhattacharyya, Dr Sarah Payne, and Professor Iain McNeish)

Oral and Maxillofacial Surgery (Edited by Mr Matthew Idle and Group Captain Andrew Monaghan)

Respiratory Medicine (Edited by Dr Lucy Schomberg, Dr Elizabeth Sage, and Dr Nick Hart)

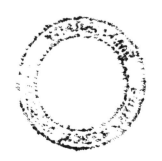

Challenging Concepts in Neurosurgery
Cases with Expert Commentary

Edited by

Mr Robin Bhatia MA PhD FRCS(SN)
Consultant Spinal Neurosurgeon, Great Western Hospitals NHS Foundation
Trust & Oxford University Hospitals NHS Trust, Oxford, UK

Mr Ian Sabin BMSc(Hons) MB ChB FRCS(Eng) FRCS(Ed)
Consultant Neurosurgeon at St Barts and the Royal London NHS Trust and at
The Wellington Hospital, London, UK

Series editors

Dr Aung Myat BSc (Hons) MBBS MRCP
BHF Clinical Research Training Fellow, King's College London British Heart Foundation
Centre of Research Excellence, Cardiovascular Division, St Thomas' Hospital, London, UK

Dr Shouvik Haldar MBBS MRCP
Electrophysiology Research Fellow & Cardiology SpR, Heart Rhythm Centre, NIHR Cardiovascular
Biomedical Research Unit, Royal Brompton & Harefield NHS Foundation Trust, Imperial College
London, London, UK

Professor Simon Redwood MD FRCP
Professor of Interventional Cardiology and Honorary Consultant Cardiologist, King's College London
British Heart Foundation Centre of Research Excellence, Cardiovascular Division and Guy's and
St Thomas' NHS Foundation Trust, Dr Thomas' Hospital, London, UK

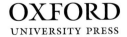

OXFORD
UNIVERSITY PRESS

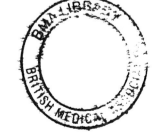

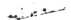

OXFORD
UNIVERSITY PRESS

Great Clarendon Street, Oxford, OX2 6DP,
United Kingdom

Oxford University Press is a department of the University of Oxford.
It furthers the University's objective of excellence in research, scholarship,
and education by publishing worldwide. Oxford is a registered trade mark of
Oxford University Press in the UK and in certain other countries

Published in the United States of America by Oxford University Press
198 Madison Avenue, New York, NY 10016, United States of America

British Library Cataloguing in Publication Data

Data available

Library of Congress Control Number: 2014957581

ISBN 978-0-19-965640-0

Printed in Great Britain by
Ashford Colour Press Ltd, Gosport, Hampshire

PREFACE

What is a challenge in neurosurgery? It might be better to ask what isn't. Of all the surgical specialties, neurosurgery is arguably the discipline with the greatest number of controversial and unresolved issues, and these confront the neurosurgeon whenever he or she manages a patient with a central or peripheral nervous problem.

For instance, one of the first and most 'basic' operations a neurosurgical trainee will learn is burr hole evacuation of a chronic subdural haematoma (CSDH). What could be challenging about this simple operation? Perhaps the training neurosurgeon should remember that the aetiology and natural history of CSDH; when (and when not) to carry out burr hole drainage; how many burr holes to drill; whether or not to leave a drain; the outcomes of burr hole versus twist drill versus craniotomy for CSDH, represent just a few of the hotly debated and largely unresolved issues to this day. Before putting knife to skin, the neurosurgeon must supply answers to these important questions, but how is this possible when the answers are not clearly known?

The purpose of this book is to present twenty-two case-based topics in neurosurgery, and our remit to contributing authors was to tackle the questions that frequently get asked, presenting evidence-based answers in an easy-to-read manner. We chose these cases after surveying both junior and senior neurosurgeons and asking 'What challenges you in your practice?' Somewhat surprisingly, the challenge was to be found in the everyday cases, rather than the atypical.

Textbooks of neurosurgery tend to contain editor bias in topic selection. *Challenging Concepts in Neurosurgery* reflects the subject matter and questions that are important to neurosurgical clinicians, both in training and as a guide to senior neurosurgeons who wish to read concise and up-to-date overviews of a broad spectrum of neurosurgical pathology.

There are clear benefits of learning by the case-based approach. Indeed, the case-based discussion has become a pivotal tool of learning and assessment laid out by the Intercollegiate Surgical Curriculum Programme in the UK, and is gaining popularity across the world. The wide scope of authors from different units in the UK and overseas helps to bring together in one book varying perspectives on patient management, and there are clear benefits of allowing trainees and expert reviewers to co-write—most notably, that one asks the questions we all want to ask and the other supplies the answers.

Robin Bhatia
Ian Sabin

CONTENTS

EXPERTS

Tipu Z. Aziz
Professor of Neurosurgery,
Nuffield Department of Surgical Sciences,
Oxford University, Oxford, UK

Rolfe Birch
Consultant in Charge,
War Nerve Injuries Clinic at the Defence Medical
Rehabilitation Centre,
Headley Court, Leatherhead, UK

Ciaran Bolger
Professor of Clinical Neuroscience, RCSI, Consultant
Neurosurgeon, Department of Neurosurgery,
Beaumont Hospital, Dublin, Ireland

Robert Bradford
Consultant Neurosurgeon, National Hospital for
Neurology & Neurosurgery, London, UK

Adrian Casey
Consultant Neurosurgeon, Royal National
Orthopaedic Hospital, Stanmore (Spinal Unit) and
National Hospital for Neurology & Neurosurgery,
London, UK

David Choi
Consultant Neurosurgeon, National Hospital for
Neurology & Neurosurgery, London, UK

Paul Gardner
Associate Professor of Neurological Surgery,
Executive Vice Chairman, Surgical Services, Co-
Director, Center for Skull Base Surgery, UPMC
Presbyterian, Pittsburgh, MA, USA

Alexander L. Green
Consultant Neurosurgeon, Nuffield Department of
Surgical Sciences, Oxford University, Oxford, UK

Nick Haden
Consultant Neurosurgeon, Derriford Hospital,
Plymouth, UK

Peter J. Hutchinson
Professor of Neurosurgery, NIHR Research
Professor, University of Cambridge, Academic
Division of Neurosurgery, Addenbrooke's Hospital,
Cambridge, UK

Michael D. Jenkinson
Consultant Neurosurgeon at The Walton Centre NHS
Foundation Trust, Liverpool, UK

Neil Kitchen
Consultant Neurosurgeon, National Hospital
for Neurology & Neurosurgery and Institute of
Neurology, London, UK

Henry Marsh
Senior Consultant Neurosurgeon, St George's
Healthcare NHS Trust, London, UK

Andrew McEvoy
Consultant Neurosurgeon, National Hospital
for Neurology & Neurosurgery and Institute of
Neurology, London, UK

Mary Murphy
Neurosurgical Tutor at the Royal College of
Surgeons, National Hospital for Neurology &
Neurosurgery, London, UK

Kevin O'Neill
Consultant Neurosurgeon, Charing Cross, St Mary's
and Hammersmith hospitals, Imperial College
Healthcare NHS Trust, London, UK

Ian Sabin
Consultant Neurosurgeon, St Barts and the Royal
London NHS Trust and at Wellington Hospital,
London, UK

George Samandouras
Victor Horsley Department of Neurosurgery,
National Hospital for Neurology & Neurosurgery,
London, UK

Thomas Santarius
Consultant Neurosurgeon, Addenbrooke's Hospital,
Cambridge University Hospitals NHS Trust,
Cambridge, UK

Patrick Statham
Consultant Neurosurgeon, Spire Edinburgh
Hospitals, Edinburgh, UK

Nigel Suttner
Consultant Neurosurgeon, Department of
Neurosurgery, Institute of Neurological Sciences,
Glasgow, UK

Dominic N. P. Thompson
Consultant in Paediatric Neurosurgery, Great
Ormond Street Hospital for Children, NHS
Foundation Trust, Great Ormond Street, London, UK

Raghu Vindindlacheruvu
Consultant Neurosurgeon, Spire Hartswood Private
Hospital, Brentwood, and Spire Roding Hospital,
Redbridge, Essex, UK

> **❝ Expert comment**
>
> It is now widely accepted that subdural haematomas (SDH) result from the rupture of a dural bridging vein into the weakly adherent dural border cell layer, allowing blood to collect between the dura and the arachnoid mater (see Figure 1.2). As a consequence of cerebral atrophy in elderly patients, head trauma results in a greater displacement of brain in relation to dura. Bridging veins are subjected to a greater degree of stretch and, thus, SDHs may develop after relatively minor head injuries.

> **✪ Learning point** Microarchitecture of the dura mater
>
> The dura mater is composed of fibroblasts and a large amount of collagen. The arachnoid barrier cells are supported by a basement membrane (black) and bound together by numerous tight junctions (red). The dural border cells layer is formed by flattened fibroblasts, with no tight junctions and no intercellular collagen. It is, therefore, a relatively loose layer positioned between firm dura mater and arachnoid. The subdural space is a potential space that can form within the dural border cell layer. (Figure 1.2).

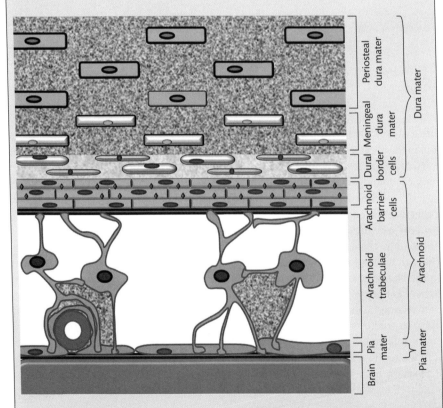

Figure 1.2 Schematic section through the dura and arachnoid mater; it is the dural border cell layer that separates in CSDH [5].

Santarius, T, et al. (2010), 'Working toward rational and evidence-based treatment of cSDH', Clinical Neurosurgery, 57.

> ✓ **Evidence base** Pathogenesis of chronic subdural haematoma
>
> The presence of blood in the subdural space elicits a complex inflammatory cascade involving proliferation of dural border cells, migration of macrophages, formation of granulation tissue, and angiogenesis [5]. In the majority of cases, this process ultimately results in resorption of the haematoma, but should this fail, the haematoma may grow and become symptomatic.
>
> Chronic subdural haematoma (CSDH) often presents in patients whose acute subdural haematoma (ASDH) was initially not symptomatic enough for the patient to seek medical attention. Many groups have studied the mechanisms underlying the evolution of ASDH into CSDH and it is likely to involve an interplay of multiple pathways, leading to an increase in the haematoma fluid volume and, consequently, mass effect. Traditionally, it was thought that the hydrolysis of acute blood products into smaller molecules increased the oncotic pressure of the haematoma, thereby drawing in water by osmosis [6]. This hypothesis fell out of favour following the publication of Markwalder's landmark paper, which first demonstrated that CSDH fluid osmolality is the same as that of blood and cerebrospinal fluid (CSF) [7].
>
> Rebleeding is one of the mechanisms that may contribute to haematoma growth. There is an abundance of coagulation inhibitors and fibrinolytic factors in the subdural fluid. High levels of tissue plasminogen activator (tPA) have been found in the subdural fluid and its concentration is predictive of recurrence [8]. Vascular endothelial growth factor (VEGF) is also found at higher concentrations in the subdural fluid [9]. VEGF is a pro-angiogenic factor and is also known to increase the 'leakiness' of capillary junctions.
>
> The hypothesis of rebleeding is supported by the frequent observation of mixed attenuation blood on CT and mixed consistency haematoma intra-operatively. Furthermore, it is hypothesized that the serial dilution of anticoagulant and fibrinolytic factors by thorough lavage may be responsible for at least some of the therapeutic efficacy of burr hole drainage.

Indications and techniques for surgical intervention

Given the relatively low morbidity and mortality associated with evacuation of CSDH, symptomatic presentation merits strong consideration for surgical evacuation. Non-surgical management is reserved for cases at both extremes in the spectrum of severity of their clinical presentation. At one end of the scale, an asymptomatic collection with minimal mass effect may be managed expectantly. At the other end, patients who are otherwise very unwell or moribund may be offered palliation.

Notably, there is a considerable variety of surgical and anaesthetic techniques that can be employed to evacuate CSDH, allowing clinicians to customize treatment to the characteristics of their patient. In the simplest of circumstances, where the patient is fit enough, general anaesthetic and burr hole evacuation is the most common technique used in most UK units. Either one or two burr holes can be used and, although there is no clear evidence supporting one over the other [5], the general consensus is that, where practicable, two burr holes allow a more complete evacuation. General anaesthetic appears to be more comfortable to patients and surgeons. It allows a higher standard of surgical technique in terms of asepsis, retention of subdural air, drain placement, wound closure, to be achieved, etc.

> ⓰ **Expert comment** One versus two burr holes
>
> While individual surgeons may have their own preference, it is generally agreed that two burr holes allow more thorough evacuation and irrigation, which in itself is probably associated with a better outcome [10]. Taussky et al. demonstrated a reduction in the incidence of recurrence where two burr holes were used [11]. Conversely, Han et al. found a 2% ($n = 51$) recurrence rate for one burr hole, compared with 7% ($n = 129$) where two burr holes were used [12]. Crucially, both of these studies were retrospective, such that there was no randomization process or equipoise. The marked disparity between them is, therefore, more likely to reflect differences in the conditions and patients being treated, rather than the technique employed.
>
> A recent systematic review has found no difference in outcome between the use of one and two burr holes [13]. As a treatment of choice we use two burr holes. One burr hole may be considered if the CSDH is more localized or the procedure is performed under local anaesthetic.

> ➕ **Clinical tip**
>
> The position of burr holes should be based on CT, in order to span as much of the haematoma as possible and allow conversion to craniotomy if required.
>
> Copious lavage with warm isotonic solution should be used until the effluent is clear. Some surgeons use a Jaques catheter to irrigate in different directions and aid complete evacuation.
>
> Over-enthusiastic advancement of the catheter into remote parts of the subdural space may result in bleeding. Irrigation with Jaques catheter alone may significantly prolong the length of the operation and it may be prudent to omit this step in high-risk surgical candidates, in whom a shorter operating time may be preferable.
>
> Closing the dependent (usually parietal) burr hole first in a strictly watertight fashion allows the subdural space to be filled with irrigation fluid, reducing the volume of pneumocephalus and the risk of recurrence.
>
> Patient positioning is important. Sandbags under the ipsilateral shoulder allow the side of the head to be almost horizontal without placing too much strain on the neck. Strapping the patient to the operating table allows safe tilting of the table, to bring the frontal burr hole to the highest point of the head prior to closure.
>
> Using a high-speed drill enables the creation of a tangential frontal burr hole, which enables passing of the drain at an angle closer to parallel than perpendicular in relation to the brain surface. This may be relevant, especially in cases with a thick skull.

In instances where the patient is unfit for general anaesthetic, but generally cooperative, infiltration with local anaesthetic and scalp block can be used. In this case, the shorter operating time of a single burr hole may be preferable.

A second surgical option for evacuation is twist drill craniostomy (TDC) and closed-system drainage. Here, a small hole is drilled, 1cm anterior to the coronal suture, above the superior temporal line or over the maximum thickness of the subdural collection. Although morbidity and mortality is similar to burr hole evacuation (apart from a higher risk of recurrence with TDC), it can be performed at the bedside under local anaesthetic, providing a safe treatment modality in unfit patients, while reducing the costs of running an operating theatre [14].

Finally, craniotomy remains an option at the surgeon's disposal in selected cases. Craniotomy was the treatment of choice until the publication of a paper in 1964, comparing craniotomy to burr hole evacuation in sixty-nine patients [15], which showed improved functional outcome and lower recurrence rate following burr hole evacuation. These findings were subsequently confirmed in a number of other studies over the following two decades. However, mini-craniotomies remain useful, particularly in the context of multiple subdural membranes, solid haematoma, re-accumulation, or failure of brain expansion. Modern minicraniotomy probably has a similar risk and benefit profile as burr hole evacuation, but thus far a direct comparison of these two techniques has not been reported in the literature.

❝ Expert comment Outcomes in modern chronic subdural haematoma surgery

Surgical treatment of symptomatic CSDH results in a rapid improvement of patient symptoms and a favourable outcome in excess of 80% of patients [16]. However, there are a number of rare, but recognized early complications, including acute subdural haematoma, tension pneumocephalus, and cerebral infarction (Table 1.2). Recurrence rates in various series are approximately between 10 and 20% [5,17], but some papers have reported rates between 5 and 30%. Post-operative seizures occur in 3–10% of patients, but there is no evidence to support prophylactic anticonvulsant use [18].

Table 1.2 Intracranial complications of CSDH drainage [32]. The overall rate of intracranial complications in this series of 500 consecutive cases was 4.6%. Recurrence is considered separately.

Complication	Rate
Acute subdural haematoma	2.6%
Tension pneumocephalus	0.8%
Cerebral infarction	0.4%
Intracerebral haemorrhage	0.2%
Extradural haematoma	0.2%
Subdural empyema	0.2%

Mori, K. and Maeda, M. (2001). 'Surgical treatment of chronic subdural hematoma in 500 consecutive cases: clinical characteristics, surgical outcome, complications, and recurrence rate', Neurologia medico-chirurgica, 41 (8), 371-81.

✪ Learning point Non-operative management

Recognition of biochemical cascades producing a localized procoagulant and angiogenic state raises the possibility of using anti-inflammatory drugs, such as corticosteroids, as an alternative or adjuvant to surgery. Steroids have been shown to inhibit tPA activity [19] and VEGF expression [20] among others. Despite multiple reports of steroid use in CSDH management [21,22], there is a distinct lack of good quality clinical studies showing any therapeutic efficacy in CSDH, and the rationale for their use is largely theoretical. At present, the further elucidation of biochemical pathways, with the promise of potential pharmaceutical targets, remains an area of important academic interest.

Anticoagulation and anti-platelet agents in CSDH

Anticoagulation with warfarin and other drugs has been associated with both occurrence [23] and recurrence of CSDH. As a consequence of widespread use among elderly patients with cardiovascular co-morbidities, therapeutic anticoagulation is frequently encountered in patients presenting with CSDH and, therefore, merits a thorough understanding and effective management.

Table 1.3 Pharmacokinetic properties of a commercially-available prothrombin complex concentrate as derived from healthy volunteers.

Component	Median half-life (h)	Range (h)
Factor II	60	25–135
Factor VII	4	2–9
Factor IX	17	10–127
Factor X	31	17–44
Protein C	47	9–122
Protein S	49	33–83

Source data from: www.medicines.org.uk

> **Expert comment**
>
> The decision as to whether to resume anticoagulant or anticoagulation therapy after evacuation is more challenging. A multi-disciplinary discussion between the neurosurgeon, general practitioner, and possibly cardiologist should consider the patients clinical status and indication for anticoagulation. It is vital that the patient understands the pros and cons of starting and withholding the anticoagulation treatment.

Warfarin inhibits vitamin K-dependent synthesis of coagulation factors II, VII, IX, and X in the liver, which in turn blocks the extrinsic coagulation cascade, thus prolonging prothrombin time (PT) and INR. The desired degree of anticoagulation is determined by the risk of thromboembolism from the underlying condition.

The principle behind reversing anticoagulation with warfarin is to restore normal circulating concentrations of coagulation factors, which can broadly be achieved in two ways. The first is to directly transfuse clotting factors, with the dose of products depending on body weight and degree of anticoagulation. This first method is quick, but expensive and its effect is short-lived (Table 1.3). The second is to supplement vitamin K, enterally or intravenously. This allows the liver to resume synthesis of vitamin K-dependent clotting factors, a process that requires hours to days. By using a combination of blood products and vitamin K, a normal coagulation profile can be achieved throughout the entire peri- and post-operative periods, allowing safe surgical intervention.

For atrial fibrillation, the risk of thromboembolic events is 2.03% per year in the absence of therapeutic anticoagulation, falling to 1.15% for patients taking warfarin [24]. Here, the target INR is 2.5 (2.0–3.0). In contrast, the risk from prosthetic heart valves may be as high as 22% [25] and the target INR is accordingly higher—3.5 (3.0–4.0). While there is no doubt that anticoagulation increases the risk of chronic subdural haematoma [5,16], there is a distinct lack of data to quantify the risks resulting from restarting anticoagulation and its timing. A recent systematic review by Chari et al summarizes the relevant evidence [26].

> **Expert comment**
>
> Antiplatelet agents, such as aspirin, clopidogrel, and dipyridamole are another important consideration in the management of CSDH [16]. While there is clear evidence that they promote occurrence, their effect on recurrence is less clear. In addition, there are no studies to determine the effect of aspirin on perioperative bleeding in intracranial surgery, but a recent survey showed neurosurgeons prefer to discontinue it's use, on average, 7 days before an elective procedure [27]. On this basis, two general principles apply. First, antiplatelet agents should be stopped the moment CSDH is diagnosed, whether the patient is likely to be a candidate for surgery or not. Secondly, if neurological status is stable, one might consider postponing surgery. In instances where early surgical intervention is required, we prefer to transfuse one pool of platelets immediately prior to surgery, with the possibility of further transfusions in the initial post-operative days.

Use of subdural drains

The reduction in pressure and/or mass effect following surgical evacuation allows the brain to gradually re-expand and fill up the space occupied by the haematoma. Filling that space with irrigation fluid reduces the amount of air trapped in the space. Fluid drained via a dependent drain facilitates brain re-expansion. The drain acts as a valve, where the forces moving the fluid out of the intracranial cavity are systolic brain expansion and the syphoning effect of the dependent drain. Both, but especially the latter are much diminished if air is trapped in the subdural space. The amount of air in the subdural space has been shown to be associated with recurrence [28–30].

Subdural drains permit continuing drainage of blood and irrigation fluid after surgical treatment. They are left in situ for an arbitrary 48 hours, which is thought to balance the risk of recurrence from inadequate brain re-expansion against the potential for infection. There is class I evidence that they reduce the incidence of recurrence and 6-month mortality, while improving functional status at discharge [3].

> ⊕ **Clinical tip** Inserting subdural drains
>
> Where drains are used, they should be inserted via the frontal burr hole and directed anteriorly, as this is an area in which the collection persists the longest. Placement of the drain via the frontal burr hole has been associated with a lower risk of recurrence [31]. It is important to direct the drain parallel to the inside of the calvarium in order to avoid inadvertent parenchymal insertion and intracerebral bleeding. Drilling the burr hole tangentially with a high-speed drill, rather than a perforator will help achieve this aim. While a dedicated subdural drain is yet to be developed, the softest and most flexible drain available should be used.
>
> Always check that drains are working at the end of the procedure and later on the ward. Drainage bags should be placed in a dependent position, and it is important to ensure that nursing staff are aware of the importance of continually maintaining dependency of the drain.

A final word from the expert

As more patients survive into their ninth and tenth decades, not only will the incidence of CSDH continue to rise, but surgeons will be faced with a patient population with an increasingly complex profile of medical co-morbidities. In particular, the issue of anticoagulation is likely to become more pertinent. Further research should be directed towards establishing evidence-based guidelines for resuming anticoagulation and antiplatelet medication after CSDH surgery. Surgery will remain the mainstay of treatment of patients with CSDH, but further work is also needed to understand the rationale efficacy of various aspects of the surgical technique, and to refine indications for the different surgical techniques used, especially for craniotomy and twist-drill craniostomy.

References

1. Evans G, Luddington R, Baglin T. Beriplex P/N reverses severe warfarin-induced overanticoagulation immediately and completely in patients presenting with major bleeding. Br J Haematol 2001; 115(4): 998–1001.

2. Santarius T, Hutchinson PJ. Chronic subdural haematoma: time to rationalize treatment? Br J Neurosurg 2004; 18(4): 328–32.

3. Santarius T, Kirkpatrick PJ, Ganesan D, et al. Use of drains versus no drains after burrhole evacuation of chronic subdural haematoma—a randomised controlled trial. Lancet 2009; 374(9695): 1067–73.

4. George J, Bleasdale S, Singleton SJ.Causes and prognosis of delirium in elderly patients admitted to a DGH. Age Ageing 1997; 26: 423–7.

5. Santarius T, Kirkpatrick PJ, Kolias AG, et al. Working toward rational and evidence-based treatment of chronic subdural hematoma. Clin Neurosurg 2010; 57: 112–22.

6. Zollinger R, Gross RE. Traumatic subdural hematoma, an explanation of the late onset of pressure symptoms. JAMA 1934; 103: 245–9.

7. Markwalder TM, Steinsiepe KF, Rohner M, et al. The course of chronic subdural hematomas after burr-hole craniostomy and closed-system drainage. J Neurosurg 1981; 55(3): 390–6.

8. Katano H, Kamiya K, Mase M, et al. Tissue plasminogen activator in chronic subdural hematomas as a predictor of recurrence. J Neurosurg 2006; 104(1): 79–84.

9. Hohenstein A, Erber R, Schilling L, et al. Increased mRNA expression of VEGF within the hematoma and imbalance of angiopoietin-1 and -2 mRNA within the neomembranes of chronic subdural hematoma. J Neurotrauma 2005; 22(5): 518–28.

10. Matsumoto K, Akagi K, Abekura M, et al. Recurrence factors for chronic subdural hematomas after burr-hole craniostomy and closed system drainage. Neurol Res 1999; 21(3): 277–80.

11. Taussky P, Fandino J, Landolt H. Number of burr holes as independent predictor of postoperative recurrence in chronic subdural haematoma. Br J Neurosurg 2008; 22(2): 279–82.

12. Han, H. J., Park CW, Kim EY, et al. One vs. two burr hole craniostomy in surgical treatment of chronic subdural hematoma. J Korean Neurosurg Soc 2009; 46(2): 87–92.

13. Smith, M.D., Kishikova, L., & Norris, J.M., Surgical management of chronic subdural haematoma: one hole or two? Int J Surg (London, England), 2012; 10(9): 450–2.

14. Chari, A., Kolias, A.G., Santarius T, et al., 2014b Twist-drill craniostomy with hollow screws for evacuation of chronic subdural hematoma. J Neurosurg 2014; 121: 176–83.

15. Svien SJ, Gelety JE. On the surgical management of encapsulated chronic subdural hematoma: a comparison of the results of membranectomy and simple evacuation. J Neurosurg 1964; 21: 172–7.

16. Ducruet AF, Grobelny BT, Zacharia BE, et al. The surgical management of chronic subdural hematoma. Neurosurg Rev 2012; 35(2): 155–69; discussion 169.

17. Weigel R, Schmiedek P, Krauss JK. Outcome of contemporary surgery for chronic subdural haematoma: evidence based review. J Neurol Neurosurg Psychiat 2003; 74(7): 937–43.

18. Ratilal B, Costa J, Sampaio C. Anticonvulsants for preventing seizures in patients with chronic subdural haematoma. Cochrane Database Syst Rev 2005 Jul 20;(3): CD004893.

19. Coleman PL, Patel PD, Cwikel BJ, et al. Characterization of the dexamethasone-induced inhibitor of plasminogen activator in HTC hepatoma cells. J Biol Chem 1986; 261(9): 4352–7.

20. Gao T, Lin Z, Jin X. Hydrocortisone suppression of the expression of VEGF may relate to toll-like receptor (TLR) 2 and 4. Curr Eye Res 2009; 34(9): 777–84.

21. Delgado-Lopez PD, Martín-Velasco V, Castilla-Díez JM, et al. Dexamethasone treatment in chronic subdural haematoma. Neurocirugia (Astur) 2009; 20(4): 346–59.
22. Berghauser Pont LME, et al., Clinical factors associated with outcome in chronic subdural hematoma: a retrospective cohort study of patients on preoperative corticosteroid therapy. Neurosurgery 2012; 70(4): 873–80; discussion 880.
23. Robinson RG. Chronic subdural hematoma: surgical management in 133 patients. J Neurosurg 1984; 61(2): 263–8.
24. Go AS, Hylek EM, Chang Y, et al. Anticoagulation therapy for stroke prevention in atrial fibrillation: how well do randomized trials translate into clinical practice? JAMA 2003; 290(20): 2685–92.
25. Liebermann A, Hass W, Pinto R. Intracranial hemorrhage and infarction in anticoagulated patients with prosthetic heart valves. Stroke 1978; 9: 18–24.
26. Chari, A., Clemente Morgado, T., & Rigamonti, D., Recommencement of anticoagulation in chronic subdural haematoma: a systematic review and meta-analysis. Br J Neurosurg 2014; 28(1): 2–7.
27. Korinth MC. Low-dose aspirin before intracranial surgery—results of a survey among neurosurgeons in Germany. Acta Neurochir 2006; 148(11): 1189–96; discussion 1196.
28. Shiomi, N., Sasajima, H., & Mineura, K., [Relationship of postoperative residual air and recurrence in chronic subdural hematoma]. No shinkei geka. Neurolog Surg 2001; 29(1): 39–44.
29. Nakajima H, Yasui T, Nishikawa M, et al. The role of postoperative patient posture in the recurrence of chronic subdural hematoma: a prospective randomized trial. Surg Neurol 2002; 58(6): 385–7; discussion 387.
30. Ohba, S., Kinoshita Y, Nakagawa T, et al., 2013. The risk factors for recurrence of chronic subdural hematoma. Neurosurg Rev 2013; 36(1): 145–9; discussion 149–50.
31. Nakaguchi H, Tanishima T, Yoshimasu N. Relationship between drainage catheter location and postoperative recurrence of chronic subdural hematoma after burr-hole irrigation and closed-system drainage. J Neurosurg 2000; 93(5): 791–5.
32. Mori K, Maeda M. Surgical treatment of chronic subdural hematoma in 500 consecutive cases: clinical characteristics, surgical outcome, complications, and recurrence rate. Neurol medico-chir 2001; 41(8): 371–81.

2 Glioblastoma multiforme

Mohammed Awad

⊕ Expert commentary Kevin O'Neill

Case history

A 59-year-old, right-handed male, with a background of hypertension and previous transient ischaemic attack (TIA), presented to his general practitioner with a 3-week history of intermittent, but progressively worsening right arm numbness. This was followed by speech disturbance a week later, and an outpatient computed tomography (CT) head scan was ordered. On examination, he was found to have a normal conscious level with a mild expressive dysphasia. He was also found to have a mild pyramidal weakness (MRC (Medical Research Council) 4/5) and sensory disturbance involving the right arm.

> **✪ Learning point** Dysphasia
>
> There are several subtypes of dysphasia, however, they broadly fall into one of three syndromes—expressive dysphasia, receptive dysphasia, or global dysphasia. **Expressive dysphasia**, also known as motor dysphasia, is a conscious difficulty in the expression of speech, including speech initiation, proper grammatical sequencing, and proper word forming and articulation. Patients can fully understand what is told to them and can fully follow commands, but speech is slow and 'forced', and features short phrases. **Receptive dysphasia** is essentially the reverse of expressive in that the patient's speech may appear quite fluent and articulate, although it may not necessarily make sense and these patients are unaware of their mistakes. They find it difficult to comprehend spoken language and or word–object relations and therefore show some difficulty in following spoken commands. Wernicke's dysphasia is the most common of the receptive dysphasias. **Conduction dysphasia**, also known as associative dysphasia, is relatively uncommon and only amounts to 10% of the presenting dysphasias. It is caused by damage to the arcuate fasciculus, essentially disconnecting Broca's from Wernicke's, and results in difficulty with repetition. Patients may also suffer the inability to describe people or objects in the proper terms. **Global aphasia** results from damage to all three regions—Broca's, the arcuate fasciculus, and Wernicke's areas, which results in total language disturbance.

> **✪ Learning point** Hemisphere dominance and language
>
> Language functions, such as vocabulary, grammar, and literal meaning are areas that reside in the dominant hemisphere of an individual. In right-handed individuals, this is the left hemisphere in approximately 90–95% of people. In left-handed people, the dominant hemisphere is still left-sided in 63–71%. The main areas of language are Broca's in the posterior inferior frontal gyrus and Wernicke's in the superior temporal gyrus. They are connected by a white matter tract, known as the arcuate fasciculus.

The CT head scan demonstrated areas of low attenuation within the left temporoparietal region that enhanced heterogeneously with surrounding mass effect and oedema (Figure 2.1). An enhanced MRI scan confirmed a left temporoparietal intrinsic space-occupying lesion. The lesion was of mixed intensity on the T2-weighted image, but predominantly iso- to hyperintense (Figure 2.2). The flair demonstrated the vasogenic oedema spreading predominantly in the white matter directed around and away from the lesion. On a T1 post-contrasted scan, the lesion showed peripheral rim enhancement with a presumed necrotic, non-enhancing centre (Figure 2.3).

In view of the perilesional oedema and mass effect, dexamethasone was administered with a proton pump inhibitor for gastric protection.

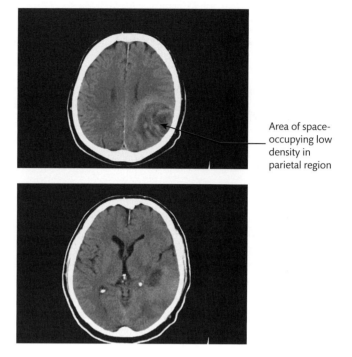

Area of space-occupying low density in parietal region

Figure 2.1 CT—axial scan images revealing a low density space-occupying lesion in the posterior temporal and parietal lobes with heterogenous contrast uptake.

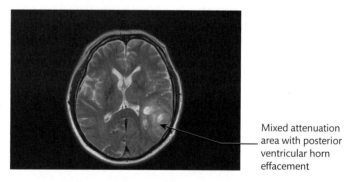

Mixed attenuation area with posterior ventricular horn effacement

Figure 2.2 T2-weighted axial MRI showing the iso-hyperintense lesion with evidence of encroachment of mass effect on surrounding eloquent areas.

⭐ **Learning point** Vasogenic oedema and dexamethasone

Vasogenic oedema occurs around tumours and inflammation as a result of a breakdown of the blood–brain barrier. This causes an influx of proteins into the extracellular space from the intravascular compartment and water follows by the process of osmosis. In normal circumstances, these proteins would not pass through tight junctions, but these are disturbed by the presence of the tumour. The exact mechanism of action of corticosteroids around tumours is unknown, but it is thought that dexamethasone works to reduce the inflammatory response around the tumour and, therefore, restore some element of normality to the blood–brain barrier. It is also thought to decrease oedema by the effect on bulk flow away from the tumour, although corticosteroids decrease capillary permeability in the tumour itself [1]. VEGF inhibitors, such as bevacizmab, as an alternative to steroids, have also been reported to reduce vascular permeability effectively and thereby brain tumour oedema in the clinical setting [2].

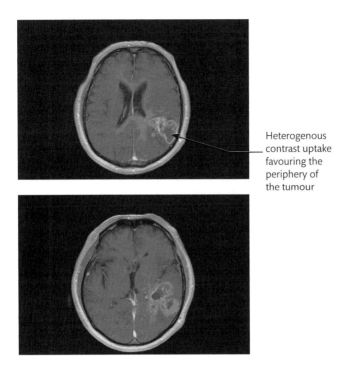

Heterogenous
contrast uptake
favouring the
periphery of
the tumour

Figure 2.3 T1-weighted images with gadolinium showing peripheral contrast uptake of the heterogeneous intrinsic lesion.

> **❝ Expert comment** The function of the multidisciplinary team
>
> The neuro-oncology multidisciplinary team (MDT) brings together all the necessary clinical expertise to optimize a brain tumour patient's care. This framework guidance was implemented by the National Institute for Health and Clinical Excellence (NICE) through its Improving Outcome Guidance (IOG) guidelines. NICE is a special health authority of the English National Health Service (NHS). NICE publishes guidelines in three areas—the use of health technologies within the NHS (such as the use of new and existing medicines, treatments, and procedures), clinical practice (guidance on the appropriate treatment and care of people with specific diseases and conditions), and guidance for public sector workers on health promotion and ill-health avoidance. The MDT's members will include neuro-oncologists (neurosurgeons, clinical oncologists), neuroradiologists, neuropathologists, psychiatrist/ psychologists, clinical nurse specialists, physiotherapists, occupational therapists, and clinical trials co-ordinators. The team should handle all neuro-oncology referrals by making recommendations about further management based on diagnosis. This will be based on current best evidence-based practice, including NICE guidance and should also provide the opportunity for eligible patients to be entered into clinical trials. The MDT may make recommendations for further investigation or clinical assessment if there are uncertainties about the case or the evidence for treatment benefit is unclear. It is now considered a core element in the patient pathway, is usually established in a designated neuro-oncology centre, and involves both inpatient care and outpatient follow-up. The overall goal of the MDT is to expedite and improve patient care, ultimately leading to better outcomes and survival. It is now mandatory to have an MDT-centric pathway to manage neuro-oncology patients in the UK.

The patient's symptoms resolved after 3 days on dexamethasone. His case was discussed in the neuro-oncology MDT meeting. The patient scored highly on the Karnofsky performance scale (90/100) and, after discussion with the patient about the management options (risks as well as benefits of surgery with adjuvant therapies versus no treatment), the decision was taken to proceed to craniotomy and debulking, with subsequent adjuvant therapy dictated by the pathology results.

> **✖ Learning point** Karnofsky score
>
> The Karnofsky performance status score is an attempt to quantify 'well-being'. It is used to determine whether patients are fit enough to withstand and benefit from standard treatments, or whether they should be exposed to less radical therapy instead. It is also used as a measure of quality of life. The Karnofsky score runs from 100 to 0, where 100 is 'perfect' health and 0 is death. This scoring system is named after Dr David A. Karnofsky, who described the scale with Dr Joseph H. Burchenal in 1949, and it is still used today.

The patient underwent craniotomy and debulking of the tumour assisted by magnetic resonance (MR)-directed image guidance with 3D intra-operative ultrasound (Sonowand™). Post-operatively he was mildly dysphasic again, but this resolved within 1 week of surgery. His post-operative CT scan showed a good clearance of the bulk of the tumour (see Figure 2.4).

> **✚ Clinical tip** Combined intra-operative MR-directed image guidance and ultrasound
>
> Sonowand™ is a combined navigation console and intra-operative ultrasound. Pre-operative DICOM magnetic resonance imaging (MRI) or CT images are uploaded and when matched with the patient can be used for flap planning, as standard with all navigation consoles. However, the Sonowand™ has the advantage of being able to update the 'road-map' being used, by providing a 3D ultrasound image as the surgery progresses, which provides real-time up-to-date images allowing for brainshift and aids with visualization of nearby vessels. The authors believe it is a great visualization surgical aid that aids with extensive and safer resections.

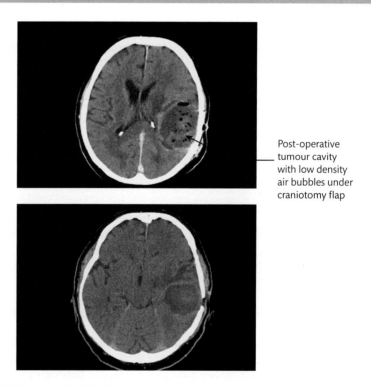

Post-operative tumour cavity with low density air bubbles under craniotomy flap

Figure 2.4 Post-operative CT axial scan showing good surgical resection of the tumour.

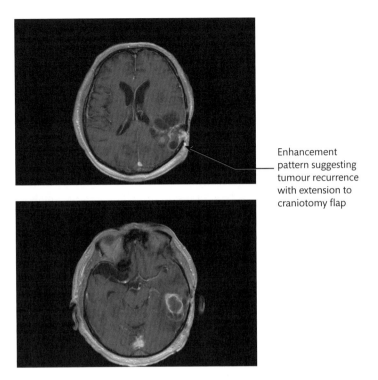

Enhancement pattern suggesting tumour recurrence with extension to craniotomy flap

Figure 2.5 T1-weighted MRI with gadolinium at 1 year post-resection, showing tumour recurrence at the site of the previous resection.

He later received standard dose conformal external beam radiotherapy (2Gy fractions daily to a total of 60Gy over 6 weeks). This is a typical regimen and each 2Gy fraction takes approximately 3 minutes. He was also given six monthly cycles of temozolomide chemotherapy. This is currently first line chemotherapy for glioblastoma multiforme (GBM) in the UK and is given for 6–12 months, depending on tumour grading, Karnofsky grade of the patient, response while undergoing treatment, and genetic marker studies. In this case, a 6-month MRI scan showed no progression, but a 12-month follow-up scan revealed significant recurrence (Figure 2.5).

Discussion

GBM is the most common form of malignant primary brain tumour. In the UK, the incidence is approximately 2–3 cases per 100,000 people per year and it accounts for approximately 20% of all primary intracranial tumours. GBM is derived from glial cells, and is thought to arise either de novo as primary GBM or secondary to malignant progression from a low-grade astrocytoma (Chapter 21). There is a greater male predilection for reasons unknown[3].

✪ Learning point Presentation times of glioblastoma

Astrocytic tumour cells may diffusely infiltrate cortex without initially affecting neuronal function. However, eventually neighbouring neurons are damaged or isolated, and patients develop neurological symptoms. In this way, GBM may be very large before patients become symptomatic, although growth in eloquent areas will manifest relatively early.

✪ Learning point The WHO classification of astrocytomas–I–IV

Grade I lesions are those with low proliferative potential and may be cured following surgical resection alone. Grade II lesions are generally infiltrative and despite showing low proliferative activity, they usually recur after surgery. Most grade II tumours transform to higher grades over time. WHO defines diffusely infiltrative astrocytic tumours with cytological atypia alone as Grade II (diffuse astrocytoma). WHO Grade III lesions (anaplastic astrocytoma) show histological evidence of malignancy, including nuclear atypia and brisk mitotic activity. Finally, WHO Grade IV lesions are cytologically malignant, mitotically active, necrosis-prone neoplasms with endovascular proliferation typically associated with rapid disease progression and a dismal prognosis. Grade IV tumours tend to show widespread infiltration of surrounding tissue and some may demonstrate craniospinal dissemination.

GBM commonly presents with neurological deficit, seizures, and signs of raised intracranial pressure. Approximately 30–50% will present with non-specific headache, which may become characteristic of raised intracranial pressure (ICP). 30–60% will present with seizures and, depending on the location, these may be simple, focal, or generalized. Focal neurological deficit is a presenting feature in 40–60% and 20–40% present with mental status changes. The location of the tumour usually delineates the neurological deficit and the time to presentation, as tumours in more eloquent areas tend to present sooner.

Intrinsic high-grade tumours may show a variety of appearances on CT and MRI. This is dependent on the presence or absence of low grade areas around the tumour, possible calcification, the rate of growth, the degree of necrosis, and the presence of any haemorrhage.

CT scans will usually demonstrate an area of low density with surrounding mass effect and after contrast administration, usually a ragged ring of enhancement, surrounded by oedema. The mass effect may be minimal and local, but may be severe enough to cause midline shift and compression of the ventricles, and may even cause hydrocephalus.

On MRI, high-grade intrinsic lesions show as low density areas on T1-weighted imaging that ring enhance, also usually in a ragged fashion, with contrast administration. On T2-weighted images they show as heterogeneous masses, usually with marked extensive surrounding oedema, predominantly in the white matter. The fluid-attenuated inversion recovery (FLAIR) sequence shows the oedema even more extensively. It is difficult, however, to distinguish between oedema and tumour infiltration, as both are of high intensity on the FLAIR sequence. The differential diagnosis of ring-enhancing lesions includes metastases, abscess, and parasitic infections. Other image sequences, such as apparent diffusion coefficient (ADC) map and gradient echo, may be helpful, with the clinical history, to differentiate between these. MR spectroscopy may also be useful.

✪ Learning point Magnetic resonance spectroscopy of glioblastoma multiformes

MR spectroscopy gives additional information to aid with diagnosis. Glioblastomas typically demonstrate high levels of choline, lactate, and lipid, and low levels of N-acetylaspartate (NAA) and creatine. Generally, the more malignant the lesion, the higher the choline-to-creatine peak ratio, with an increased lactate peak, and decreased NAA peak ratio. A typical graph of a sampled glioblastoma is shown in Figure 2.6.

(continued)

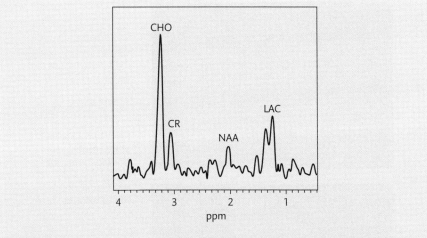

Figure 2.6 A typical MR spectroscopy graph of sampled glioblastoma tumour tissue.

CHO: choline; CR: creatine; NAA: N-acetylaspartate; LAC: lactate; ppm: parts per million.

❝ Expert comment Imaging glioblastoma multiformes

When imaging all gliomas, including GBM, I will always require a structural MRI, which will include a T1-weighted series of images, with and without contrast to determine the enhancing bulk of the tumour. I will also want, as standard, a T2 sequence with a T2 FLAIR to get an estimate of the extent of tumour and or any oedema within the surrounding parenchyma. In essence, one has to assess the location and extent of the tumour. From this I can assess its contribution to local mass effect and estimate the degree of diffuse invasion. Ultimately, we know that radical resection can improve the patient's outlook and response to adjuvant treatments, but this has to be balanced against inflicting morbidity or deficit that could worsen their prognosis. In certain cases, where tumours look resectable, but are close to eloquent areas or tracts, I will request functional MRI and/or tractography. Most tumours, particularly the lower grade gliomas, undergo physiological scanning with spectroscopy and cerebral blood volume maps to build a database of MRI biomarkers, particularly, if we are following tumours for any length of time. Again, all gliomas that require surgery will have a neuronavigation thin slice acquisition scan to be able to use this now standard technology. I incorporate as much imaging information into that system as I can for the purposes of accurate navigation. In addition, my preferred mode of intra-operative imaging to update the pre-operative image data is 3D ultrasound, which provides similar, but complimentary information to the MRI, and will take into account resection and brain shift. In addition to intra-operative imaging, awake craniotomy and cortical mapping are useful adjuncts to avoid neurological deficit during surgery near eloquent cortex.

Gliomas are composed of a heterogeneous mix of poorly differentiated neoplastic astrocytes. Glioblastomas are distinguished from WHO grade III astrocytomas by the presence of necrosis and endothelial hyperplasia. Both usually form in the cerebral white matter. In adults, this is usually in the cerebral hemispheres supratentorially, but in children it is not unusual for the primary location to be the brainstem. Approximately, half of the supratentorial tumours occupy more than one lobe or are bilateral. The classic 'butterfly appearance' (Figure 2.7) develops as a result of growth across the corpus callosum. Grade III and IV tumours most commonly can develop de novo or can be the result of a transformation from a lower grade astrocytoma (less than 10%). These secondary GBMs are more common in a younger age

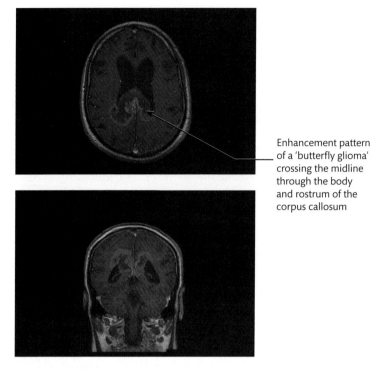

Enhancement pattern of a 'butterfly glioma' crossing the midline through the body and rostrum of the corpus callosum

Figure 2.7 T1-weighted MRI with gadolinium. Axial and coronal sections showing the classic appearance of a butterfly glioma.

group (average age 45) versus primary GBMs (average age 62) [4]. Rarely, high-grade gliomas may seed through the CSF to distant cranial or spinal sites. They can cause meningeal gliomatosis and, indeed, may be found in CSF, resulting in high protein content.

High-grade gliomas are invariably difficult to treat due to the degree of diffuse infiltration in the surrounding brain making surgical resection incomplete, the lack of efficacy of standard radiotherapy, and a lack of effective chemotherapy. As a result they are currently considered incurable. Treatment is ultimately palliative and aimed at increasing the length of survival and quality of life.

The options are:

- Purely conservative and supportive (palliative care).
- Radiotherapy with or without chemotherapy.
- Surgery with or without radio and/or chemotherapy.

Surgery may be used simply to achieve a histological diagnosis through a biopsy or may reduce the tumour bulk, either to reduce mass effect, or to allow adjuvant therapy its best chance by reducing the tumour cell load.

Clinical research is emerging that shows that radically extensive volume resections have a greater impact on length of survival and, therefore, in the UK the trend is moving towards radical debulking of high-grade lesions with subsequent adjuvant radio- or chemotherapy if the patient is fit enough.

★ Learning point Risk factors for glioblastoma multiformes

- Male.
- Older age: over 50 years old.
- Caucasians and Asians.
- Low-grade astrocytoma.
- Having one of the following genetic disorders is associated with an increased incidence of gliomas: neurofibromatosis, tuberous sclerosis, von Hippel–Lindau (VHL) disease, Li–Fraumeni syndrome, Turcot syndrome.

✪ Learning point Extent of resection

A landmark paper that assessed the length of survival of patients with glioblastomas according to the extent of resection was a multivariate analysis of 416 patients [5]. The conclusion was that a significant survival advantage was associated with resection of 98% or more of the tumour volume (median survival 13 months), compared with 8.8 months for resections of less than 98%. Many other studies have reached similar conclusions. Stummer et al. [6] looked at the extent of glioblastoma resections with the aid of 5-ALA fluorescence. This was a randomized study of 270 patients. Half underwent surgical resection guided by fluorescence achieved with 5-ALA and the remainder under white light. They found that 65% of the 5-ALA patients had complete resections of the pre-operative MRI-enhancing areas versus only 36% under white light. They also found that 41% of the 5-ALA resected patients had progression-free survival at 6 months compared with 21% for the control group. Vuorinen et al. [7] found a survival advantage of >2 months for craniotomy and surgical resection versus biopsy for GBM patients. They also concluded that craniotomy and debulking offered a modest survival advantage over biopsy in elderly patients with a poor Karnofsky score, unsuitable for other adjuvant therapies. In a study of 500 patients with newly-diagnosed glioblastoma operated between 1997 and 2009. Evidence has emerged from studies showing that the extent of resection at repeat craniotomy for recurrent glioblastoma predicted overall survival. They concluded that even if initial resection had not been optimal, the repeat craniotomy should attempt to achieve macroscopic complete resection if at all possible, as this significantly improved survival benefit

✛ Clinical tip Maximizing resection, while minimizing neurological deficit

Following the advice of Lacroix et al. [5], the evidence suggests that attempting a radical (>98%) resection will significantly increase life expectancy. However, this should not be at the expense of quality of life. In order to avoid or minimize damage to surrounding functioning brain and en-passant vessels, one should always use the adjuncts of image guidance, Moreso, the use of intra-operative ultrasound, or MRI will allow for a larger resection, while keeping within the tumorous tissue and not beyond in eloquent areas. The use of the 'angio mode' on intra-operative ultrasound (Sonowand™) will also allow for the visualization of en-passant vessels and help keep them intact, thereby potentially reducing the incidence of post-operative deficit. Stummer et al. [8] also demonstrated that operating on high-grade tumours with the aid of 5-ALA microscopy greatly aided the surgeon in visualizing abnormal tissue, and therefore in obtaining an extensive resection. The crucial point with surgery for glioblastomas is not to attempt a complete resection if there is a risk of leaving permanent damage, given that these are currently incurable tumours. Many surgeons will now obtain intra-operative histology (smear, frozen section), in order to confirm the diagnosis and decide how aggressive they will be with their resections.

❝ Expert comment Intracavity chemotherapy

Gliadel® wafers represent an alternative approach to the delivery of chemotherapy in malignant glioma. Gliadel® wafers contain Carmustine® and are designed to release this agent over a 2–3-week period. Gliadel® wafers are placed on the surface of the resected tumour. For recurrent malignant glioma one randomized control trial (RCT) compared the efficacy of Gliadel® with that of placebo in patients with recurrent glioma. No significant survival advantage was seen in the primary analysis, however, a survival advantage for Gliadel® was observed in patients with GBM after adjustment for prognostic factors. This suggests that Gliadel® may increase overall survival in some patients with recurrent resectable malignant glioma. As such patients generally have a poor outlook, any treatment that has the potential for prolonging life without significant adverse events should be considered an option. However, given that no subgroups had been identified beforehand, the results of the subgroup analysis of GBM patients in that trial should be interpreted with caution.

(continued)

The strongest evidence for their use involves trials in newly-diagnosed malignant glioma. Two RCTs compared the efficacy of Gliadel® with placebo in patients with newly-diagnosed gliomas. In the largest RCT to date, patients who received Gliadel® for newly-diagnosed malignant glioma were reported to have experienced a 2-month improvement in median survival compared with patients who received placebo ($p = 0.017$). In addition, analysis of the survival curves revealed a significant 27% reduction in risk of mortality for patients who received Gliadel® ($p = 0.018$). A survival advantage with Gliadel® in patients with GBM was not detected, but the trial was not designed to make comparisons between histological subgroups. Because the researchers in another randomized trial were unable to obtain sufficient Gliadel®, that trial included only 32 patients newly diagnosed with malignant glioma, instead of the anticipated 100. Although a survival benefit was reported for Gliadel® in the overall patient population and in patients with GBM, no conclusions could be reached, based on the small number of patients enrolled. Both studies reported similar adverse events in the treatment and control arms. The most common adverse events associated with Gliadel® were hemiplegia, convulsions, confusion, and brain oedema. The most commonly reported adverse events among patients who received placebo were convulsions, confusion, brain oedema, and aphasia. A significantly higher number of patients experienced intracranial hypertension in the Gliadel® arm of the Westphal trial. Because neither trial included a comparison with systemic therapy, the possible contrast between the adverse event rates associated with interstitial chemotherapy wafers and the rates expected with systemic chemotherapy is unclear. Given that the largest trial demonstrated a survival advantage in the Gliadel® treatment arm, Gliadel® may be considered an option in the subgroup of patients with newly-diagnosed resectable malignant gliomas. However, the exact patient population (based on age, histology, performance status, and so on) that may benefit from Gliadel® is unclear; further investigation is needed. In addition, no comparison has been performed between the efficacy of interstitial and systemic chemotherapy; clinicians should therefore review the latest evidence for the benefit of systemic chemotherapy in patients with newly-diagnosed malignant glioma.

As a result of these studies Carmustine® wafers (Gliadel®) are now recommended for use by NICE for selected patients, provided the following criteria are satisfied:

- Pre-operative MRI suggestive of newly-diagnosed high-grade glioma (HGG).
- Discussion before surgery in a neuro-oncology MDT.
- Surgical resection by a specialist neurosurgical oncologist.
- Surgical resection of more than 90% of the tumour.
- Intra-operative pathological confirmation of HGG.
- The ventricle is not widely opened.

A recent national audit yet to be published suggested that brain tumour surgeons are not considering the use of wafers in many patients that may be eligible. I believe that most surgeons are concerned about potential complications, such as brain oedema, wound healing and infection rates, and perhaps also cost in a period of reducing spending cuts in healthcare.

The prognosis for these high-grade tumours is very poor, although over the last 10 years, it has improved somewhat due to improved surgery and better chemotherapy agents. The average survival without any treatment is 3–6 months, but with aggressive treatment in the form of surgery, radiotherapy and chemotherapy, this can commonly be 1–2 years [9]. Older patients and patients with neurological deficit at presentation carry a worse prognosis. Conversely, younger patients, under 50 years, with a good initial Karnofsky Performance score of >70, and those with surgical resections >98% carry a better prognosis [5].

Death from GBM is usually secondary to raised ICP or severe neurological deterioration allowing opportunistic infections or thromboembolic events to supercede.

There are several molecular markers associated with outcome prediction in glial tumours. The 1p/19q codeletion strongly predicts response to treatment and survival in oligodendroglial tumours. The Methylguanine-methyltransferase promoter methylation, which is thought to render the cells more vulnerable to alkylating chemotherapy agents is also associated with a better outcome. Hegi et al. [10] tested the relationship between MGMT silencing in the tumour and the survival of patients enrolled in a randomized trial comparing radiotherapy alone with radiotherapy and adjuvant temozolomide. They concluded that patients with glioblastoma containing a methylated MGMT promoter benefitted from temozolomide, whereas those who did not have a methylated MGMT promoter did not have such a benefit. Their work has led to significant changes in oncological practice. Finally, and more recently, mutations of the *IDH1* gene have been found in 40% of gliomas and are inversely correlated to grade. *IDH1* mutation is a strong and independent predictor of survival [11]. These are all DNA characteristics intrinsic to the patient and currently cannot be altered externally.

Long-term disease-free survival is possible, but these tumours usually reappear, often within 3cm of the original site, and 10–20% may develop new lesions at distant sites (termed multifocal GBM). Further radical surgery, perhaps supplemented with adjuvant radiosurgery and/or suitable chemotherapy may lead to additional prolongation of life, but the benefits of such treatment need to be assessed realistically and quality of life must also be taken into account.

A final word from the expert

Clearly, the prognosis for patients with malignant glioma remains poor, with median survival in the region of 12–14 months. This has only changed marginally over the last few decades with the use of systemic chemotherapy alongside surgical resection and radiotherapy. There are outliers who do better or worse than the median, and 3-year survival percentages do seem to be increasing with current treatment regimes. The results tell us that these tumours are very heterogenous in their genetics and response to therapy. Laboratory research has not only identified abnormal genes, but also abnormal epigenetic control of normal gene expression, which may be even more important. More and more pathways are being discovered that relate to biological behaviour and prognosis. The problem is that the cellular targets differ from tumour to tumour. That is why I believe the future of GBM management will become much more tailored to the individual patient. This will mirror the trend in surgery with improved tumour identification techniques already seen with fluorescent markers and intra-operative imaging technology. As research is broadening there will also be an increasing use of physical treatments, such as particle beam and other forms of electromagnetic energy, as well as nanotechnology to deliver targeted therapy. The therapy will need to be effective against all cell types, rather than selecting out resistant populations. There is currently a resurgence of interest in the immunology and metabolism of these tumours in the search for magic bullets. The future holds many challenges, but much potential for improvement.

References

1. Molnar P, Lapin GD, Groothuis DR. The effects of dexamethasone on experimental brain tumors: I. Transcapillary transport and blood flow in RG-2 rat gliomas. Neuro Oncol 1995; 25(1): 19–28.
2. Gerstner ER, Duda DG, di Tomaso E, et al. VEGF inhibitors in the treatment of cerebral edema in patients with brain cancer. Nat Rev Clin Oncol 2009; 6(4): 229–36.

3. Ohgaki H, Kleihues P. Population-based studies on incidence, survival rates, and genetic alterations in astrocytic and oligodendroglial gliomas. J Neuropath Exp Neurol 2005; 64(6): 479–89.

4. Ohgaki H, Kleihues P. Genetic alterations and signaling pathways in the evolution of gliomas. Cancer Sci 2009; 100(12): 2235–41.

5. Lacroix M, Abi-Said D, Fourney DR, et al. A multivariate analysis of 416 patients with glioblastoma multiforme: prognosis, extent of resection, and survival. J Neurosurg 2001; 95(2): 190–8.

6. Stummer W, Pichlmeier U, Meinel T, et al. Fluorescence-guided surgery with 5-aminolevulinic acid for resection of malignant glioma: a randomised controlled multicentre phase III trial. Lancet Oncol 2006; 7(5): 392–401.

7. Vuorinen V, Hinkka S, Färkkilä M, et al. Debulking or biopsy of malignant glioma in elderly people—a randomised study. Acta Neurochir (Wien) 2003; 145: 5–10.

8. Stummer W, Pichlmeier U, Meinel T, Wiestler OD, Zanella F, Reulen HJ, ALA-Glioma Study Group, Fluorescence-guided surgery with 5-aminolevulinic acid for resection of malignant glioma: a randomised controlled multicentre phase III trial. Lancet Oncol. 2006; 7(5): 392–401.

9. Krex D, Klink B, Hartmann C et al. Long-term survival with glioblastoma multiforme. Brain 2007; 130(Pt 10): 2596–606.

10. Hegi ME, Diserens AC, Gorlia T, et al. MGMT gene silencing and benefit from temozolomide in glioblastoma. N Engl J Med 2005; 352: 997–1003.

11. Ducray F, del Rio MS, Carpentier C, et al. Up-front temozolomide in elderly patients with anaplastic oligodendroglioma and oligoastrocytoma. Journal of Neuro-oncology. 2011; 101(3): 457–462.

12. Westphal M, Hilt DC, Bortey E, et al. A phase 3 trial of local chemotherapy with biodegradable carmustine (BCNU) wafers (Gliadel wafers) in patients with primary malignant glioma. Neuro Oncol 2003; 5: 79–88.

13. Westphal M, Ram Z, Riddle V, et al. Gliadel wafer in initial surgery for malignant glioma: long-term follow-up of a multicenter controlled trial. Acta Neurochir (Wien) 2006; 148: 269–75.

3 Spondylolisthesis

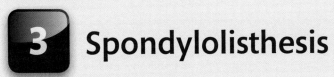

Eoin Fenton

🕮 **Expert commentary** Ciaran Bolger

Case history

A 43-year-old woman was referred to the neurosurgical unit from the pain clinic. She complained of severe unremitting lower back pain radiating to both buttocks and lower limbs for the previous 4 years. By the time she was seen by the neurosurgical team she had received multiple bilateral facet joint injections and a caudal epidural, but derived no relief from these. She had also taken part in a physiotherapy programme, which she rigorously adhered to, and an exercise regime that included swimming.

❂ **Learning point** The role and effectiveness of conservative measures in the treatment of spondylolisthesis

The non-operative measures quoted in the Spine Patient Outcomes Research Trial (SPORT) were active physiotherapy, education, and counselling, with instructions regarding home exercise and non-steroidal anti-inflammatories (NSAIDs) if tolerated [1]. Injection techniques were also used. Conservative treatment does not address any underlying anatomic abnormality, but aims to relieve pain, restore function, and reduce the number of painful exacerbations. The rehabilitation programme must be tailored to suit each patient individually, according to the nature and severity of their symptoms. Factors such as age, occupation, and degree of disability are also relevant. Only a few RCTs exist with regard to drugs and injection techniques [2]. While there is a lack of evidence in the literature to support one non-operative technique over another [3], they appear to complement one another as part of an holistic approach to symptomatic relief.

The patient complained of heaviness in her legs in the evenings. She felt her back pain was worse than her leg pain. She intermittently took paracetamol, anti-inflammatories, and amitriptyline at night.

On assessment in the outpatient clinic, a visual analogue for pain scale (VAS) and a short-form 36 health survey (SF-36) were carried out. Her VAS score for back pain was 7/10 and leg pain was 3/10. Her SF-36 physical functioning score was 40/100 and her mental health score was 45/100. Severe restrictions were noted in physical, emotional, and mental health, as well as social and physical activities. She was unable to work due to back trouble and rated her overall general health as somewhat worse compared with 12 months previously. She had no neurological deficit on examination, but experienced back pain during the assessment.

> **⊗ Learning point** Outcome measures in lumbar spine surgery
>
> There are various questionnaires available that are suitable for measuring adult pain and are useful for both clinicians and researchers [4]. The pain VAS is available in the public domain at no cost. The SF-36 is available free of charge from the RAND corporation. It references eight health concepts:
>
> - Physical functioning.
> - Bodily pain.
> - Role limitations due to physical functioning.
> - Role limitations due to personal and emotional problems.
> - Emotional well-being.
> - Social functioning.
> - Energy/fatigue.
> - General health perceptions.
>
> The Oswestry Disability Index (ODI) is also commonly used to measure lumbar spine surgery outcomes. The ODI is considered a valid and vigorous measure [5]. The validity of VAS for pain is questionable [6]. The SF-36 has been validated for use in measuring morbidity and surgical outcomes in common spinal disorders [7].

MR imaging of her lumbar spine revealed a Grade 1 isthmic spondylolisthesis at L5/S1 (see Figure 3.1). Flexion and extension plain radiographs of the lumbar spine were also performed. These demonstrated dynamic instability at L5/S1.

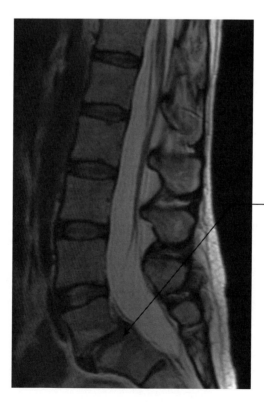

L5-S1 spondylolisthesis (grade 1) with endplate Modic changes, but no overt canal stenosis

Figure 3.1 Sagittal T2-weighted MRI of the lumbar spine demonstrates Grade 1 anterolisthesis of L5 on S1 with resultant disc uncovering. Associated Modic end-plate changes, disc desiccation, and disc height loss are also noted.

Given the symptoms, findings on imaging, and the fact that the patient had completed an exhaustive trial of non-operative management, it was felt that she was a candidate for lumbosacral fusion surgery. This option was fully discussed with her pre-operatively, particularly with respect to her expectations of symptomatic improvement. She was admitted for surgery and underwent a mini-open posterolateral fusion at L5/S1. Following the induction of general anaesthesia, she was given cefuroxime 1.5g intravenously and positioned prone on rolls (one at chest level and one at the level of her pelvis) on the operating table. Through a bilateral Wiltse paraspinal approach, pedicle screws and rods were placed at L5 and S1 with osteo-inductive synthetic bone graft (silicate substituted calcium phosphate). She made a good post-operative recovery, and was mobilizing independently on day 1. She was discharged on post-operative day 2.

> ➕ **Clinical tip** The Wiltse approach
>
> In 1968, Wiltse et al. described the paraspinal sacrospinalis-splitting approach to the lumbar spine [8] (see Figure 3.2). The approach was felt to be particularly valuable in young people with spondylolisthesis. It involves making two incisions, each about 3cm lateral to the midline. The muscle is split with the index finger and the lumbar transverse processes are found (or the sacrum, depending on the level of fusion). Retractors are inserted and the landmarks for pedicle screw insertion can be visualized. Transverse processes are fully decorticated and bone graft placed into the lateral gutter. This approach leaves the supraspinous and interspinous ligaments intact, and avoids the laminar strip of the paraspinal muscle, which is believed to compromise vascularity, and lead to atrophy of the muscle, and increased post-operative back pain.
>
>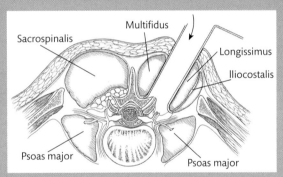
>
> **Figure 3.2** Wiltse approach for in situ fusion of spondylolisthesis (arrow). Through a paramedian longitudinal fascial incision and muscle-splitting approach, the pars, facet, and transverse process of the involved levels are exposed, creating a large space for posterolateral grafting and fusion. The midline is left undisturbed.
>
> Wiltse LL, Bateman JG, Hutchinson RH, Nelson WE. The paraspinal sacrospinalis-splitting approach to the lumbar spine. J Bone Joint Surg Am. 1968 Jul;50(5):919–26

At her 6-week post-operative check, her skin incisions had healed well, and the patient had no new neurological deficit. At 6 months, her VAS score for back pain was now 4/10 and her lower limb symptoms had completely resolved. Her SF-36 physical functioning score and mental health score had both improved by 20%. Flexion-extension X-rays revealed satisfactory instrumentation and no overt dynamic slip (Figure 3.3). She reported that she was essentially pain free apart from when doing strenuous activities for long periods of time. She felt that she had returned to normal activities.

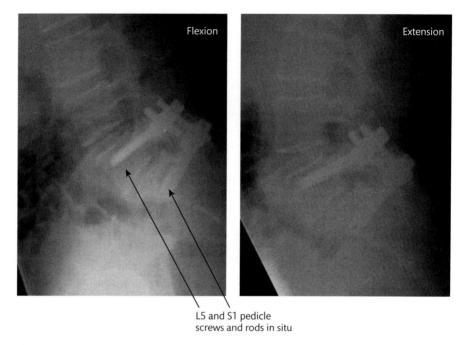

Flexion

Extension

L5 and S1 pedicle
screws and rods in situ

Figure 3.3 6-month imaging (flexion and extension views) show no movement at the fused level. Post-operative flexion/extension views demonstrate resolution of dynamic instability. There is loss of disc space height and early incorporation of graft material.

Discussion

Lumbosacral vertebral slip was first described by Herbiniaux, a Belgian obstetrician in 1782, as a factor likely to hinder the delivery process during childbirth [9]. The term spondylolisthesis was first defined by Kilian (1854) as forward displacement of a lumbar vertebral body relative to the vertebral body or sacrum below it [10,11].

Following separation or elongation of the pars, there may be a tendency for anterior slippage to occur. This has never been reported as being present at birth (the foetal incidence of spondylolisthesis is 0% according to Fredrickson [12]). The incidence is 4.4% at 6 years of age, rising to 6% in adulthood [13]. Most childhood and adolescent spondylolisthesis is associated with spondylolysis of the pars interarticularis at the L5/S1 motion segment [14]. Although typically considered a paediatric condition, isthmic spondylolisthesis is more symptomatic in the adult population. Slip progression is more common in the paediatric population and rarely occurs in adulthood. The younger the patient is on diagnosis, the higher the risk of progression. Although most paediatric patients respond to conservative therapy, those that do require surgery have a lower rate of pseudarthrosis than the adult population [15]. The incidence of degenerative spondylolisthesis increases as the population ages, and is five or six times more likely to occur in women than in men [16]. In adulthood, the lesion is most likely to occur at the L4/L5 motion segment [16]. The natural history of degenerative spondylolisthesis is generally favourable, however, with only 10–15% of patients seeking treatment actually proceeding to surgery [17].

Several classifications have been described, but the most widely used classification is that of Wiltse, Newman, and MacNab [18]. They described five types. **Dysplastic spondylolisthesis** (Type I) is associated with congenital abnormalities of the upper sacrum or the arch of L5. Incomplete formation of the anatomic elements may be present. Sagittally-orientated facets can also result in instability, most prominently at the lumbosacral junction. **Isthmic spondylolisthesis** (Type II) refers to bilateral pars defects, and this type is subdivided into Types IIA, IIB, and IIC. In Type IIA, there is lysis of the pars, i.e. a fatigue fracture. In Type IIB, the pars is elongated but intact, due to repeated fracture. Type IIC refers to an acute fracture of the pars. **Degenerative spondylolisthesis** (Type III) is acquired and occurs later in life, secondary to motion segment degenerative change (facet joint and disc degeneration). It is more common in females and usually occurs at L4/L5. **Traumatic spondylolisthesis** (Type IV) results form a fracture anywhere other than the pars. **Pathologic spondylolisthesis** (Type V) occurs when a pathological condition affects the bone, such as Paget's disease, tumours, or infection. The aetiology is therefore multifactorial, and can include a congenital predisposition and/or various biomechanical conditions.

> ✪ **Learning point** Lumbar spondylolisthesis can be classified according to the underlying aetiology or degree of slip
>
> *Aetiological classification* [18]
>
> - *Type I*: dysplastic.
> - *Type II*: isthmic.
> - *Type IIA*: lytic fatigue fracture of the pars.
> - *Type IIB*: elongation, but intact pars.
> - *Type IIC*: acute fracture.
> - *Type III*: degenerative.
> - *Type IV*: traumatic.
> - *Type V*: pathologic.
>
> In an article published in 1938, Meyerding described a method for grading the degree of subluxation in cases of spondylolisthesis [19].
>
> - *Grade 1*: 0–25% slip.
> - *Grade 2*: 26–50% slip.
> - *Grade 3*: 51–75% slip.
> - *Grade 4*: 76–100% slip.
> - *Grade 5*: >100%—spondyloptosis (not part of Meyerding's original classification).

Spondylolysis and spondylolisthesis tend to occur in the lower lumbar spine. Lumbar lordosis means that the angle of the vertebrae relative to the ground increases moving from L1 to L5. The facet joints also become more vertical. Lower levels are therefore more susceptible to shear forces. Shear forces are primarily countered by intact posterior elements by means of a tension band principle and by the ligamentous function of the annulus fibrosus [14]. It is estimated that the posterior elements carry approximately 20% of the total load when standing upright [20]. In the presence of bilateral pars defects, the posterior tension band loses its integrity. This can result in anterior slippage and potential development of symptoms.

There is a diverse spectrum of symptoms associated with spondylolisthesis. It can be asymptomatic, although the prevalence of asymptomatic spondylolisthesis

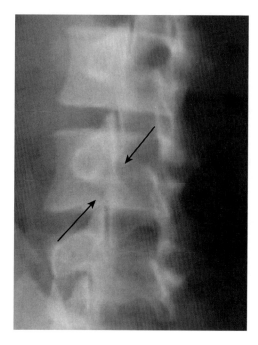

Figure 3.4 Arrows indicate the intact 'neck of scotty dog' on oblique lumbar radiograph.

in the population is not accurately known. Otherwise, it can cause low back pain, radicular symptoms, or both. Symptoms vary depending on the age of the patient and the degree of slippage. Patients can present with gait disturbance, neurogenic claudication, radicular pain, or referred pain from facet joint pathology. The neuropathic pain can originate from central canal stenosis or foraminal stenosis secondary to the slippage itself, or from flaval or facet joint hypertrophy, or both in the setting of degenerative disease. Disc prolapse can also produce symptoms. Cauda equina syndrome can also be a presenting complaint.

A number of imaging modalities can be used to assess and diagnose spondylolisthesis. It can be visualized on plain lateral lumbar spine radiographs in the upright position, but may decrease or disappear in the supine position. Spondylolysis can be seen on oblique views (commonly referred to as the broken neck of the Scotty dog - Figure 3.4). However, modern CT scanners can deliver much lower radiation doses and have a much higher diagnostic yield. There is, therefore, a trend against the use of oblique lumbar plain films, particularly in young patients. Flexion/extension radiographs are used to assess for instability. For the assessment of the thecal sac or neural compression, MR imaging or CT myelography is required.

Conservative treatment should be employed initially in the management of spondylolisthesis (unless signs and symptoms of cauda equina syndrome are present). It is important to note that conservative treatment refers to active non-operative management of the patient with the aim of reducing pain and increasing quality of life. Pain specialists and physiotherapists should be involved. Pain specialists may prescribe various analgesics and/or perform nerve root, joint, or epidural injections. Physiotherapy involves exercises, education on ergonomics, transcutaneous electrical nerve stimulation (TENS), and/or acupuncture. Cognitive intervention should be sought if available. Weight loss and smoking cessation should be encouraged. Flexion and extension core-strengthening exercises may increase the stability of the lumbar spine, and reduce pain and functional disability [14].

Patients who do not improve with appropriate conservative therapy, whose symptoms progress despite conservative therapy, or who initially present with worsening neurological deficit or significant instability are candidates for surgery. The aim of surgery is to stabilize the affected segment and, in the presence of neural compression, decompress the relevant neural elements. Surgical options range from simple decompression without fusion to posterolateral fusion to lumbar interbody fusion supplemented with posterolateral instrumentation. Simple decompression may be considered in patients with degenerative spondylolisthesis showing no evidence of spinal instability. A laminotomy should be the operation of choice if neural decompression is required, keeping excision of the facet joints and posterior ligaments to a minimum. The rationale behind decompression alone is based on early studies reporting satisfactory results from decompression alone. There are also studies that report high satisfactory rates following decompression and fusion in patients with pseudarthrosis (presumably the symptomatic relief was as a result of the decompression as the fusion failed). Simple decompression also eliminates the increased morbidity associated with fusion [2]. Complications of fusion include blood loss, dural tear, infection, rod or screw fracture, and neural injury.

Where instability is present or where it is felt that the decompression may further destabilize the patient, fusion is indicated. Posterior lumbar interbody fusion (PLIF) [21] and transforaminal lumbar interbody fusion (TLIF) [22] are surgical options. Interbody fusion involves the replacement of the intervertebral disc with some form of a spacer (cage or bone graft). In a PLIF procedure, discectomy, and cage insertion involves nerve root retraction to access the disc space. In a TLIF, the disc space is accessed through Kambin's triangle and minimizes nerve root retraction. Both approaches should always be supplemented by posterolateral instrumentation [23]. There is debate in the literature about whether to perform an interbody fusion with posterolateral instrumentation or a posterolateral fusion alone in spondylolisthesis Some surgeons contend that interbody fusion is the gold-standard for lumbar fusion surgery due to the relative area of vertebral apposition and axial load through this region [24]. Some report superior mechanical strength with interbody fusion, but no difference in clinical outcome [25]. Others contend that interbody fusion should be reserved for higher grades of slippage [26] and posterolateral fusion has better outcome in low grades [27], while others recommend posterolateral fusion over interbody fusion, on the basis of clinical outcome and lower morbidity [28]. A recurring theme in the literature is that no significant clinical difference has been noted in many studies when interbody fusion is compared with posterolateral fusion in spondylolisthesis [14, 29]. The second major debate concerns fusion in situ versus reduction of spondylolisthesis. The level of evidence does not support a clear-cut answer to this question—reduction of high-grade spondylolisthesis aims to return that region of the spine to a normal alignment (which may improve global pan-spinal sagittal balance in the long-term), and increases the area for interbody fusion to take place. Conversely, increased rates of nerve damage and instrumentation failure have been reported with high-grade spondylolisthesis reduction. One must also inform the patient of approximately 30% chance of adjacent segment disease after spinal fixation in this context.

Expert comment Assessing solidity of fusion

There is no reference standard for non-invasive imaging of evaluation of fusion [30]. The criteria for assessing solidity of fusion radiographically as defined by Ray [31] are listed here. They have not been externally validated, but have gained clinical acceptance [32].

- Less than 3 degrees of intersegmental position change on lateral flexion and extension views.
- No lucent area around the implant.
- Minimal loss of disc height.
- No fracture of the device, graft, or vertebra.
- No sclerotic changes in the graft or adjacent vertebra.
- Visible bone formation in or about the graft material.

66 Expert comment Exhaust conservative treatment before considering surgery for Grade 1 and 2 disease

66 Expert comment Exhaust conservative treatment before considering surgery for Grade 1 and 2 disease

- Decompression of the L5 root, under the pars defect is usually necessary, as well as fusion. This is essential if a reduction of the slip is planned.
- If you do want to reduce, distract before retracting L5.
- Spondylolisthesis can be treated with minimally invasive techniques.

66 Expert comment

The authors' group performed an audit of their practice and have largely abandoned interbody fusion. A retrospective study of thirty-two patients (twenty-one females and eleven males) was performed. Indications for surgery were low back pain, with or without sciatica, and all patients had undergone unsuccessful conservative therapies for at least 6 months prior to surgery. Twelve patients had undergone mini-open posterolateral fusion (PLF) with pedicle screw fixation and twenty had undergone interbody fusion (PLIF or TLIF) supplemented with unilateral pedicle screws. The average age was 45 years. Functional outcomes were assessed using SF-36, ODI, and pain VAS. The mini-open PLF group fared significantly better than the interbody fusion group at 2 years.

✓ Evidence base Surgical compared with non-operative treatment for lumbar degenerative spondylolisthesis

Four-year results in the SPORT randomized and observational cohorts. Weinstein et al. [1].

This study involved two cohorts of patients from thirteen centres, with symptoms of at least 12 weeks duration, and radiological evidence of degenerative spondylolisthesis with spinal stenosis. In the randomized cohort, patients were randomized to receive surgery or randomized to receive non-operative care. In the observational cohort, the choice of treatment was made by the patients and their doctors. A total of 304 patients were enrolled in the randomized cohort and 303 patients enrolled in the observational cohort. Primary outcome measures were the SF-36 and the modified ODI at 6 weeks, 3 months, 6 months, and yearly for up to 4 years. The results were as follows. Clinically relevant advantages of surgery were reported with treatment effects of 15.3 for bodily pain, 18.9 for physical function, and –14.3 for the ODI. Early advantages (at 2 years) of surgical treatment in terms of the secondary measures of how troublesome back and leg symptoms are, overall satisfaction with current symptoms, and self-rated progress were also maintained at 4 years. The study concluded that, compared with patients who are treated non-operatively, patients in whom degenerative spondylolisthesis and associated spinal stenosis are treated surgically maintain substantially greater pain relief and improvement in function for 4 years.

A final word from the expert

Fusion surgery for spondylolisthesis in a patient with chronic back pain is surgery of last resort—all other conservative measures should exhausted first

There is much debate as to whether the slippage needs to be reduced or not. I favour fusion in situ for a number of reasons.

- There is no evidence that reducing the slip is associated with a better outcome.
- What is known is that reducing the slip carries a greater risk of damage to the L5 nerve roots.
- Many patients with spondylolisthesis have reached a state of sagittal balance. If you restore the normal anatomy by reducing the slip, it is possible to destroy the sagittal balance and make matters worse for the patient.

Concepts such as the slip angle of the sacrum, and the presence of a rounded sacral dome and/or trapezoidal L5 (grade of dysplasia) may also be important considerations in the surgical management of spondylolisthesis.

References

1. Weinstein JN, Lurie JD, Tosteson TD, et al. Surgical compared with nonoperative treatment for lumbar degenerative spondylolisthesis. Four-year results in the Spine Patient Outcomes Research Trial (SPORT) randomized and observational cohorts. J Bone Jt Surg Am 2009; 91(6): 1295–304.

2. Gunzburg R, Szpalski M (eds.) Spondylolysis, spondylolisthesis, and degenerative spondylolisthesis. Sydney: Lippincott Williams and Wilkins, 2005.

3. Kalichman L, Hunter DJ.Diagnosis and conservative management of degenerative lumbar spondylolisthesis. Eur Spine J 2008; 17(3): 327–35.

4. Hawker GA, Mian S, Kendzerska T, et al. Measures of adult pain: Visual Analog Scale for pain (VAS pain), Numeric Rating Scale for pain (NRS pain), McGill Pain Questionnaire (MPQ), Short-Form McGill Pain Questionnaire (SF-MPQ), Chronic Pain Grade Scale (CPGS), Short Form-36 Bodily Pain Scale (SF-36 BPS), and Measure of Intermittent and Constant Osteoarthritis Pain (ICOAP). Arthritis Care Res (Hoboken) 2011; 63 (Suppl. 11): S240–52.

5. Fairbank JC, Pynsent PB. The Oswestry Disability Index. Spine 2000; 25(22): 2940–52 ; discussion 2952.

6. Boonstra AM, Schiphorst Preuper HR, Reneman MF, et al. Reliability and validity of the visual analogue scale for disability in patients with chronic musculoskeletal pain. Int J Rehabil Res. 2008; 31(2): 165–9.

7. Guilfoyle MR, Seeley H, Laing RJ. The Short Form 36 health survey in spine disease— validation against condition-specific measures. Br J Neurosurg 2009; 23(4): 401–5.

8. Wiltse LL, Bateman JG, Hutchinson RH, et al. The paraspinal sacrospinalis-splitting approach to the lumbar spine. J Bone Jt Surg Am 1968; 50(5): 919–26.

9. Herbiniaux G. Traité sur divers accouchemens laborieux et sur les polypes de la matrice. Bruxelles: J. L. de Boubers. 1782.

10. Kilian H. De spondylolisthesi gravissimae pelvagustiae caussa nuper detecta. Commentario anatomico-obstetrica. Bonn: C Georgii Co; 1854.

11. The American Heritage The American Heritage Dictionary of the English Language. Entry: spondylolisthesis. Available at: http://ahdictionary.com/word/search. html?q=spondylolisthesis (accessed 1 September 2012.

12. Fredrickson BE, Baker D, McHolick WJ, The natural history of spondylolysis and spondylolisthesis. J Bone Jt Surg Am 1984; 66(5): 699–707.

13. Beutler WJ, Fredrickson BE, Murtland A, et al. The natural history of spondylolysis and spondylolisthesis: 45-year follow-up evaluation. Spine 2003; 28(10): 1027–35; discussion 1035.

14. Metz LN, Deviren V. Low-grade spondylolisthesis. Neurosurg Clin N Am 2007; 18(2): 237–48.

15. Agabegi SS, Fischgrund JS. Contemporary management of isthmic spondylolisthesis: pediatric and adult. Spine J 2010; 10(6): 530–43.

16. Rosenberg NJ. Degenerative spondylolisthesis. Predisposing factors. J Bone Jt Surg Am 1975; 57(4): 467–74.

17. Vibert BT, Sliva CD, Herkowitz HN. Treatment of instability and spondylolisthesis: surgical versus nonsurgical treatment. Clin Orthop Relat Res 2006; 443: 222–7.

18. Wiltse LL, Newman PH, Macnab I. Classification of spondylolisis and spondylolisthesis. Clin Orthop Relat Res 1976; (117): 23–9.

19. Meyerding HW. Spondylolisthesis: surgical treatment and results. J Bone Jt Surg Am 1943; 25(1): 65–77.

20. Gatt CJ Jr, Hosea TM, Palumbo RC, et al. Impact loading of the lumbar spine during football blocking. Am J Sports Med 1997; 25(3): 317–21.

21. Cloward RB. The treatment of ruptured lumbar intervertebral disc by vertebral body fusion. III. Method of use of banked bone. Ann Surg 1952; 136(6): 987–92.

22. Lowe TG, Tahernia AD, O'Brien MF, et al. Unilateral transforaminal posterior lumbar interbody fusion (TLIF): indications, technique, and 2-year results. J Spinal Disord Tech 2002; 15(1): 31–8.

23. Lund T, Oxland TR, Jost B, et al. Interbody cage stabilization in the lumbar spine: biomechanical evaluation of cage design, posterior instrumentation and bone density. J Bone Jt Surg Br 1998; 80(2): 351–9.

24. Müslüman AM, Yılmaz A, Cansever T, et al. Posterior lumbar interbody fusion versus posterolateral fusion with instrumentation in the treatment of low-grade isthmic spondylolisthesis: midterm clinical outcomes. J Neurosurg Spine 2011; 14(4): 488–96.

25. La Rosa G, Conti A, Cacciola F, et al. Pedicle screw fixation for isthmic spondylolisthesis: does posterior lumbar interbody fusion improve outcome over posterolateral fusion? J Neurosurg 2003; 99 (Suppl. 2): 143–50.

26. Dehoux E, Fourati E, Madi K, et al. Posterolateral versus interbody fusion in isthmic spondylolisthesis: functional results in 52 cases with a minimum follow-up of 6 years. Acta Orthop Belg 2004; 70(6): 578–82.

27. Madan S, Boeree NR. Outcome of posterior lumbar interbody fusion versus posterolateral fusion for spondylolytic spondylolisthesis. Spine 2002; 27(14): 1536–42.

28. Inamdar DN, Alagappan M, Shyam L, et al. Posterior lumbar interbody fusion versus intertransverse fusion in the treatment of lumbar spondylolisthesis. J Orthop Surg (Hong Kong) 2006; 14(1): 21–6.

29. Endres S, Aigner R, Wilke A. Instrumented intervertebral or posterolateral fusion in elderly patients: clinical results of a single center. BMC Musculoskelet Disord 2011; 12: 189.

30. Rutherford EE, Tarplett LJ, Davies EM, et al. Lumbar spine fusion and stabilization: hardware, techniques, and imaging appearances. Radiographics 2007; 27(6): 1737–49.

31. Ray CD. Threaded fusion cages for lumbar interbody fusions. An economic comparison with 360 degrees fusions. Spine 1997; 22(6): 681–5.

32. Young PM, Berquist TH, Bancroft LW, et al. Complications of spinal instrumentation. Radiographics 2007; 27(3): 775–89.

4 Intramedullary spinal cord tumour

Ruth-Mary deSouza

⊕ Expert commentary David Choi

Case history

A 52-year-old right-handed woman was referred by her general practitioner to the neurosurgical outpatient department with an 8-month history of neck and left arm pain. She had been involved in a minor traffic accident a few weeks before attending her GP and reported a worsening of her symptoms after this. Further direct questioning revealed progressive neck pain, left arm pain, and weakness, which impaired tasks such as carrying shopping. She also complained of tiredness after walking, and feeling pins and needles in her toes intermittently. Her only medical history was hypothyroidism. The patient worked as a school music teacher and had noticed a gradual decline in her dexterity, which impaired her ability to teach classes that required demonstration of technique.

On examination, she had increased tone in the left upper limb, MRC (Medical Research Council) grade 4/5 left hemiparesis, and hyperreflexia in both arms and legs. MR imaging of her whole spine revealed a well-defined homogenous gadolinium-enhancing mass within the spinal cord extending between the C4 and C6 levels. A small syrinx and cord oedema was associated with the mass on T2 sequences (Figure 4.1).

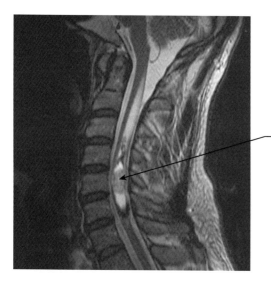

Intrinsic space occupying spinal cord lesion, with syrinx and oedema extending superiorly and inferiorly

Figure 4.1 T2-weighted sagittal MRI scan through the cervical spine revealing an intrinsic space-occupying lesion centred between C4 and C6. A combination of syrinx and cord oedema extend above and below the lesion from C1 down to C7.

Image courtesy of David Choi.

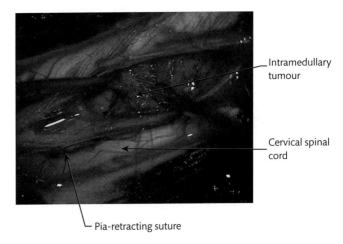

Intramedullary tumour

Cervical spinal cord

Pia-retracting suture

Figure 4.2 Intra-operative photograph of a spinal cord ependymoma resection. The cord is split in the midline and the tumour resected using micro-instruments, with neurophysiological monitoring of both the sensory and the motor tracts.

After discussion in the spinal oncology MDT meeting and at length with the patient, a decision was made to attempt resection of this intramedullary cord lesion. After C4–6 laminectomies, a midline durotomy was carried out and, under the microscope, a midline myelotomy revealed a cavity containing tumour. A clear plane of dissection was identified between the tumour and the surrounding spinal cord, allowing complete macroscopic excision of the lesion (Figure 4.2). Intra-operative neurophysiological monitoring comprising motor- and somatosensory-evoked potentials remained stable throughout the procedure.

Histopathological analysis revealed a WHO Grade 2 ependymoma. Post-operatively the patient had no new neurological deficit. She developed a CSF leak

❝ Expert comment Intra-operative neuromonitoring

Intra-operative potentials are recorded from the thenars, hypothenars, tibialis anterior, and flexor hallucis brevis, as these have strong pyramidal innervation. The sensitivity of motor-evoked potentials (MEPs) for post-operative motor deficit approaches 100% and is about 90% specific.

Recent guidelines provide level A evidence that intra-operative neurophysiology during spinal cord predicts an increased risk of paraparesis, paraplegia, and quadriplegia. All twelve studies included in this analysis demonstrated that every incident of paraparesis, paraplegia, and quadriplegia was associated with changes in monitoring output and no paralysis occurred without changes in the monitoring output. The role of intra-operative monitoring in the prevention of mild motor deficits was not studied [1].

✪ Learning point Histopathology and World Health Organization grading of ependymomas

Histological characteristics of ependymomas typically include the presence of perivascular and ependymal rosettes (Figure 4.3), and positive immunohistochemical staining for glial fibrillary acidic protein (GFAP), CD56, and epithelial membrane antigen (EMA).

According to the 2007 WHO classification of tumours of the central nervous system, there are three grades of ependymal tumours [2]:

● *Grade I*: subependymoma and myxopapillary ependymoma.
● *Grade 2*: ependymoma without the malignant features that define Grade 3 (the most common type).
● *Grade 3*: anaplastic ependymoma, revealing malignant features of increased cellularity, brisk mitotic activity, microvascular proliferation, and pseudopalisading necrosis.

There are four recognized histological subtypes of ependymona—cellular, papillary, clear cell, and tanycytic. The subtypes generally apply to Grades 2 and 3 ependymomas.

A controversy in the grading of ependymomas arises in the distinction between Grades 2 and 3 [3]. Poor correlation with clinical progression and lack of biological usefulness in distinguishing Grades 2 and 3. The current grading system does not take account of factors such as location, segments involved, age, and clinical features.

(continued)

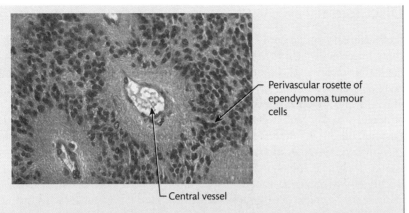

Perivascular rosette of ependymoma tumour cells

Central vessel

Figure 4.3 A characteristic feature of ependymoma tumours is the presence of perivascular rosettes or pseudorosettes as shown in this histology slide, that is tumour cells arranged around central vessels with anuclear zones in between (H&E stain).

Taken from 'Pubcan: A Public Database of Human Cancers' http://www.pubcan.org/printicdotopo.php?id=4715

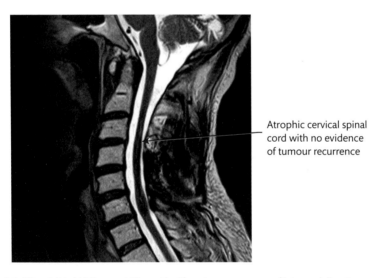

Atrophic cervical spinal cord with no evidence of tumour recurrence

Figure 4.4 T2-weighted MRI scan at 12 months. There is no recurrence of intramedullary tumour and post-operative cord atrophy.

Images courtesy of David Choi.

from the wound 2 days after the operation, which terminated after a mattress suture was placed at the leaking point. She was referred for spinal rehabilitation, and made a good recovery, although she was not able to regain employment as a music teacher, due to continuing problems with fine motor tasks of the left hand. At 12 months, no recurrence was seen on follow-up MRI (Figure 4.4). Motor function remained stable in the left hand with grade 4/5 power and improved in the left leg to 4+/5. The patient was independent with all daily activities, except complex fine motor tasks.

Discussion

Intramedullary spinal cord tumours (IMSCT) are rare, constituting about 2–4% of central nervous system (CNS) tumours. In adults, they represent about a fifth of spinal malignancies and a higher proportion in children (approaching 40%). The main body of evidence for surgery in IMSCTs comes from retrospective series. The lack of level 1 and 2 evidence available with regard to IMSCTs, and the high-risk nature of surgery, makes this a challenging area of neurosurgery. Interestingly, Harvey Cushing, during his time at Johns Hopkins, remarked that there was 'No performance in surgery more interesting and satisfactory' [4]. The most common type of IMSCT in adults is ependymoma (about 70%), followed by astrocytoma (about 20%). In children astrocytoma is the most common tumour type (70%), with low grade being more common than high grade astrocytoma [5]. Other IMSCTs include haemangioblastoma, cavernoma, oligodendroglioma, and glioblastoma. Intramedullary metastases are extremely rare, have a poor prognosis, and are typically managed with palliative radiotherapy.

Clinical features of IMSCTs are insidious at onset, and can mimic degenerative spinal pathology. This, in addition to their rarity, means that diagnosis can be delayed. Common presentations are of radicular pain, sensory disturbances, and mild motor weakness leading to gait problems. Sphincter involvement is less common. Children also present with pain and sensorimotor disturbance, and they appear more likely to have a deformity, such as scoliosis and torticollis, at the time of initial presentation [6]. Up to 15% of children have hydrocephalus with an IMSCT. In children too young to report symptoms, the parents may report falls, inadvertent injuries, nocturnal pain, and motor regression [6].

> **🗨 Expert comment** Presentation of intramedullary spinal cord tumours
>
> Patients with large intramedullary tumours often present with relatively mild symptoms from slowly-growing tumours. Persistent, progressive atypical symptoms or signs in young patients should raise alarm bells.
>
> MRI can provide high quality definition of the lesion and associated features, such as cord oedema, nerve root involvement, syrinx, and local extension. Currently, MRI cannot reliably differentiate between ependymoma and astrocytoma, although ependymomas are often better defined than diffuse astrocytomas. Reported differential diagnoses for an IMSCT include abscess, tuberculoma, sacroid, cysts, and plaques of demyelination. Preliminary evidence is emerging that Diffusion Tensor Imaging may be useful in predicting the resectability of IMSCTs [7]. In the work up of IMSCT, other investigations include:
>
> • Screening CT of the chest, abdomen, and pelvis.
> • MRI of the head (posterior fossa tumours can occasionally produce 'drop metastases' in the spine).
> • Dynamic X-rays of the spine, in case the presence of instability requires adjunctive surgical instrumentation.
>
> Factors affecting outcome in surgically-treated IMSCTs have been identified from retrospective series. One of the largest series is by Raco et al., reporting the outcome of 202 patients with surgically-treated IMSCTs, and reports that the key factors affecting outcome are histological type of lesion, completeness of excision, and pre-operative neurological status [8]. Other factors show a weaker association with outcome. These include multilevel involvement, thoracic location, and age [9, 10, 11, 12].
>
> There is some evidence of pre- and peri-operative factors that may impair recovery and ambulation after surgery. These include hyperglycaemia and pre-operative radiation [13]. Some of these factors, namely those elucidated by Raco et al. [8], generate debate in neurosurgery and are discussed in greater depth below.

Surgical options for infiltrative tumours include biopsy, debulking, or subtotal resection. Biopsy only is an appropriate choice in patients not fit to tolerate extensive surgery, or when the diagnosis is uncertain and the lesion could represent non-malignant athology. The extent of resection in infiltrative tumours is guided by microscopy and intra-operative MEPs, somatosensory-evoked potentials (SSEPs) and occasionally D-wave (epidural) monitoring. Some papers suggest a role for intra-operative ultrasound in defining the margins of the tumour, its relation to the spinal cord, vascular relations, and its consistency [15]. Karikari et al. point out that the extent of resection is dependent on the plane of dissection, which is somewhat variable in the literature [14], with some series such as Garcés-Ambrossi et al. describing a fairly high rate (up to 40%) of gross total resection of spinal cord astrocytomas [10]. McGirt et al. point out that aggressive resection of astrocytoma can lead to substantial motor deficits and this risk needs to be balanced against the option of a more conservative resection, followed by radiotherapy [16]. Complete resection is, however, associated with a lower recurrence risk [17, 18]. While some papers show the degree of resection to be an independent risk factor in recurrence, it may be that those tumours that are easier to resect are also the ones that are benign. A series of 100 IMSCTs showed that 45% had an associated syrinx [19]. The authors suggested that the presence of a syrinx may be a favourable prognostic sign as it suggests displacement, rather than infiltration of the cord [19]. The presence of a syrinx may also facilitate resection by creating natural planes within the cord and improve outcome compared with cases without a syrinx [10].

Another area of controversy in the management of IMSCTs is the optimal timing of surgery. Since most authors advocate aiming for complete excision, it can be argued that early surgery on a small mass is desirable. However, in patients who are not functionally impaired by their neurological deficit and who have a slow growing tumour on serial imaging, the risks of surgery may not be acceptable. Since pre-operative neurological deficit is an established determinant of outcome, it is important to operate before neurological deficits that affect mobility and function appear. Whether surgery should be performed in an asymptomatic patient, or whether to risk the development of neurological deficits in time from an expanding tumour, is a difficult decision to make. Patients should be counselled about the risks and benefits of early or delayed surgery. Evolving neurological deficit is a definite indication for surgery.

It is known that intra-operative monitoring is effective in reducing neurological deficit. However, the interpretation of intra-operative monitoring is not a clear-cut matter. Various grading systems have been proposed to quantify loss of potentials intra-operatively. No widely-accepted system is available. Intra-operative monitoring is of limited value in patients with pre-operative neurological deficits. Differences in intra-operative monitoring waveforms in infiltrating versus well-defined tumours, especially towards the tumour margins, have not been defined.

Surgery for IMSCTs is high risk and the patient should be counselled about this. The main risks include infection, CSF leak [17], transient and permanent neurological deficits, and chronic pain post-operatively. Hydrocephalus can occur in about 1% of patients by an unknown mechanism [22]. IMSCTs are not uncommon in the over-60 age group, which can lead to some concerns about the suitability of these patients for surgical management. Reports in the literature on neurosurgery in elderly patients suggest that elective procedures in the absence of diffuse neurological disturbance does not lead to poor outcomes [23, 24, 25]. Neuropathic pain in IMSCTs is described pre- and post-operatively in the literature for neural and vascular tumours [26, 27, 28], and can be the cause of significant disability and depression

Expert comment Resecting intramedullary tumours

A challenge in the surgical management of IMSCTs is how aggressively to resect tumours, especially those without a clear plane of dissection. Tumour histology has been found to influence ease of resection and ability to achieve complete resection [14]. For ependymomas and vascular tumours with well-defined margins, the gold standard is total resection. Astrocytoma and other infiltrative tumours, however, are more difficult to resect as there is no clear dissection plane and, here, the aim may not be complete resection, but rather subtotal resection without causing new neurological deficits.

Clinical tip Loss if motor-evoked potentials / somatosensory-evoked potentials signal intra-operatively

Diminishing signals are a warning that neurological deficit may occur and gives the surgeon an opportunity to react. Should signals be lost, stop surgery and assess for spontaneous recover of potentials. Irrigate the operative field with warm saline and increase the blood pressure to increase spinal cord perfusion [20]. Sala et al. reported that surgery may need to be stopped for up to 30 minutes in some cases, before potentials reappear and surgery can progress. If potentials fail to recover, it may be appropriate to perform the operation as a two-stage procedure or even to abandon surgery completely [20, 21].

Expert comment Minimizing the risk of cerebrospinal fluid leak

Perfect primary closure is important, for example, by using a running 4/0 prolene or nylon suture (vicryl can tear the dura), supplemented with a dural patch and tissue adhesive. Lumbar drains are seldom required, and should be reserved for troublesome persistent leaks.

for patients. Pain and spinal deformity are two long-term sequelae after surgery for IMSCTs, the latter being more common in children. A retrospective series of 52 IMSCTs in children showed that fusion or instrumentation at the time of tumour excision was associated with a significantly lower risk of post-operative deformity [29]. Removal of more than three laminae was associated with significantly increased risk of kyphotic deformity.

In terms of adjuvant treatment, radiotherapy is used variably. It can be used for all high-grade tumours, high-grade tumours with incomplete resection margins, and recurrence of high-grade tumours. There is currently no level 1 or 2 evidence investigating the role of adjuvant radiotherapy in IMSCTs, so the decision is made on a case-by-case basis. Typically, external beam radiotherapy has been reserved for recurrence, inoperable tumours, and palliatively [30]. Cyberknife radiotherapy has been attempted for IMSCTs, but there are no long-term outcome data on its effectiveness as yet. Chemotherapy can be considered in patients with progression of disease following radiotherapy, but data are limited [31, 32]. Vascular intramedullary tumours broadly comprising spinal cord cavernomas and haemangioblastomas, present specific challenges. They are benign, usually well-defined, and typically can be shelled out en bloc.

> **✔ Evidence base** Surgery for IMSCTs
>
> The literature on IMSCTs is comprised of retrospective series, which represents NHS Class C evidence. Two of the larger series are:
>
> - Raco et al. review the outcome of 202 IMSCTs. Sixty-one (30%) were cervical tumours (30%), sixty (29%) thoracic, and fifty-one (25%) cervicothoracic. Astrocytoma (eighty-six patients, 42%) and ependymoma (sixty-eight patients, 34%) were the main tumour types. Long-term functional outcome was determined by histology, degree of resection and pre-operative neurological status [8].
> - Kucia et al. [17] review sixty-seven spinal ependymomas. Like Raco et al. [8], cervical and thoracic location predominated. Complete resection was achieved in fifty-five patients. The findings of note in this paper were that pre- and post-operative neurological outcome correlated significantly (P < 0.001). Early post-operative neurological worsening was found at 3-month follow-up to have improved in a significant number. This series reported a high complication rate of 34%, mainly wound infections and cerebrospinal fluid leaks

Spinal cavernomas mainly affect the cervical and thoracic cord. A recent literature review suggests that just over a quarter of these have a co-existing cranial cavernoma and a tenth have a family history of cavernoma [33]. Mutations in the cerebral cavernous malformation (CCM) one, two, and three genes have been described in cavernoma development. Clinical features can be secondary to expansion and/or to recurrent haemorrhaging, and progressive deterioration follows an acute, stepwise, or progressive nature [27]. Gross et al. [33] discussed surgical management based upon whether the lesion is exophytic or deep, and whether it is symptomatic or not. They recommended intervention for symptomatic lesions and for accessible lesions, while recommending observation for deep and asymptomatic or mildly symptomatic lesions [33]. This approach is supported by a retrospective review of 96 intramedullary cavernomas, where 91% of operated cases were stabilized or improved, and none of the twelve conservatively-managed patients deteriorated [34]. Radiologically, cavernomas are commonly described as having a 'popcorn' appearance, due to the hyperdense vascular component surrounded by a hypodense haemosiderin ring on MRI with gradient echo sequencing. Operatively, this translates into the presence of a well-defined gliotic plane along the outside of the cavernoma.

Haemangioblastmas can be sporadic or occur in the setting of VHL disease, where they are more likely to be multiple. Mehta et al. reported on 218 spinal haemangioblastoma surgeries in 108 VHL patients, where 99.5% were completely resected and 96% improved clinically post-operatively [35]. Later decline was due to VHL disease progression unrelated to the operated cavernoma.

> ✪ **Learning point** Von Hippel–Lindau disease
>
> VHL disease is an autosomal dominant syndrome with a defect on chromosome 3 (*3p25-p26*), which is a tumour suppressor gene. VHL is associated with renal cell carcinoma, pheochromocytoma, hemangioblastomas of the CNS, retinal angiomas, epididymal cysts, endolymphatic sac tumours, and pancreatic cysts and solid lesions.

> ➕ **Clinical tip** Pre-operative preparation of vascular intramedullary spinal cord tumours
>
> Haemangioblastomas can cause massive intra-operative haemorrhage! Ensure there are blood products available and consider pre-operative endovascular embolization.

A final word from the expert

Intramedullary spinal tumours are relatively uncommon, but can result in severe neurological deficit if left untreated. Gross total resection (GTR) should be the goal for the majority of benign pathologies. Surgery on intramedullary tumours should be performed by neurosurgeons who deal with these lesions on a regular basis; considerable experience is required to achieve high GTR rates and to limit rates of permanent morbidity. Intra-operative monitoring with MEPs and/or SSEPs are utilized to facilitate optimal tumour resection.

References

1. Nuwer MR, Emerson RG, Galloway G, et al. Evidence-based guideline update: intraoperative spinal monitoring with somatosensory and transcranial electrical motor evoked potentials. J Clin Neurophysiol 2012; 29(1): 101–8.
2. Louis DN, Ohgaki H, Wiestler OD, et al. The 2007 WHO classification of tumours of the central nervous system. Acta Neuropathol 2007; 114(2): 97–109. Erratum: Acta Neuropathol 2007; 114(5): 547.
3. Godfraind C. Classification and controversies in pathology of ependymomas. Childs Nerv Syst 2009; 25(10): 1185–93.
4. Dasenbrock HH, Pendleton C, Cohen-Gadol AA, et al. 'No performance in surgery more interesting and satisfactory': Harvey Cushing and his experience with spinal cord tumors at the Johns Hopkins Hospital. J Neurosurg Spine 2011; 14(3): 412–20.
5. Benes V 3rd, Barsa P, Benes V Jr, et al. Prognostic factors in intramedullary astrocytomas: a literature review. Eur Spine J 2009; 18(10): 1397–422.
6. Chatterejee S, Chatterjee U. Intramedullary tumours in children. J Pediatr Neurosci 2011; 6 (Suppl. 1): S86–90.
7. Setzer M, Murtagh RD, Murtagh FR, et al. Diffusion tensor imaging tractography in patients with intramedullary tumors: comparison with intraoperative findings and value for prediction of tumor resectability. J Neurosurg Spine 2010; 13(3): 371–80.
8. Raco A, Piccirilli M, Landi A, et al. High-grade intramedullary astrocytomas: 30 years' experience at the Neurosurgery Department of the University of Rome 'Sapienza'. J Neurosurg Spine 2010; 12(2): 144–53.
9. Matsuyama Y, Sakai Y, Katayama Y, et al. Surgical results of intramedullary spinal cord tumour with spinal cord monitoring to guide extent of resection. J Neurosurg Spine 2009; 10(5): 404–13.

10. Garcés-Ambrossi GL, McGirt MJ, Mehta VA, et al. Factors associated with progression-free survival and long-term neurological outcome after resection of intramedullary spinal cord tumours: analysis of 101 consecutive cases. J Neurosurg Spine 2009; 11(5): 591-9.

11. Constantini S, Miller DC, Allen JC, et al. Radical excision of intramedullary spinal cord tumours: surgical morbidity and long-term follow-up evaluation in 164 children and young adults. J Neurosurg 2000; 93 (Suppl. 2): 183-93.

12. Ebner FH, Roser F, Falk M, et al. Management of intramedullary spinal cord lesions: interdependence of the longitudinal extension of the lesion and the functional outcome. Eur Spine J 2010; 19(4): 665-9.

13. Woodworth GF, Chaichana KL, McGirt MJ, et al. Predictors of ambulatory function after surgical resection of intramedullary spinal cord tumors. Neurosurgery 2007; 61(1): 99-105; discussion 105-6.

14. Karikari IO, Nimjee SM, Hodges TR, et al. Impact of tumour histology on resectability and neurological outcome in primary intramedullary spinal cord tumours: a single-center experience with 102 patients. Neurosurgery 2011; 68(1): 188-97 ; discussion 197.

15. Zhou H, Miller D, Schulte DM, et al. Intraoperative ultrasound assistance in treatment of intradural spinal tumours. Clin Neurol Neurosurg 2011; 113(7): 531-7.

16. McGirt MJ, Goldstein IM, Chaichana KL, et al. Extent of surgical resection of malignant astrocytomas of the spinal cord: outcome analysis of 35 patients. Neurosurgery 2008; 63(1): 55-60 ; discussion 60-1.

17. Kucia EJ, Bambakidis NC, Chang SW, et al. Surgical technique and outcomes in the treatment of spinal cord ependymomas, part 1: intramedullary ependymomas. Neurosurgery 2011; 68 (Suppl. 1, Operative): 57-63 ; discussion 63.

18. Boström A, von Lehe M, Hartmann W, et al. Surgery for spinal cord ependymomas: outcome and prognostic factors. Neurosurgery 2011; 68(2): 302-8; discussion 309.

19. Samii M, Klekamp J. Surgical results of 100 intramedullary tumors in relation to accompanying syringomyelia. Neurosurgery 1994; 35(5): 865-73 ; discussion 873.

20. Sala F, Bricolo A, Faccioli F, et al. Surgery for intramedullary spinal cord tumors: the role of intraoperative (neurophysiological) monitoring. Eur Spine J 2007; 16 (Suppl. 2): S130-9.

21. Kothbauer KF. Intraoperative neurophysiologic monitoring for intramedullary spinal-cord tumor surgery. Neurophysiol Clin 2007; 37(6): 407-14.

22. Mirone G, Cinalli G, Spennato P, et al. Hydrocephalus and spinal cord tumors: a review. Childs Nerv Syst 2011; 27(10): 1741-9.

23. Maurice-Williams RS, Kitchen N. The scope of neurosurgery for elderly people. Age Ageing 1993; 22(5): 337-42.

24. Sacko O, Haegelen C, Mendes V, et al. Spinal meningioma surgery in elderly patients with paraplegia or severe paraparesis: a multicenter study. Neurosurgery 2009; 64(3): 503-9; discussion 509-10.

25. Chibbaro S, Di Rocco F, Makiese O, et al. Neurosurgery and elderly: analysis through the years. Neurosurg Rev 2010; 34(2): 229-34.

26. Cerda-Olmedo G, De Andrés J, Moliner S. Management of progressive pain in a patient with intramedullary chordoma of the spine. Clin J Pain 2002; 18(2): 128-31.

27. Deutsch H. Pain outcomes after surgery in patients with intramedullary spinal cord cavernous malformations. Neurosurg Focus 2010; 29(3): E15.

28. Saito N, Yamakawa K, Sasaki T, et al. Intramedullary cavernous angioma with trigeminal neuralgia: a case report and review of the literature. Neurosurgery 1989; 25(1): 97-101.

29. Anakwenze OA, Auerbach JD, Buck DW, et al. The role of concurrent fusion to prevent spinal deformity after intramedullary spinal cord tumor excision in children. J Pediat Orthop 2011; 31(5): 475-9.

30. Jallo GI, Danish S, Velasquez L, et al. Intramedullary low-grade astrocytomas: long-term outcome following radical surgery. J Neuro Oncol 2001; 53(1): 61-6.

31. Chamberlain MC. Temozolomide for recurrent low-grade spinal cord gliomas in adults. Cancer 2008; 113(5): 1019–24.

32. Lowis SP, Pizer BL, Coakham H, et al. Chemotherapy for spinal cord astrocytoma: can natural history be modified? Childs Nerv Syst 1998; 14(7): 317–21.

33. Gross BA, Du R, Popp AJ, et al. Intramedullary spinal cord cavernous malformations. Neurosurg Focus 2010; 29(3): E14. Review.

34. Liang JT, Bao YH, Zhang HQ, et al. Management and prognosis of symptomatic patients with intramedullary spinal cord cavernoma: clinical article. J Neurosurg Spine 2011; 15(4): 447–56.

35. Mehta GU, Asthagiri AR, Bakhtian KD, et al. Functional outcome after resection of spinal cord hemangioblastomas associated with von Hippel-Lindau disease. J Neurosurg Spine 2010; 12(3): 233–4.

5 Surgery for temporal lobe epilepsy

Victoria Wykes and Anna Miserocchi

Expert commentary Andrew McEvoy

Case history

A 30-year-old, left-handed woman was referred to the epilepsy service with frequent seizures occurring three or four times per month, which had proved refractory to medication. She described daily episodes of gradual onset of 'butterflies in the stomach' followed by 'a bitter taste' lasting several minutes. Witnesses stated that she would lose awareness. Sometimes she turned her head to the right prior to flexing both elbows to 90 degrees, with clenching of her left hand. The episodes lasted several minutes and occurred once per week. After the event, she would rub her nose with her right hand, had speech difficulty for up to 5 minutes and experienced left arm weakness, which fully recovered after several hours. Triggers included sleep deprivation and the menstrual cycle. Seizures have resulted in four recent episodes of skin burns. Two secondary generalized tonic clonic seizures (GTCS) had occurred 8 years ago, but no episodes of status epilepticus.

> **✪ Learning point**
>
> In 1981, the International League Against Epilepsy (ILAE) established a standardized classification and terminology based on seizure manifestations and electroencephalography (EEG) to aid diagnosis, and communication between health professionals and patients [1]. With ongoing advances, new proposals are being made to this classification scheme [2]. Both ILAE classifications are based on the widely-accepted concept that seizures may be generalized or focal.
>
> Generalized seizures arise from large areas of cortex, and consciousness is lost. However, focal seizures arise in specific small areas of the cortex in one hemisphere, can spread within the same hemisphere or cross to the contralateral side, and may progress into a generalized seizure. Focal seizures can be further divided into simple partial seizures (SPS), which occur without alteration in consciousness and complex partial seizures (CPS) in which consciousness is impaired (see Tables 5.1 and 5.2 for characteristics). CPS arising in the temporal lobe typically demonstrates a tripartite seizure pattern with aura, loss of awareness and automatisms
>
> **Table 5.1 Simple partial seizure characteristics**
>
> | Manifestations | Ictal semiology | Hemispheric localisation |
> |---|---|---|
> | Motor | Clonus, spasms, or posturing
Jacksonian march
Progression of seizure along primary motor cortex affecting corresponding muscles
Todd's paresis
Post-ictal unilateral motor weakness fully reversible within 24 hours | Contralateral to side of seizure semiology |
>
> (continued)

Table 5.1 Simple partial seizure characteristics (continued)

Manifestations	Ictal semiology	Hemispheric localisation
Somatosensory	Epigastric rising	Mesial temporal lobe
	Tingling, numbness, electrical shock sensation, burning	Contralateral central or parietal region
	Simple visual phenomena, flashing lights or colours	Calcarine cortex
Autonomic	Change in pupil size, skin colour, blood pressure, heart rate, pilo-erection	May be isolated to simple partial seizures, but more common in CPS and GTCS

Table 5.2 Complex partial seizure characteristics

Manifestation	Ictal semiology	Hemispheric localization
Aura	Short-lived event lasting seconds (may last days) occurring in isolation or proceed into CPS or GTCS	
Altered consciousness	Absence with motor arrest	
Automatism, involuntary motor action. May be purposeful, complex activity with interaction with the local environment.	**Oro-alimentry:** chewing, lip smacking, swallowing drooling	Mesial temporal lobe
	Gestural: fiddling hand movements, tapping/ patting/ rubbing. Complex actions include undressing and genital-directed actions	Contralateral temporal and frontal lobe
	Verbal: meaningless sounds, whistling, word repetition or formed sentences.	
	Mimicry: excitement, laughter, anger, or fear	
	Ambulatory: walking, running, circling	
	Responsive: semi-purposeful *behaviour*, with interaction with environment	
	Violence: consider as acutely confused patient. Never premeditated, remembered, skilful, and rarely goal direct (important features in forensics)	

Her past medical history revealed a normal birth and achievement of normal developmental milestones. There was no history of infection of the CNS or head injury. She had suffered a single febrile convulsion, at age 18 months

❝ Expert comment

Childhood febrile seizures (FS) are common, occurring in approximately 5% of children. Simple FS are unlikely to be associated with long-term sequelae. Complex FS are defined as prolonged (greater than 15 minutes), multiple within 24 hours, lateralized, or associated with post-ictal neurological deficits, in the absence of a defined cause. Overall, the risk of developing long-term epilepsy following atypical FS is reported as 6% (ten times higher than average). 40–60% of patients with temporal lobe epilepsy (TLE) will report an atypical FS. It is unclear as to whether this reflects a causal association or indicates pre-existing neurological disease, which is responsible for both the complex febrile seizure and later epilepsy [3].

Seizures re-emerged when she was 18 years old and she was started on anti-epileptic drugs (AED). When seen, she was taking three AED: carbamazepine 1600mg, levetiracetam 4000mg and pregabalin 300mg daily; however she had tried five other AED, which either did not improve her symptoms or caused intolerable side effects.

ᏮᏮ Expert comment

There is debate regarding what constitutes an 'adequate trial of therapy' before a patient is diagnosed with medically refractory epilepsy. The current consensus is failure of two first-line AED at an appropriate dose, appropriate to the type of epilepsy, over 2 years [4]. Patients presenting for epilepsy surgery assessment have frequently had extensive and prolonged medication trials. There is a drive to identify medically refractory epileptic patients early, especially children, and offer them surgery.

Her additional past medical history was unremarkable. She felt that both her short- and long-term memory had deteriorated since commencing AED. There was no family history of seizures or neurological abnormality. General and neurological examinations were unremarkable. There were no psychiatric contraindications to surgery. Her neuropsychology assessment demonstrated that she functioned intellectually at an average level. Her episodic memory for both verbal and non-verbal material was good. Most noteworthy was the finding of relative weakness in verbal reasoning, working memory, and literacy skills. This profile suggested dominant hemisphere cerebral dysfunction.

ᏮᏮ Expert comment

Favourable outcome from surgery relies on accurate pre-surgical evaluation of the ictal onset zone, through a variety of investigations including:

- Clinical semiology (localizing signs).
- Structural and functional radiological imaging.
- Electrical localization with inter-ictal and ictal EEG, performed most commonly via video-telemetry.
- Detailed neuropsychological profiling to ascertain any localizing functional deficit.

T2-weighted coronal MRI head scans demonstrated hyperintensity in a shrunken right hippocampus consistent with hippocampal sclerosis (Figure 5.1). Other associated findings may include loss of hippocampal head digitations, dilatation of the ipsilateral temporal horn of the lateral ventricle, and atrophy of the fornix and mammillary bodies. Hippocampal volumetric analysis was calculated by measuring the cross-sectional area from successive volumetric T1-weighted MRI coronal images. The right hippocampus was measured to be 40% smaller in comparison with the left.

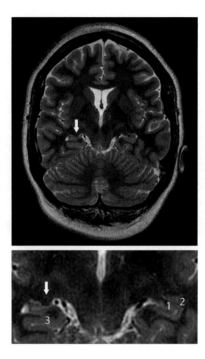

Figure 5.1 T2-weighted coronal MRI head (3 Tesla) demonstrating severe diffuse right hippocampal sclerosis (arrow). Structure 1: cornu ammonis (CA) 1–4, structure 2: subiculum, structure 3: parahippocampal gyrus.

The patient was admitted for a period of video telemetry.

⊗ **Learning point**

The EEG measures changes in voltage over the scalp resulting from summed post-synaptic potentials in cortical neurons. The international 10–20 electrode placement (Figure 5.2) allows standardization and reproducibility of electrode placement and naming. The '10' and '20' refer to the fact that the actual distances between adjacent electrodes are either 10 or 20% of the total nasion–inion distance of the

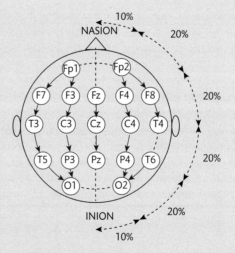

Figure 5.2 Electrode placement according to the 10–20 international system. 'Double banana' longitudinal bipolar montage represented in purple.

(continued)

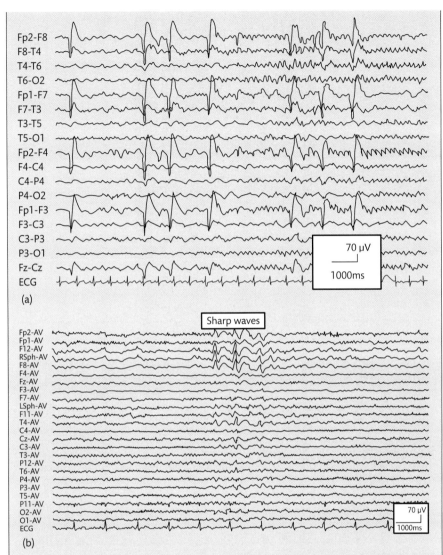

Figure 5.3 (a) Ictal EEG with longitudinal bipolar 'double banana' montage demonstrating epileptiform discharges over the right frontal and temporal areas with spread to left fronto-temporal regions. (b) Inter-ictal awake EEG with average reference montage demonstrates a run of sharp waves seen maximally over the right anterior inferior temporal and frontal areas extending into the left temporal and frontal area.

Courtesy of Dr B. Diehl, Department of Neurophysiology, NHNN, London, UK.

skull. The letter describes anatomical location (Fp = frontopolar, F = frontal, T = temporal, P = parietal, O = occipital, C = central). Electrodes placed over the right hemisphere are represented by even numbers, over the left hemisphere by odd numbers, and midline represented by 'z' (zero). Lower numbers indicate more medial placement, while higher numbers indicate more lateral placement. Additional electrodes may be useful, e.g. superficial sphenoidal electrodes when recording from the anterior or mesial temporal lobe.

The display montage represents the way the electrodes are connected and referenced. In the 'longitudinal bipolar' montage, also known as the 'double banana', each channel represents the difference between two adjacent electrodes (Figure 5.3). Whereas in the 'average reference' montage, the outputs of all of the electrodes are summed and averaged, and this averaged signal is used as the common reference for each channel.

Sharp waves 70–200msec and spikes lasting less than 70ms duration indicate epileptiform activity.

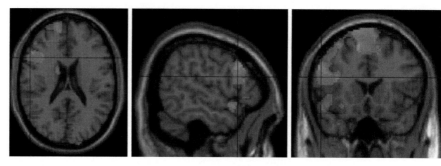

Figure 5.4 Language fMRI paradigms for verbal fluency (orange) and verb generation (yellow) provided evidence for right-sided language dominance (for colour version of this figure please see online edition).

Courtesy of Dr C. Micallef & Mr J. Stretton Department of Neuroradiology, NHNN, London, UK.

In this left-handed patient with right-sided hippocampal sclerosis and post-ictal dysphasia functional MRI (fMRI) was performed with language paradigms to lateralize language dominance (Figure 5.4).

> ### ✪ Learning point
>
> The incidence of language hemisphere dominance has been investigated using fMRI studies in healthy populations. In the right-hand dominant group, 94% were considered left hemisphere language dominant, with 6% demonstrating bilateral language representation [5]. A similar study in a non-right-hand dominant group demonstrated only that 8% were right hemisphere language dominant, with 78% demonstrating left hemisphere language dominance [6].
>
> The language system is variable in location across individuals, influenced by handedness, and in patients with TLE may reorganize with bilateral representation or transfer to the contralateral hemisphere [5].
>
> Anterior temporal lobe resection (ATLR) may impair both language and memory functions. Dominant hemisphere ATLR may impair naming and verbal memory, while non-dominant hemisphere ATLR may impair visual memory. Precise pre-operative assessment of language and memory lateralization is essential prior to surgery, to predict risk of post-operative deficits allowing informed consent of the patient.
>
> The Wada test has been, and in some centres still is, considered to be the Gold standard investigation of both language and memory functions. Reversible pharmacological deactivation of one cerebral hemisphere is achieved by injection of the barbiturate sodium amobarbital into the internal carotid artery, while the patient is awake, allowing evaluation of functions in the opposite hemisphere. The inherent risks of this invasive procedure and the emergence of non-invasive alternatives, particularly fMRI has led to replacement in many centres [7–9].

To summarize, this 30-year-old, left-handed woman had presented with complex motor seizures since the age of 18 years. MRI demonstrated right hippocampal sclerosis. Inter-ictal EEG showed right anterior temporal spikes and the ictal EEG showed a right hemisphere seizure with maximal activation in the temporal region. Semiology indicated right hemisphere lateralizing signs of seizure onset including:

- Head deviation to the right at seizure onset.
- Left tonic fist posturing.
- Post-ictal nose rubbing with right hand.
- A left Todd's paresis.
- Post-ictal speech difficulty, supporting right hemisphere language dominance.

Table 5.3 Specific operative risks of anterior temporal lobe resection (ATLR) depending on hemisphere dominance:

ATLR dominance	Risk
Dominant	Impairment of language, particularly naming and verbal memory (20–30%)
Non-dominant	Impairment of visual memory (10%)
Both	Infection (<3%) Hemiparesis and speech disturbance (<1%) Visual field loss (10%), visual field deficit resulting in driving ban (5%) Neuropsychiatric deficit: mood disturbances, including emotional lability, depression, and anxiety may occur on up to 1:5 patients. Rarely (1%) acute psychosis can occur.*

Neuropsychological assessment is consistent with dominant cortical hemisphere dysfunction. fMRI demonstrated right hemisphere language localization. Importantly, she had no psychiatric contraindications to surgery.

This data was presented in a multidisciplinary epilepsy surgery planning meeting, which concluded that the findings were concordant with a presumed epileptogenic zone in the right temporal lobe secondary to right hippocampal sclerosis. A success rate of seizure freedom was predicted at 60%t, with an additional 20% of significant improvement in seizure frequency following a standard right-sided ATLR. Pre- and peri-operative counselling is essential for all patients undergoing epilepsy surgery. Risk–benefit discussions with the patient and their family should be performed and documented, and given to the patient in written format. The standard operative risks and specific risks of a dominant hemisphere ATLR were discussed with the patient (see Table 5.3).

Temporal lobe resection for epilepsy

The patient was placed supine in the Mayfield head clamp. The head was rotated 90 degrees, with the zygoma parallel to the floor. A temporal question mark skin incision (Figure 5.5a) and myocutaneous flap were made (Figure 5.5b). Two burr holes were made, one over the pterion and the other above the root of the zygoma (Figure 5.5c), allowing a craniotomy (Figure 5.5d). The craniotomy should be made as low as possible to allow access to the floor of the middle cranial fossa with minimal retraction. The dura was opened in a C-shape to expose the Sylvian fissure.

ATLR involved resection of the lateral neocortex, facilitated by identification of the temporal horn of the lateral ventricle, followed by resection of the mesial temporal structures (amygdala, hippocampus, parahippocampal gyrus).

To achieve the neocortical resection, 4cm was measured from the temporal pole over the long axis of the middle temporal gyrus and the posterior border marked on the cortical surface using irrigating bipolar forceps. This was extended along the superior temporal gyrus approximately 5mm below the Sylvian vessels creating an 'L shape'. The arachnoid of the L shape was divided with microscissors and subpial dissection performed using a Rhoton dissector.

Using intra-operative navigation, the temporal horn of the lateral ventricle was located. The approach to the ventricle was along the middle fossa floor, identifying the collateral sulcus. Dissection perpendicular to the floor, following the collateral

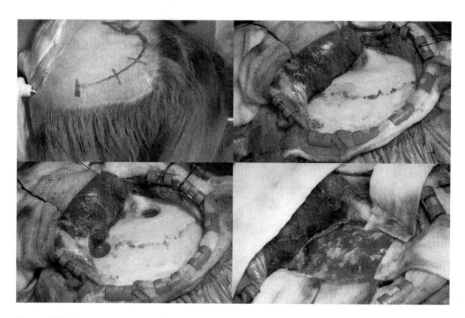

Figure 5.5 Right anterior temporal lobe exposure.

sulcus, enabled the ventricle to be entered inferiorly. This reduced the risk of damage to the optic radiation, in particular Meyer's loop (which is lateral and superior to the ventricle). A cottonoid patty was inserted into the temporal horn of the ventricle to prevent CSF loss, and blood entering the ventricular system as the temporal pole was removed.

The temporal stem was disconnected by passing a blunt hook from the tip of the temporal horn towards the previously dissected superior temporal gyrus, allowing removal of the lateral temporal neocortex.

The mesial temporal structures were then resected. The uncus and amydala were removed using a low-powered Cavitron Ultrasonic Aspirator (CUSA). On removal of the uncus along its pial boundary, the third cranial nerve, posterior communicating artery and the edge of the tentorium could be visualized. The anterior choroid point is an important anatomical landmark as it represents the most anterior aspect of the choroid plexus, localizes entry of the anterior choroidal artery, and demarcates the posterior part of the hippocampal head.

The amygdala can be resected anteriorly and lateral to an imaginary line drawn from this anterior choroid point to the Sylvian fissure. Care must be taken not to go too deep during amygdala resection to avoid entering the frontal lobe.

A blunt hook was used to gently separate the choroid plexus from the hippocampus to reveal the fimbria. Gentle dissection of the fimbria off the underlying arachnoid revealed the hippocampal artery arcade lying within the hippocampal sulcus, which supplies the hippocampal head. The vessels were cauterized and the hippocampus resected. The parahippocampal gyrus and pes were finally resected, taking care not to damage the underlying adjacent cerebral peduncle. The craniotomy was closed and all samples sent to pathology.

Post-operatively, the patient continued her AEDs, experienced no neurological deficit, and was seizure-free at 1 year follow-up.

➕ **Clinical tip** Anterior temporal lobe resection

- When positioning, the neck must be both extended and flexed to allow the ventricular approach along the middle temporal fossa.
- When positioning the patient, care should be taken that the neck is not over-flexed, reducing the risk of brachial plexus injury. All bony prominences must be well padded to avoid pressure sores.
- During the craniotomy, if the mastoid air cells are opened, these must be packed off with bone wax or biological sealant to prevent CSF leak or encephalocoele.
- The vein of Labbe is located over the dominant posterior temporal lobe with variable anatomy. Dissection should proceed anterior to the vein as damage to this vessel may produce venous infarction in cortical and subcortical speech areas.
- Subpial dissection of the superior temporal gyrus exposes the arachnoid overlying the insular cortex and branches of the middle cerebral artery. These landmarks can facilitate dissection of the temporal stem, but care must be taken not to penetrate the arachnoid layer and enter the Sylvian Fissure.
- The CUSA is used on low power to ensure no breech of the pial boundary into the basal cisterns. If blood enters these cisterns chemical meningitis may ensue, resulting in headache, neurological irritation, and a prolonged hospital stay.
- Meyer's loop lies lateral and superior to the temporal horn of the lateral ventricle and damage will result in superior temporal visual field defect.
- When resecting the amygdala, care must be taken, particularly at the superior medial aspect, as there are no clear anatomical landmarks. Amygdala resection below an imaginary line taken from the anterior choroidal point to the anterior superior arachnoid of the limen insulae and uncus is deemed safe. Above this line lies the globus pallidus and branches of the middle cerebral artery en route to the basal ganglia, which if damaged may result in hemiplegia and hemianopia.

Discussion

The estimated incidence of epilepsy is 50 per 100,000 in the general population [10] and 20% are estimated to become refractory to medication [11]. A UK study reported that the commonest surgical procedure for epilepsy was temporal resection for hippocampal sclerosis [12]. Brain tumours represent a common finding in patients with intractable focal epilepsies. Approximately 60% are dysembryoplastic neuroepithelial tumours and gangliomas [13]. Other lesions include glioma, focal cortical dysplasia, heterotopia, arteriovenous malformation, cavernoma, infarct, granuloma (e.g. secondary to cysticercosis, tuberculosis), and traumatic intraparenchymal brain injury. Dual pathology exists in up to 30% of surgical specimens of patients operated on for TLE, with the most common extrahippocampal lesion abnormality reported as cortical dysplasia. The pathogenesis of dual pathology is poorly understood [14]. Cryptogenic or paradoxical TLE refers to patients in whom no pathology is identified in the resected temporal lobe and constitutes less than 10% of cases [15].

💬 **Expert comment** Hippocampal sclerosis

The pathological diagnosis of HS is characterized by gliosis and neuronal loss (especially pyramidal neurons) predominantly in CA1, but also in the CA3 and CA4 subfields. Typically, there is an accompanying loss of excitatory mossy cells, neuropeptide Y-secreting neurons and GABAergic neurons [16]. There may be associated gliosis and similar neuronal loss in the ipsilateral amygdala and entorhinal cortex (Figure 5.6). A recent classification of Hippocampal Sclerosis (HS) suggests that a non-classical histological pattern (although occurring less frequently) has a worse outcome in relation

(continued)

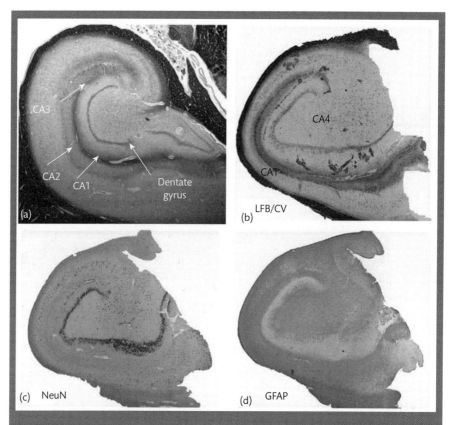

Figure 5.6 Sections demonstrating (a) healthy hippocampus; (b, c, d) classical hippocampal sclerosis. Sections are stained with: (a) Luxol Fast Blue (LFB); (b) LFB and cresyl violet (CV). (c) Neuronal nuclei (NeuN) stained section demonstrating neuronal loss mainly in CA1 and CA4. (d) Glial fibrillary acidic protein (GFAP) demonstrating the diffuse fibrillary gliosis in CA4 and CA1, (for colour version of this figure please see online edition).

Images courtesy of Dr Thom, Department of Neuropathology, Institute of Neurology, London.

Table 5.4 Characteristics of classical and non-classical features of HS and post-operative seizure freedom

	Percentage in a series of 178 patients	Neuronal loss	Post-operative seizure freedom at 1 year (%)
No Mesial temporal sclerosis (MTS)	19	Nil	59
MTS 1a (classical)	19	CA1 predominantly with some neuronal loss in all other subfields excluding CA2	72
MTS 1b (classical)	53	All hippocampal subfields	73
MTS 2 (non-classical)	6	CA1	67
MTS 3 (non-classical)	4	End folium sclerosis in hilar area	29

Summarized from Blümcke I, Pauli E, Clusmann H et al. A new clinico-pathological classification system for mesial temporal sclerosis. *Acta Neuropathol* 2007; 113: 235–44. Distributed under the terms of the Creative Commons Attribution License 2.0 [17].

to seizure freedom 1 year post-operatively (Table 5.4) [17]. Although HS was identified nearly 200 years ago [18], it is still an area of active research, particularly with regard to identifying the cause and mechanism of seizure generation in this region of mesial neuronal loss.

> **❂ Learning point**
>
> A MDT and systematic approach to investigations is essential in evaluating candidates for epilepsy surgery [19].
>
> **Clinical evaluation**
>
> Birth and developmental history, epilepsy history, current seizure pattern, drug history (failure of two AEDs), co-morbidities preventing surgery, clinical examination (with emphasis on neurological, cardiovascular, skin systems (stigmata of epilepsy syndromes), ECG.
>
> **Initial investigations**
>
> MRI head, prolonged inter-ictal EEG, video-EEG, neuropsychology, and neuropsychiatry.
>
> **Multi-disciplinary meeting**
>
> If concordant data: surgical planning is required—fMRI for language/motor function, visual fields, if surgical resection is in proximity to these areas.
>
> If discordant, but a potential surgical candidate, further imaging techniques can be used to derive the target for intracranial EEG using depth electrode, subdural grids, and strips.
>
> It is imperative that patients and their families are given realistic expectations and associated risks of surgery, and to ensure that long-term post-operative follow-up is maintained.

Neurophysiology

The aim of prolonged scalp inter-ictal and ictal EEG in pre-surgical work-up for resective epilepsy procedures includes:

- Demonstration of an electrophysiological-clinical seizure: up to 10% of candidates undergoing pre-surgical work up for epilepsy surgery have psychogenic non-epileptic attacks.
- Characterization of electro-clinical seizures to ensure concordance that all seizures are arising from the same location.
- If there is discordance due to other epileptogenic areas (e.g. dual pathology), this will reduce the chance of seizure freedom.

> **❝ Expert comment** If dual epileptogenic areas are present, invasive EEG can be considered
>
> Depth electrodes are multiple contact wires inserted under stereotactic MRI guidance and are most useful for investigating deep epileptogenic zone. Their disadvantage is they sample only small areas of brain. Subdural grid and strip electrodes record from large superficial cortical areas and are inserted via a craniotomy. Electrical stimulation to map function can also be performed through both types of electrodes.

Neuroimaging in temporal lobe epilepsy

A 3-Tesla MRI brain scan consisting of T1- and T2-weighted, and FLAIR imaging in axial and coronal planes, can reveal lesions that were not identified on previous imaging. Gradient-echo imaging may be useful to detect a vascular abnormality. Hippocampal volumetric analysis can provide evidence of HS. If imaging does not yield a structural cause for the epilepsy, or there is discordance between clinical and EEG data, functional imaging can be considered: positron emission tomography (PET), single-photon emission CT (SPECT) with ictal–inter-ictal subtraction, simultaneous EEG and fMRI [20] and magneto-encephalography (MEG). Cortical regions can be highly variable in terms of size and location, and stereotactic atlases fail to take into account this intrinsic variability. Eloquent functions can be mapped with fMRI, using language, memory, primary motor, and somatosensory paradigms with diffusion tensor imaging for white matter tracts [21]. Co-registration of multi-modal imaging can facilitate surgical planning and intra-operative MRI can aid surgical resection.

> ✪ **Learning point**
>
> ATLR for TLE may be complicated by a visual field deficit (VFD), typically a contralateral superior quadrantinopia caused by damage to the anterior optic radiation (Meyer's loop). Despite being seizure free, post-operative patients may have significant VFD to prevent driving [22].
>
> There is significant anatomical variability in Meyer's loop and integration of tractography of optic radiation and real-time neuronavigation is currently being characterized [23].

Neuropsychological assessment

Pre-operative neuropsychological assessment is performed using the Wechsler Adult Intelligence Scale. The full-scale intelligence quotient (IQ) is made up from scores obtained by testing verbal IQ comprising verbal comprehension and working memory, and performance IQ comprising perceptual organization, and processing speed. The results may aid localization and lateralization of cerebral dysfunction—impaired memory functions suggest localization to the temporal lobes. Comparison of visual IQ to performance IQ can help with lateralization, impaired verbal memory lateralizes to the dominant temporal lobe (usually the left), whereas impaired visual memory lateralizes to the non-dominant temporal lobe. fMRI memory paradigms are now also providing information that helps predict post-operative cognitive deficit [8,9]. The extent of any post-operative deficit depends both on the functionality of the removed tissue and the functional reserve of the non-resected structures. Pre-operative assessment can help predict the risk for post-surgical cognitive decline, allowing appropriate pre-operative counselling and post-operative support. Assessment of the cognitive baseline is useful, as this may be deleteriously affected by the seizures themselves, as part of the spectrum of epilepsy syndromes, AED, and is of paramount importance to ensure the patient has a high enough IQ for informed consent.

Neuropsychiatry assessment

Psychiatric morbidity (particularly depression, anxiety, and psychosis) is common with lifetime prevalence rates of up to 50% in TLE. 25% of patients post-surgery for TLE, report transient mood disturbances, including emotional lability, depression, and anxiety during the first 3 months with 10% experiencing more persistent symptoms. Post-operative de novo psychosis has been reported to occur in 1% of patients. The risk factors for developing post-operative psychiatric disorders include pre-operative psychiatric history, pre-operative bilateral epileptiform discharges, and poor post-operative seizure control [24].

Surgery for temporal lobe epilepsy

Sir Victor Horsley (National Hospital of Neurology and Neurosurgery, London, UK) was one of the pioneers of epilepsy surgery in the 1800s, correlating clinical observation and seizure semiology to plan lesionectomy. With the invention of the EEG by Hans Berger in 1924, pre- and intra-operative recordings allowed resection to include areas that gave rise to epileptiform activity, even though the area to be removed may have appeared grossly normal. Wilder Penfield (Montreal Neurological Institute, Canada) first identified that, for patients with TLE, the temporal lobe, hippocampus, and amygdala could be removed safely and with good result in terms of reduction in seizure frequency. In the 1950s, Murray Falconer (Maudsley Hospital, London, UK) pioneered the en bloc anatomical temporal lobectomy. However, this led to significant deficits especially with regard to neuropsychological and superior quadrantanopia visual field deficits. Alternative procedures aiming to reduce the size of the neocortical resection include the Spencer-type technique and the selective amygdalohippocampectomy [25,26]. The Spencer technique was developed to preserve the function of the lateral temporal cortex and to access the medial temporal structures through a temporal corridor. The selective amygdalohippocampectomy can be approached transcortically, transylvian, and subtemporally with the perceived advantage that the adjacent temporal neocortex remains intact. It has been difficult to compare the various surgical techniques, as there has been a lack of standardized operative outcome criteria, and the optimal size of temporal resection is still controversial and requires further study [27,28].

In the late 1990's, a Canadian trial randomly assigned 80 patients with medically refractory TLE, to surgery or 1 year of AED therapy [29]. The primary outcome was freedom of seizures that impair awareness of self and surroundings. Wiebe et al. demonstrated that surgery afforded 58% seizure freedom in comparison with 8% in the medical therapy arm. Similarly, a cohort study of consecutive patients undergoing anterior temporal lobe resections or temporal lesionectomies for TLE at a single UK centre, demonstrated that approximately 60% of 537 patients were seizure free (excluding simple partial seizures) at 5 years [30].

A RCT was recently started to compare the outcome of standard surgical temporal lobe resection with the results of gamma knife radiosurgery of the same surgical target. The main study hypothesis of the Radiosurgery or Open Surgery for Epilepsy (ROSE) trial was that radiosurgery (which requires no hospital stay), is as safe and effective as open surgery in treating patients with seizures arising from the medial temporal lobe. The study was abandoned in 2012 due to difficulty in patient recruitment.

Palliative procedures exist for medically refractory patients that are either not suitable for resective surgery, or who do not improve following resective surgery. These adjunctive therapies include continuous stimulation with deep-brain stimulation of the anterior thalamus (DBSANT; Medtronic Inc.), intermittent stimulation with vagal nerve stimulation (VNS; Cyberonics Inc.), and responsive neurostimulation (RNS; Neuropace Inc.). To date, only VNS is licensed for use in both Europe and the USA.

VNS provides a third of patients with greater than 50% reduction in seizures, a third experience less than 50% reduction, and no improvement is seen in the remaining third [31]. Spiral-shaped bipolar electrodes are wrapped around the left vagal nerve, the distal ends are tunnelled over the clavicle into a subcutaneous pocket above the pectoral fascia in which an implantable pulse generator (IPG) is sited. Stimulation parameters can be adjusted via a programming device, using radio-frequency signals. Typically, patients slowly have their stimulation parameters increased until individual optimal seizure control and side effect tolerance is reached. The patient can also trigger the stimulator by resting a magnet (often worn as a bracelet) over it, allowing extra stimulation during an aura, which may arrest progression into a seizure.

> ✪ **Learning point**
>
> The left vagus nerve is stimulated due to concerns that bradycardias or arrhythmias may be induced on stimulating the right vagal nerve.
>
> The vagus is approximately 80% afferent and composed of unmylinated fibres. The fibres project to the nucleus tractus solitarius in the brainstem and then on to other structures including hypothalamus, thalamus, and cortex. The exact mechanism of action for seizure reduction is unknown.
>
> Insertion and stimulation may be associated with a hoarse voice, cough, throat pain, or paraesthesia and dyspnoea.

A final word from the expert

- Operative safety may be improved with the development of surgical image guidance systems, allowing reliable integration of structural and functional data available in real time as surgery progresses.
- Neuromodulation is a rapidly evolving field. DBS of different targets are being investigated, e.g. centromedian thalamic nucleus [32]. Seizure prediction devices are also under development. Implantable electrodes communicate to a hand-held device, indicating the likelihood of seizure activity in the coming hours and allow direct electrical stimulation to prevent or reduce severity of the seizure.
- Electrically-active drug release implants may allow direct access of drugs to epileptogenic areas avoiding systemic metabolism, and impermeability of the blood–brain barrier.
- Optogenetic tools comprise a variety of different light-sensitive proteins that, via a viral vector, can be expressed in mammalian neurons to effectively control their excitability. Expression of the inhibitory halorhodopsin in hippocampal principal cells has recently been used as a tool to effectively control chemically- and electrically-induced epileptiform activity in animal slice preparations [33]. Optogenetic tools represent a novel way of manipulating neural networks at a molecular level and may offer a future strategy in epilepsy treatment [34].
- Cell transplantation therapies with either mature cells or stem cells derived from foetal tissue or genetically-engineered cells that enhance synaptic inhibition, and so reduce seizures or protect neurons from damage, are being investigated in animal models [35].

References

1. Commission on Classification, International League Against Epilepsy. Proposed provisions of clinical and electroencephalographical classification of epileptic seizures. Epilepsia 1981; 22: 489–501.
2. Berg AT, Berkovic SF, Brodie MJ, et al. Revised terminology and concepts for organization of seizures and epilepsies: report of the ILAE Commission on Classification and Terminology, 2005–2009. Epilepsia 2010; 51: 676–85.
3. Annegers JF, Hauser WA, Shirts SB, et al. Factors prognostic of unprovoked seizures after febrile convulsions. N Engl J Med 1987; 316: 493–8.
4. Brodie MJ, Kwan P. Staged approach to epilepsy management. Neurology 2002; 58: S2–8.

5. Springer JA, Binder JR, Hammeke TA, et al. Language dominance in neurologically normal and epilepsy subjects. A functional MRI study. Brain 1999; 122: 2033–45.

6. Szaflarski JP, Binder JR, Possing ET, et al. Language lateralization in left-handed and ambidextrous people fMRI data. Neurology 2002; 59: 238–44.

7. Arora J, Pugh K, Westerveld M, et al. Language lateralization in epilepsy patients: fMRI validated with the Wada procedure. Epilepsia 2009; 50: 2225–41.

8. Bonelli SB, Powell RHW, Yogarajah M, et al. Imaging memory in temporal lobe epilepsy: predicting the effects of temporal lobe resection. Brain 2010; 133: 1186–99.

9. Bonelli SB, Thompson PJ, Yogarajah M, et al. Imaging language networks before and after anterior temporal lobe resection: results of a longitudinal fMRI study. Epilepsia 2012; 53: 639–50.

10. Sander JWAS. Some aspects of prognosis in the epilepsies: a review. Epilepsia 1993; 34: 1007–16.

11. Hart YM.Shorvon SD. The nature of epilepsy in the general population: I. Characteristics of patients receiving medication for epilepsy. Epilepsy Res 1995; 21: 43–9.

12. Lhatoo SD, Soloman JK, McEvoy AW, et al. A prospective study of the requirement for and the provision of epilepsy surgery in the United Kingdom. Epilepsia 2003; 44: 673–6.

13. Blümcke I. Epilepsy-associated brain tumors. Handb Clin Neurol. 2012; 108: 559–68.

14. Harroud A, Bouthillier A, Weil AG, et al. Temporal lobe epilepsy surgery failures: a review. Epilepsy Res Treatment 2012. Available at: http://dx.doi.org/10.1155/2012/201651

15. Thom M. Hippocampal sclerosis: progress since Sommer. Brain Pathol 2008; 19: 565–72.

16. Thom M, Sisodiya SM, Najm I. Epilepsy. In: S Love, DN Lewis, DW Ellison (eds), Greenfield's neuropathology 8th edn. (pp. 833–87). London: Hodder-Arnold, 2008.

17. Blümcke I, Pauli E, Clusmann H, et al. A new clinico-pathological classification system for mesial temporal sclerosis. Acta Neuropathol 2007; 113: 235–44.

18. Bouchet C, Cazauvieilh C.A. De l' épilepsie considerée dans ses rapports avec aliénation mentale. Recherche sur la natur et le siège de ces maladies. Arch Gén Méd 1825; 9: 510–42.

19. Duncan JS. Selecting patients for epilepsy surgery: synthesis of data. Epilepsy Behav 2011; 20: 230–2.

20. Vulliemoz S, Thornton R, Rodionov R, et al. The spatio-temporal mapping of epileptic networks: combination of EEG-fMRI and EEG source imaging. Neuroimage 2009; 46: 834–43.

21. Duncan JS. Imaging in the surgical treatment of epilepsy. Nat Rev Neurol 2010; 6: 537–50.

22. Yogarajah M.Focke NK, Bonelli S, et al. Defining Meyer's loop—temporal lobe resections, visual field deficits and diffusion tensor tractography. Brain 2009; 132: 1656–68.

23. Winston GP. Epilepsy surgery, vision, and driving: what has surgery taught us and could modern imaging reduce the risk of visual deficits? Epilepsia 2013; 54: 1877–88.

24. Foong J, Flugel D. Psychiatric outcome of surgery for temporal lobe epilepsy and presurgical considerations. Epilepsy Res 2007; 75: 84–96.

25. Harkness W. Temporal lobe resections. Childs Nerv Syst 2006; 22: 936–44.

26. Campero A, Tróccoli G, Martins C, et al. Microsurgical approaches to the medial temporal region: an anatomical study. Neurosurgery 2006; 59: 279–308.

27. Schramm J. Temporal lobe epilepsy surgery and the quest for optimal extent of resection: a review. Epilepsia 2008; 49: 1296–307.

28. Al-Otaibi F, Baeesa SS, Parrent AG, et al. Surgical techniques for the treatment for temporal lobe epilepsy. Epilepsy Res Treat 2012; 2012: 374848.

29. Wiebe S, Blume WT, Girvin JP, et al. A randomized controlled trial of surgery for temporal lobe epilepsy. N Engl J Med 2001; 345: 311–18.

30. De Tisi J, Bell, GS, Peacock JL, et al. The long-term outcome of adult epilepsy surgery, patterns of seizure remission, and relapse: a cohort study. Lancet 2011; 378: 1388–95.

31. Janszky J, Hoppe M, Behne F, et al. Vagus nerve stimulation: predictors of seizure freedom. J Neurol Neurosurg Psychiat 2005; 76: 384–9.

32. Velasco F, Velasco AL, Velasco M, et al. Deep brain stimulation for treatment of the epilepsies: the centromedian thalamic target. Acta Neurochir Suppl. 2007; 97: 337–42.
33. Tønnesen J.Sørensen AT, Deisseroth K, et al. Optogenetic control of epileptiform activity. Proc Natl Acad Sci 2009; 106: 12162–7.
34. Kokaia M.Andersson M.Ledri M. An optogenetic approach to epilepsy. Neuropharmacology 2013; 69: 89–95.
35. Boison D. Cell and gene therapies for refractory epilepsy. Curr Neuropharmacol 2007; 5: 115–25.

Management of lumbosacral lipoma in childhood

Martin M. Tisdall and Greg James

Expert commentary Dominic N. P. Thompson

Case history

A 13-month-old girl was referred to a tertiary paediatric neurosurgical centre from a paediatric orthopaedic service. At birth she had been noted to have a lumbosacral cutaneous lesion and bilateral foot deformity. The feet remained weak, with a tendency to collapse inward. Proximal muscle power had shown reasonable development, with sitting attained at 8 months and crawling at 1 year. There was no indication of pain relating to the lumbar lesion.

She had persistently wet nappies, with a tendency to urinary dribbling. There had been no urinary tract infections. Urodynamic studies had revealed a neurogenic bladder with weak detrusor activity, but reasonable volume and no vesico-ureteric reflux. She had been commenced on intermittent urinary catheterization. There was some evidence of neurogenic bowel dysfunction with constipation requiring aperient medication.

On examination, a midline lumbosacral lipoma was found. There was reasonable muscle bulk in all major muscle groups of the lower limbs. The feet were held in equinus. Motor examination revealed MRC Grade 5 hip extension, Grade 3 hip extension, Grade 4 knee extension and flexion, and absent plantar flexion and extension bilaterally. Sensation appeared reduced around both feet, and lower limb reflexes could not be elicited.

Expert comment

The lumbosacral lipomas are considered under the term 'occult spinal dysraphism' or spina bifida occulta, a category that includes, amongst others, split cord malformations, dermal sinus tracks, and fatty filum terminale. These are skin covered lesions and the term distinguishes this group of disorders from 'open spinal dysraphism' or spina bifida aperta (myelomeningocele), in which there is a deficiency in the skin with exposure of the incompletely developed neural tube. The word 'occulta' is misleading as, in the majority of cases, there is an abnormality of the overlying skin, such as a lipomatous swelling, haemangioma, or hairy patch. These are referred to as the stigmata of spinal dysraphism. Such a finding should always alert the clinician to the possibility of an underlying spinal cord abnormality, even if there are no obvious neurological symptoms or signs.

MRI revealed a complex dysraphic malformation with an extensive transitional type lipoma extending from L2 to the sacral spinal canal (Figure 6.1).

At this stage, it appeared that the observed changes in ankle power were related to a severe motor deficit associated with the congenital dysraphic defect, rather than the effects of mechanical spinal cord tethering. As the proximal muscle groups,

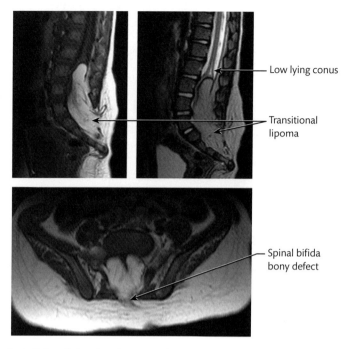

Low lying conus

Transitional lipoma

Spinal bifida bony defect

Figure 6.1 Sagittal T1 and T2, and axial T1 MRIs of lumbosacral spine, demonstrating large transitional type spinal lipoma. The lipoma extends from L2 to the caudal sacral canal, and involves the conus and cauda equina extensively.

whose innervation was partly involved in the lipomatous mass, appeared to be developing. Given the complex nature of the surgical target, the inherent risks of surgical resection, and the lack of clear evidence of deterioration relating to spinal cord tethering, the initial plan was to follow-up with radiological and clinical surveillance.

The subsequent review took place at age 16 months. At this stage she had deteriorated, with evidence of lumbar pain and reduced left leg function. On examination, she had anti-gravity movements in the hips and knees, but the left leg was now weaker than the right. MRI appearances were stable. Given that she had now developed progressive symptomatology, it was decided to proceed to surgical resection of the lipomatous lesion and spinal cord detethering.

> **☉ Learning point** Tethered cord syndrome
>
> Spinal lipomas may result in terminal spinal cord and cauda equina dysfunction [1–3]. The clinical manifestations of this dysfunction may be:
>
> - **Neurological:** pain, sensory disturbance and neuropathic ulceration.
> - **Urological:** impaired bladder emptying, urinary dribbling, and failure to attain continence—the neuropathic bladder.
> - **Orthopaedic:** foot or ankle deformity, asymmetric muscle wasting, and gait disturbance.
>
> These consequences of spinal dysraphism are sometimes termed the 'neuro-orthopaedic syndrome' or, more commonly, the tethered cord syndrome. The latter is probably best used to describe the clinical syndrome, rather than the radiological appearance. A low ('tethered') spinal cord on MRI may have no clinical sequelae.

At operation, the subcutaneous component of the lipoma was initially mobilized to delineate the defect in the lumbosacral fascia. A paraspinal muscle reflection was then performed, and a wide laminectomy performed to ensure adequate exposure of the interface between the lipoma and the dura. After dural opening, the relationship of the dorsal root entry zone (DREZ) to the lipoma was established (Figure 6.2) and electrophysiological mapping was used to identify functional nerve roots. Microdissection was then used to dissect along the plane between the lipoma and the neural placode (Figure 6.3). The exposed neural placode was then neuralated (sutured in the midline) (Figure 6.4) and, finally, an expansion duraplasty was performed (using dural substitute) in an attempt to increase the volume of the thecal sac and thus reduce the risk of future retethering (Figure 6.5).

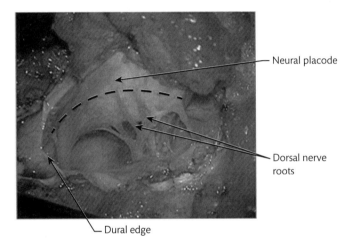

Figure 6.2 Operative view of transitional lipoma after dural opening. Dorsal root entry zone depicted by dotted line.

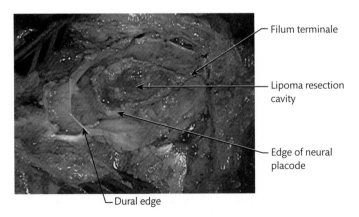

Figure 6.3 Operative appearance after resection of lipoma.

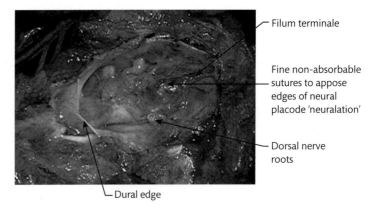

Filum terminale

Fine non-absorbable sutures to appose edges of neural placode 'neuralation'

Dorsal nerve roots

Dural edge

Figure 6.4 Operative appearance following neuralation of the placode.

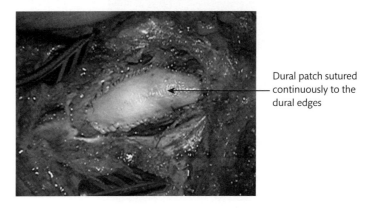

Dural patch sutured continuously to the dural edges

Figure 6.5 Operative appearance following expansion duraplasty with dural substitute.

Post-operatively, she made a good recovery. Neurological function was unchanged, although her pain appeared to be reduced. MRI at 2 months post-operatively showed near total lipoma resection. She remains under review with regular radiological, clinical, and urological surveillance.

> **❝ Expert comment**
>
> The anatomy of spinal lipomas is complex. Achieving a safe and durable untethering with minimal risk to neurological function, and avoiding post-operative wound-related complications, represents a major surgical challenge. Important principles include:
>
> - **Wide bony exposure:** the attachment between the lipoma and the dura may be very lateral and a wide exposure is needed to access the dural margin
> - **Working from normal anatomy:** the identification of normal spinal cord immediately rostral to the lesion will aid orientation and early identification of the interface between the normal spinal cord and lipoma
> - **Identifying the dorsal nerve roots over normal spinal cord and following the DREZ into the lesion:** the spinal cord is splayed open and the lipomatous placode means that the dorsal roots are displaced laterally.
> - **Nerve root mapping is essential:** identification of the sphincteric innervation is of particular importance.

- **Lipoma resection:** sharp micro-dissection is continued along the interface between the lipoma and the neural placode. The aim is maximal lipoma removal in order to reduce the risk of retethering
- **Neuralation of the placode:** the edges of the placode are sutured in the midline, thus reconstituting the terminal spinal cord
- **A duraplasty is performed:** the aim is to achieve a watertight and capacious terminal thecal sac.

Discussion

Up until the beginning of the twenty-first century, the perceived surgical wisdom has been that all lumbosacral lipomas should be treated with surgical debulking and spinal cord detethering in an attempt to prevent neurological deterioration [4]. This philosophy is based on the assumptions that inevitable deterioration will occur without surgery, and that surgery is safe and effective [5–8]. Over the last decade, evidence has emerged to challenge these assumptions. Data from paediatric neurosurgery groups at Necker-Enfants Malades, Paris [9] and Great Ormond Street, London [10] have suggested that, in the absence of neurological or urological deterioration, conservative management may have a similar or even superior outcome when compared with traditional surgical techniques.

Conversely, a single group from the United States headed by Dachling Pang have reported the results of radical total, or near total, lipoma removal, guided by meticulous neurophysiological monitoring, reconstruction of the neural placode, and duraplasty [11,12]. Their results suggest that this approach may be superior to both conservative management and traditional surgical technique.

Classification

The most widely recognized classification is that proposed by Chapman [5]. It is based on the anatomical position of the attachment of the lipoma to the spinal cord, and is divided into dorsal, caudal, and transitional types. The **dorsal type** is attached exclusively to the dorsal surface of the spinal cord rostral to the conus. The **caudal type** is attached to the termination of the spinal cord and involves the tip of the conus. The complex **transitional type** is intermediate between the two, and extends from the dorsal surface of the cord to the conus and cauda equina.

Epidemiology and embryology

Lumbosacral lipomas occur in approximately 1:4000 births and have a female:male ratio of 2:1 [13]. Their embryological basis remains unclear. It has been proposed that premature dysjunction, comprising early separation of neuro- and cutaneous ectoderm, prior to closure of the neural tube, could expose the developing neural structures to underlying mesoderm, which adheres to it and subsequently differentiates into fat [14]. While this hypothesis has some merit and might explain the anatomy of the dorsal type lipoma, it fails to account for the formation of the more caudally-attached transitional and caudal lipomas. These subtypes have some attachment at or below the level of the conus.

❝ Expert comment

The management of lumbosacral lipoma sits at a fascinating crossroads with different groups advocating diametrically opposed strategies. This debate will only be settled with the acquisition of more data. Here, we will examine the current evidence supporting these various management strategies and present our current treatment algorithm.

❝ Expert comment

The anatomy may be further distorted by rotation of the neural placode resulting in shortening of the nerve roots on one side. Pang et al. have suggested the term **chaotic lipoma** as a subtype of the transitional type, in which the lipoma blends with the roots of the cauda equina and extends to lie ventral to the roots [13].

> **✪ Learning point**
>
> Formation of the conus and cauda equina results from the incompletely understood and later-occurring process of secondary neuralation, in which pluripotent cells situated in the tail bud, coalesce to form the secondary neural tube before attaching to the distal spinal cord. Therefore, dysjunction plays no part in the formation of the conus and, thus, an alternative pathogenesis must be considered for the caudal and transitional types of lipoma [15–17]. Co-existing malformations of the ano-rectal region and lower urinary tract are not uncommon and are in keeping with the concept of a loco-regional disorder of caudal cell mass development [18].

Natural history

The traditional view that untreated lumbosacral lipoma leads to inevitable neurological, urological, or orthopaedic deterioration has little scientific basis and, until recently, the natural history of the condition has not been accurately reported. The literature has been hampered by the inclusion of various lipomatous anomalies within the same studies, the lack of distinction between asymptomatic and symptomatic cases and a dearth of cases managed without surgical intervention. Those advocating surgical treatment for all, point to data showing that outcome for patients treated before symptom onset is superior to that for patients treated in the presence of neurological deficit and to a diminished number of asymptomatic patients in the older age groups [8,19]. Both of these arguments are inherently flawed. First, it cannot be assumed that the asymptomatic patient is simply at an earlier time point in the same disease process as the symptomatic patient and, secondly, it is not possible to know the true prevalence of asymptomatic disease in the older patient, who may not seek medical attention [20]. Surgery for an asymptomatic child is a prophylactic undertaking and so potential surgical morbidity must be carefully weighed against the perceived long-term gain.

> **❝ Expert comment** Causes of neurological deterioration
>
> That children with spinal lipomas can develop neurological deterioration is beyond doubt [1–3], but the mechanisms underlying that deterioration are less clear. Fixation of the lower spinal cord by the lipoma may result in tractional forces as the spine grows. Experimental evidence has shown that these tractional forces can result in spinal cord ischaemia and neuronal dysfunction [21]. This mechanical explanation, known as 'tethering', is the basis upon which surgical treatment is based, but other factors, which have received less attention are also likely to be involved. Histological evaluation of spinal lipomas frequently reveals much more than just adipocytes. Tissues from each of the germ cell layers have been isolated from spinal 'lipomas', suggesting a true malformation process [22]. Particularly in the complex transitional forms of lipoma, it is possible, if not probable, that there is some associated neural dysgenesis. This may account for some of the congenital neurological deficits seen in patients, such as the one described in the case history above. The consequences of neural dysgenesis, for example, on bladder function may be difficult to detect in an infant and may only emerge as the child grows. Thus, what might appear to be a progressive deficit might simply be the consequences of abnormal spinal cord development unveiled by the passage of time. Finally, mass effect may have some role. The intraspinal component of the lipoma can be large and cause compression of the underlying spinal cord and nerve roots [22].

While neurological, urological, and orthopaedic deterioration in the context of spinal lipoma is well described, the natural history appears more benign than previously thought, particularly in those cases (up to 30% of lipomas) that appeared to be asymptomatic at the time of presentation. Based on the suspicion that the traditional surgical approach of lipoma debulking and spinal cord detethering was yielding unsatisfactory results, Kulkarni et al. reported that outcome for asymptomatic patients managed conservatively with close neurological and urological surveillance [9]. Fifty-three asymptomatic cases with spinal lipoma were followed over a mean period of 4.4 years. During this period, only 25% exhibited neurological deterioration. The authors calculated that the actuarial risk of deterioration at 9 years was 33% compared with 46% for an earlier series of asymptomatic patients treated with surgery. The cohort was subsequently followed for 10 years and the rate of deterioration remained at 33%.

The group from Great Ormond Street Hospital in London has recently collected similar data from 56 asymptomatic patients [10]. They found a cumulative risk of deterioration at 2 and 10 years of 18 and 40%, respectively. Sixteen patients developed neurological symptoms and underwent subtotal resection of the lipoma with attempted detethering of the spinal cord, guided by electrophysiological monitoring. At a median post-operative follow-up of 2.5 years, nine patients experienced improvement in their pre-operative deficit and seven remained symptomatic.

> **❝ Expert comment**
>
> Many studies have documented the risks of late deterioration following conventional partial resection of asymptomatic spinal lipomas and, allowing for variations in the surgical series, a 40% rate of deterioration at 8 years can be anticipated [12,23,24]. These results appears no better than the natural history and suggest, therefore, that conventional surgery for asymptomatic lipomas is of questionable benefit, particularly as initial surgery not only has its own morbidity, but might increase the risk of secondary deterioration due to re-tethering.

The surgical results published by Pang et al. suggest that a more radical surgical approach might prove far more valuable. They advocate a technique comprising total or near-total resection of the lipoma, guided by meticulous neurophysiological mapping, followed by reconstruction of the neural placode and expansion duraplasty. They report progression free survival of 82.8% at 16 years for all patients and 98.4%, if only the asymptomatic cases are considered [11,12]. These results are not only far superior to previously reported surgical series, but also significantly better than the natural history.

Clearly, if these results can be reproduced by other centres, it heralds a major advance. However, the technique relies heavily on neurophysiological monitoring, which may not be available in all centres. Furthermore, it is technically demanding and carries a potentially significant risk of inflicting neurological or urological deficit, in addition to the risk of wound related complications, such as CSF leakage or pseudomeningocele formation [1,8]. As the incidence of this condition is low, it may take considerable time to develop the necessary surgical skills.

Given that a significant number of asymptomatic cases will not deteriorate, the Great Ormond Street group has tried to risk-stratify their patients. They found that, within the asymptomatic cases, female sex, transitional type lipoma, and presence of a syrinx cavity were associated with a greater risk of deterioration [10].

Toward a management algorithm

Initial assessment comprises clinical history, motor examination, MRI, and urological evaluation to include bladder function assessment.

Based on this evaluation, patients are divided into asymptomatic or symptomatic (i.e. with evidence of a deficit attributable to the dysraphic anomaly). Symptomatic patients are further sub-divided into those who are symptomatic with a fixed deficit (e.g. an ankle or foot deformity, present since birth), termed 'symptomatic static', and those who are symptomatic with a new or worsening deficit, termed 'symptomatic progressive'. For the latter group with a progressive deficit (e.g. the child with new pain or new onset bladder symptoms), an attempted radical surgical intervention, as described by Pang [11,12] is undertaken. For the asymptomatic patients, a policy of close neurological and urological surveillance is pursued 6-monthly until continence is established, when surveillance is reduced to annually. If, at any stage, new changes are identified and then the child is considered as symptomatic progressive and treated accordingly. For the child with a fixed deficit (symptomatic static), our present policy is to treat along the same lines as being asymptomatic, accepting that this is a particularly controversial group. Any evidence of progression would again lead us to recommend radical surgery.

Further data collection will permit evaluation of this management approach and provide valuable information as to the reproducibility of the excellent results of Pang et al [11,12].

A final word from the expert

One is left asking how to best manage these patients? Conventional partial debulking of asymptomatic lipomas appears to be no better than the natural history of the disease, but conservative management also carries a significant risk of deterioration. If the results of Pang [11,12] are reproduced by other groups, their radical surgical approach may become standard care for all spinal lipomas, yet we currently lack the data to endorse this fully. We suggest a management algorithm for newly-diagnosed patients with spinal lipomas, which aims to recognize the benign course of the disease in many asymptomatic patients and to provide effective long-term treatment results for those who deteriorate (Figure 6.6).

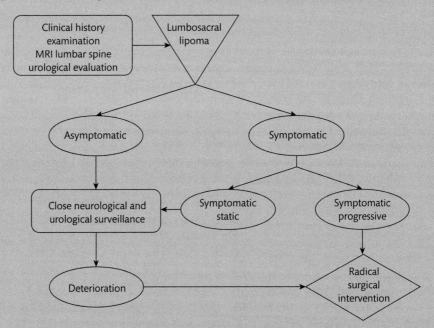

Figure 6.6 Proposed management algorithm for treatment of spinal lipomas.

Taken from Wykes V, Desai D, Thompson DN. Asymptomatic lumbosacral lipomas—a natural history study. Childs Nerv Syst, 2012; epub ahead of print.

References

1. Pierre-Kahn A, Zerah M, Renier D, *et al*. Congenital lumbosacral lipomas. Child's Nervous System 1997; **13**: 298–334.
2. Gourineni P, Dias L, Blanco R, Muppavarapu S. Orthopaedic deformities associated with lumbosacral spinal lipomas. Journal of Pediatric Orthopaedics 2009; **29**: 932–6.
3. Kang J-K., Lee K-S., Jeun S-S., Lee I-W., Kim M-C. Role of surgery for maintaining urological function and prevention of retethering in the treatment of lipomeningomyelocele: experience recorded in 75 lipomeningomyelocele patients. Child's Nervous System 2003; **19**: 23–9.
4. Bassett RC. The neurologic deficit associated with lipomas of the cauda equina. Annals of Surgery 1950; **131**: 109–16.
5. Chapman PH. Congenital intraspinal lipomas: anatomic considerations and surgical treatment. Child's Brain 1982; **9**: 37–47.
6. Hoffman HJ, Taecholarn C, Hendrick EB, Humphreys RP. Management of lipomyelomeningoceles. Experience at the Hospital for Sick Children, Toronto. Journal of Neurosurgery 1985; **62**: 1–8.
7. McLone DG, Naidich TP. Laser resection of fifty spinal lipomas. Neurosurgery 1986; **18**: 611–15.
8. La Marca F, Grant JA, Tomita T, et al. Spinal lipomas in children: outcome of 270 procedures. Pediatric Neurosurgery 1997; **26**: 8–16.
9. Kulkarni AV, Pierre-Kahn A, Zerah M. Conservative management of asymptomatic spinal lipomas of the conus. Neurosurgery 2004; **54**: 868–73.
10. Wykes V, Desai D, Thompson DN. Asymptomatic lumbosacral lipomas—a natural history study. Child's Nervous System, 2012; 28 (10): 1731–9.
11. Pang D, Zovickian J, Oviedo A. Long-term outcome of total and near-total resection of spinal cord lipomas and radical reconstruction of the neural placode: Part I-surgical technique. Neurosurgery 2009; **65**: 511–28.
12. Pang D, Zovickian J, Oviedo A. Long-term outcome of total and near-total resection of spinal cord lipomas and radical reconstruction of the neural placode, part II: outcome analysis and preoperative profiling. Neurosurgery 2010; **66**: 253–72.
13. Finn MA, Walker ML. Spinal lipomas: clinical spectrum, embryology, and treatment. Neurosurgery Focus 2007; **23**: E10.
14. Naidich TP, McLone DG, Mutluer S. A new understanding of dorsal dysraphism with lipoma (lipomyeloschisis): radiologic evaluation and surgical correction. AJR American Journal of Roentgenology 1983; **140**: 1065–78.
15. Copp AJ, Brook FA. Does lumbosacral spina bifida arise by failure of neural folding or by defective canalisation? Journal of Medical Genetics 1989; **26**: 160–6.
16. Müller F, O'Rahilly R. The primitive streak, the caudal eminence and related structures in staged human embryos. Cells Tissues Organs 2004; **177**: 2–20.
17. Saitsu H, Yamada S, Uwabe C, Ishibashi M, Shiota K. Development of the posterior neural tube in human embryos. Anatomy and Embryology 2004; **209**: 107–17.
18. Qi BQ, Beasley SW, Arsic D. Abnormalities of the vertebral column and ribs associated with anorectal malformations. Pediatric Surgery International 2004; **20**: 529–33.
19. Oi S, Nomura S, Nagasaka M, et al. Embryopathogenetic surgicoanatomical classification of dysraphism and surgical outcome of spinal lipoma: a nationwide multicenter cooperative study in Japan. Journal of Neurosurgery: Pediatrics 2009; **3**: 412–19.
20. Dorward NL, Scatliff JH, Hayward RD. Congenital lumbosacral lipomas: pitfalls in analysing the results of prophylactic surgery. Child's Nervous System 2002; **18**: 326–32.
21. Tani S, Yamada S, Knighton RS. Extensibility of the lumbar and sacral cord. Pathophysiology of the tethered spinal cord in cats. Journal of Neurosurgery 1987; **66**: 116–23.

22. Hirsch JF, Pierre-Kahn A. Lumbosacral lipomas with spina bifida. Child's Nervous System 1988; **4**: 354–60.
23. Xenos C, Sgouros S, Walsh R, Hockley A. Spinal lipomas in children. Pediatric Neurosurgery 2000; **32**: 295–307.
24. Colak A, Pollack IF, Albright AL. Recurrent tethering: a common long-term problem after lipomyelomeningocele repair. Pediatric Neurosurgery 1998; **29**: 184–90.

7 Idiopathic intracranial hypertension

David Sayer

ⓘ **Expert commentary** Raghu Vindindlacheruvu

Case history

A 20-year-old lady presented to her local Accident and Emergency (A&E) department with a history of gradual onset headache over a period of 6 months, associated with visual disturbance. The headache was global, dull, and worse when she was lying flat. It increased when she laughed and coughed. The patient described blurring of her vision with onset at the same time as her headache. Her body mass index (BMI) was 32. There was no family history of headaches, she had previously had one child, and there were no risks factors for thrombosis.

Her previous medical history was otherwise unremarkable and she took no regular medication. Neurological examination was unremarkable, but fundoscopy revealed bilateral papilloedema.

A non-contrasted CT head scan was normal. At a lumbar puncture, the opening pressure was $50cmH_2O$ and 50mL of CSF was drained to bring the pressure down to $18cmH_2O$. The protein content of the CSF was 0.25g/L and the glucose was 3.6mmol/L (both normal). She initially complained of a post-lumbar puncture headache, but this settled after a few hours. Over the next few weeks her headache and visual disturbance improved. She was advised to lose weight, although this was never achieved.

ⓘ **Expert comment** Initial work-up and management of idiopathic intracranial hypertension (IIH)

The natural history of IIH is variable. It may be self-limiting, intermittent, or become progressively worse. Approximately one-third of patients are in each of these categories [1]. The worst complication is visual loss and can be severe in up to 25% of patients [2].

> ★ **Learning point** Cerebrospinal fluid constituents and pressure (Table 7.1)
>
> **Table 7.1 CSF constituents and pressure**
>
> | CSF constituent | Normal range |
> | --- | --- |
> | CSF pressure | 5–15mmHg (7–20cmH₂O) |
> | Protein | 0.15–0.45g/L |
> | Glucose | 3.3–4.4mmol/L |
> | White cell count (WCC) | 0–5 × 106/L |
> | Red cell count (RCC) | 0–10 × 106/L |

The neurological diagnosis was IIH. Over the next 12 months her condition was managed medically with repeated lumbar punctures and acetazolamide, starting at 250mg daily and escalating by 250mg weekly to a maximum dose of 1000mg/day. Unfortunately, while acetazolamide gave her some symptomatic relief she had to discontinue it as she found the side effects of gastrointestinal upset and fatigue intolerable. To compound this, after every lumbar puncture, she suffered for a number of weeks with low pressure headaches. These were followed by a quiescent period, then a gradual return of her pressure symptoms.

> ✪ **Learning point** Diagnostic criteria for idiopathic intracranial hypertension
>
> *Modified Dandy Criteria for the Diagnosis of Idiopathic Intracranial Hypertension [3]*
> - Signs and symptoms of increased intracranial pressure (ICP).
> - No localizing focal neurological signs except unilateral or bilateral sixth nerve paresis.
> - CSF opening pressure >25cmH$_2$O, without cytological or chemical abnormalities.
> - Normal neuroimaging adequate to exclude cerebral venous thrombosis.

> ✪ **Learning point** Acetazolamide
>
> Acetazolamide is a carbonic anhydrase inhibitor that is believed to work by decreasing the rate of CSF production. CSF is formed as an ultrafiltrate of plasma and active secretion of CSF in the choroid plexus. This process is energy dependent and requires the enzyme carbonic anhydrase. This enzyme converts carbon dioxide and water into carbonic acid. Acetazolamide inhibits this enzyme and thus the reaction. This reaction takes place in the epithelial cells of the choroid plexus [4]. As a sulphonamide derivative potential side effects of acetazolamide are blood disorders, such as leukopenia, leading to infections and rashes. Other side effects and nausea/vomiting, headache, fatigue, and GI disturbances including taste disturbance [5].

At this point, she was referred for a neurosurgical opinion. An MRI scan demonstrated engorgement and dilatation of the optic nerve sheath complexes bilaterally (Figure 7.1). A small incidental lesion in the left parietal lobe was found to be an unrelated cavernoma. A CT venogram pre- and post-lumbar puncture demonstrated static narrowing of the tranverse sinuses (Figure 7.2). At this point, the opening pressure was 40cmH$_2$O and after drainage of 32mL of CSF, and the closing pressure was 12cmH$_2$O.

In view of the significant post-lumbar puncture headaches, it was recommended that lumbar peritoneal or ventricular peritoneal shunting should be avoided if possible in the first instance. Instead, she was assessed for venous sinus stenting and

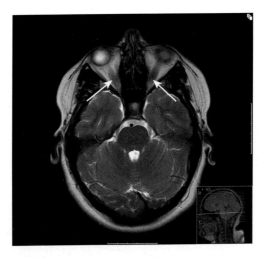

Figure 7.1. T2-weighted axial MRI imaging demonstrating bilateral optic nerve engorgement (arrows).

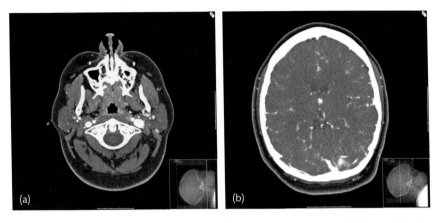

Figure 7.2. CTA (delayed filling of venous structures) demonstrating asymmetry of the internal jugular veins (a), and narrowed transverse venous sinuses (b).

offered venous pressure measurements of the transverse sinus, but she declined this treatment, preferring the option of shunting. At this time, she was undergoing approximately one lumbar puncture every 3 months to control her symptoms.

She underwent insertion of a valveless lumbar peritoneal shunt. In the immediate post-operative period she experienced low pressure headaches, which resolved over the ensuing week. She then had a number of weeks of complete symptom resolution, but high pressure symptoms subsequently recurred. A further lumbar puncture revealed an opening pressure of $32cmH_2O$. Ophthalmological assessment showed an acuity of 6/5 in the right eye and 6/9 on the left, with papilloedema and mild enlargement of the blind spot in both eyes, unchanged from before.

After careful counselling, she was offered VP shunting on the basis that she had benefitted from repeated lumbar punctures and the lumbar peritoneal shunt had initially resolved symptoms. At this point she became pregnant and her treatment was deferred. After delivery, the patient's symptoms had improved to a tolerable level and she decided that she did not wish to proceed with the shunt.

Discussion

Idiopathic intracranial hypertension has also been called benign intracranial hypertension (despite not running a benign course) and pseudotumour cerebri. The clinical and imaging features of the syndrome are of raised ICP, without dilated ventricles or intracranial mass lesions, but with evidence of papilloedema [6]. In 90% of cases this affects obese women with an incidence of 3.5/100 000 in the 20–44 years age group [7].

The commonest symptom is headache. This tends to be a non-specific global headache that is aggravated by actions that increase the cerebral venous pressure, e.g. coughing, sneezing, and straining on defaecation. It can be accompanied by features associated with migraine, such as photosensitivity, nausea, and vomiting [1]. Visual disturbance is also common and can manifest as blurring or transient visual obscurations. These may be postural. Other symptoms include diplopia, visual field deficits, and pulsatile tinnitus. Focal neurology is rare and should prompt a search for another cause. Papilloedema is the diagnostic hallmark of this condition and, indeed, it is sometimes an incidental finding in an otherwise asymptomatic patient.

A diagnostic lumbar puncture should be performed and, by definition, the opening pressure should be above 25cmH$_2$O [7]. The CSF analysis should also be normal.

In the first instance, a non-contrasted CT head scan is performed to exclude hydrocephalus and ensure safety of lumbar puncture. A contrasted MRI scan is normally also performed to exclude mass lesions or meningeal infiltration, which may be responsible for raised pressure. Additional imaging may include MRI of the spine to exclude abnormalities such as Chiari malformation, imaging of the venous sinuses, either by CT venography, MR venography, or angiography, to exclude venous sinus thrombosis or to demonstrate narrowing of the sinuses that may present a therapeutic target [1].

IIH is primarily a diagnosis of exclusion. A careful history and examination must be performed to rule out any other potential causes for the headaches. Imaging as described above excludes any mass lesions and ensures that ventricles are of normal size. Lumbar puncture confirms raised pressure and CSF analysis further excludes any other secondary causes. Treatment is typically medical in the initial setting. Visual deterioration will lead to more aggressive and earlier treatment. Once treatment has been started, it is reasonable to review the patient regularly and gradually decrease the dosage of acetazolamide, as the condition stabilizes and improves. Management, however, is often difficult and protracted.

The patient should be advised to lose weight and strategies put in place to help the patient achieve this, including bariatric surgery where necessary [8]. Pregnancy may worsen symptoms and patients must be aware of the implications of this, particularly with regard to vision [1].

❝ **Expert comment** The efficacy of conservative measures

With regard to the control of headache, analgesia is frequently prescribed, but is not usually helpful and may lead to 'analgesic abuse' headaches. Acetazolamide can be added as described above, although side effects may be an issue. Other medication, which may be useful includes topiramate [9], which has a weak carbonic anhydrase inhibitor action, steroids, and octreotide, an inhibitor of insulin like growth factor [10]. The mainstay of conservative management, however, is therapeutic lumbar puncture.

It must be stressed that, while conservative/medical approaches are effective in many patients, if vision is deteriorating, then other options must be explored urgently, primarily CSF diversion. If repeated lumbar punctures are giving satisfactory relief, but are undesirable, shunting should be considered. Either lumboperitoneal (LP) or ventriculo-peritoneal (VP) shunts may be used, depending on surgeon/ patient preference.

➕ **Clinical tip** Lumboperitoneal shunts—valve or valveless?

Recently, LP shunts can incorporate valves, allowing for pressure or flow control of CSF transit. There is no doubt that adopting an erect posture will increase CSF pressure in the lumbar cistern and increase flow into the peritoneal cavity: this may underlie the development of the low pressure headache and occasionally iatrogenic Chiari malformation (chronic hindbrain herniation). However, the development of LP valves and, in particular, the science behind flow- and pressure-adjustments is in its infancy, and further research is required.

> ✪ **Learning point** Intracranial venous sinus stenting [12]
>
> Transverse sinus stenosis may be focal or diffuse. The exact nature of the stenosis is ascertained by MR venography, particularly the auto-triggered elliptic centric-ordered (ATECO sequence) technique, giving excellent anatomical detail. If amenable to stenting, this is performed under general anaesthesia. Stenting requires heparin cover and pre-treatment with clopidogrel, with aspirin and clopidogrel therapy for a number of months following procedure to prevent thrombosis. Increasing the flow in the transverse sinus reduces venous hypertension and thus relieves symptoms.

A final word from the expert

The complex nature of this disease often necessitates a multi-disciplinary approach and referral to an ophthalmic surgeon should be considered as fenestration of the optic nerve sheath [13] allows direct drainage of CSF away from the optic nerve providing protection against visual deterioration with a significant chance of visual improvement.

If there is narrowing of the transverse sinus, stenting is another option [14]. This is a new treatment, but shows promise. Another potential treatment option is bilateral subtemporal craniectomies [15].

To summarize, IIH is a poorly understood condition. Patients who develop it often have a prolonged course with a risk of severe loss. The variety of management options available demonstrates that there is no single therapy that works for all patients and treatment needs to be directed by the patient's response.

References

1. Winn H. Youman's neurological surgery, 6th edn. Amsterdam: Elsevier.
2. Krajewski KJ, Gurwood AS. Idiopathic intracranial hypertension: pseudotumor cerebri. Optometry 2002; 73(9): 546–52.
3. Biousse V, Bruce B, Newman N. Update on the pathophysiology and management of idiopathic intracranial hypertension. Journal of Neurology, Neurosurgery & Psychiatry 2012; **83**: 488–94.
4. Brown PD, Davies SL, Speake T, et al. Molecular mechanisms of cerebrospinal fluid production. Neuroscience 2004; 129(4): 957–70.
5. Joint Formulary Committee. British national formulary, 62nd edn. London: Pharmaceutical Press.
6. Durcan FJ, Corbett JJ, Wall M. The incidence of pseudotumor cerebri. Population studies in Iowa and Louisiana. Archives of Neurology 1988; 45: 875–7.
7. Friedman DI, Jacobson DM. Diagnostic criteria for idiopathic intracranial hypertension. Neurology 2002; 59: 1492e5.
8. Ko MW, Chang SC, Ridha MA, et al. Weight gain and recurrence in idiopathic intracranial hypertension: a case-control study. Neurology 2011; 76: 1564e7.
9. Celebisoy N, Gokcay F, Sirin H, et al. Treatment of idiopathic intracranial hypertension: topiramate vs acetazolamide, an open-label study. Acta Neurologica Scandinavica 2007; 116: 322e7.

10. Deftereos SN, Panagopoulos G, Georgonikou D, et al. Treatment of idiopathic intracranial hypertension: is there a place for octreotide? Cephalalgia 2011; 31: 1679e80.
11. Yadav YR, Prihar V, Agarwal M, et al. Lumbar periotenal shunting in idiopathic intracranial hypertension. Turkish Neurosurgery 2012, 22(1): 21–6.
12. Ahmed RM, Wilkinson M, Parker GD, et al. Transverse sinus stenting for idiopathic intracranial hypertension: a review of 52 patients and of model predications. AJNR American Journal of Neuroradiology 2011; 32(8): 1408–14.
13. Thambisetty M, Lavin PJ, Newman NJ, et al. Fulminant idiopathic intracranial hypertension. Neurology 2007; 68: 229e32.
14. Ahmed R, Friedman DI, Halmagyi GM. Stenting of the transverse sinuses in idiopathic intracranial hypertension. Journal of Neuroophthalmology 2011; 31: 374e80.
15. Werndle MC, Newling-Ward E, Rich P, et al. Patient controlled intracranial pressure for treating idiopathic intracranial hypertension. Proceedings of the 2012 Spring Meeting of the Society of British Neurological Surgeons. British Journal of Neurosurgery 2012; 26(2): 132–74.

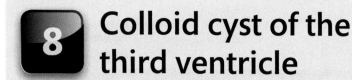

Colloid cyst of the third ventricle

Robin Bhatia

Expert commentary Ian Sabin

Case history

A 41-year-old, right-handed man presented to his local A&E department with a 2-week history of progressively worsening headache. The pain was global, dull in nature, and worse on waking in the morning; in the 2 days before admission additional symptoms included vomiting and transient visual obscurations.

Direct questioning revealed that this patient had been experiencing episodic headaches for the last 5 months, but could not attribute these to any particular activity or time of day, and had not sought medical advice.

His previous medical history was unremarkable. Family history included an older sister who had 5 years previously presented to the same hospital with similar symptoms, and had undergone resection of a colloid cyst. On examination, he was neurologically intact. Fundoscopy revealed Frisen Stage 1 papilloedema bilaterally.

Learning point Papilloedema staging

Lars Frisen proposed a staging scheme based on the ophthalmological signs of disturbed axoplasmic flow underlying papilloedema [1]. This scheme showed good reproducibility between different observers. Stage 0 represented a normal optic disc; Stage 1, blurred nasal margin of the optic disc; Stage 2, blurred nasal and temporal disc margins; Stage 3, elevated borders obscuring segments of major retinal vessels; Stage 4, obliteration of the optic cup; Stage 5, anterior expansion of the entire nerve head. Added to each stage is the presence of hyperaemia/pallor, haemorrhages, or cotton wool spots.

CT imaging of his brain revealed an $8 \times 8 \times 10$-mm hyperdense space-occupying lesion in the anterosuperior aspect of the third ventricle. MRI revealed a T2 hyperintense lesion, with central low intensity, reversing on T1 sequencing, as shown in Figure 8.1. The lesion did not enhance post-contrast administration.

Given his symptoms and the appearances on imaging, the patient was offered surgical resection of the lesion. Five days after admission he underwent right frontal craniotomy and a transcortical transventricular approach to the mass, which was a colloid cyst (see Figure 8.2). The cyst contents were evacuated, and the cyst wall resected in a piecemeal fashion until complete clearance was achieved. An ipsilateral external ventricular drain (EVD) was sited at the end of the operation.

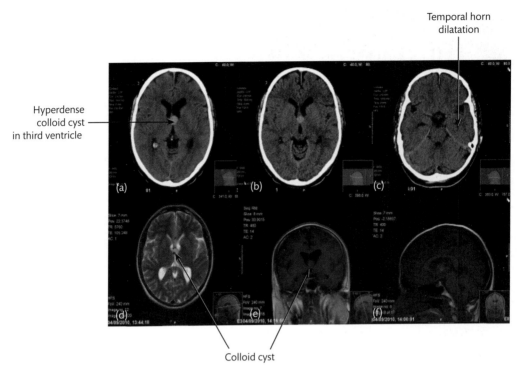

Temporal horn dilatation

Hyperdense colloid cyst in third ventricle

Colloid cyst

Figure 8.1 Upper panel: Sequential axial non-enhanced CT images revealing a cystic hyperdense lesion within the anterior part of the third ventricle, with associated moderate hydrocephalus (temporal horn dilatation on image c). Lower panel: T2-weighted axial MR imaging shows largely hyperintense lesion with a central region of lower intensity (d), reversed on T1 coronal and sagittal images (e and f).

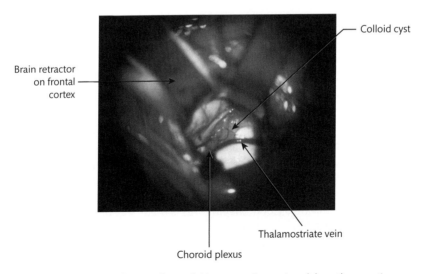

Colloid cyst

Brain retractor on frontal cortex

Thalamostriate vein

Choroid plexus

Figure 8.2 Transfrontal cortical approach to colloid cyst resection as viewed down the operating microscope. There is choroid plexus overlying the cyst. The thalamostriate vein runs inferiorly.

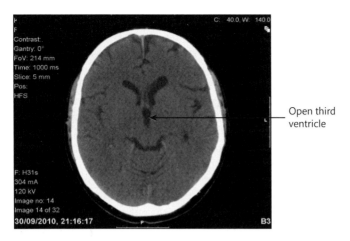

Open third
ventricle

Figure 8.3 Axial unenhanced CT imaging 2 days post-operatively, showing total cyst excision.

Histology revealed fragments of a cyst lined by ciliated pseudostratified epithelium with mild hyalinization and chronic inflammation of the wall. The second specimen consisted of amorphous cyst content and a diagnosis was made of colloid cyst of the third ventricle, with no evidence of malignancy.

Post-operative recovery was unremarkable, headaches resolved, and post-operative CT imaging revealed total cyst resection (Figure 8.3). The patient had no new neurological deficit. The EVD was removed day 3 post-operatively.

Follow-up after 3 months revealed an asymptomatic patient with no deficit who had returned to full-time employment.

Discussion

Colloid cysts are benign intracranial cysts which were first described by Wallmann in 1858 [2]. Formerly, they were a part of the World Health Organization classification of CNS tumours, incorporated within the category of 'Cysts and tumour-like lesions'.

Neuropathologists still debate the origin of colloid cysts. They may stem from the neuroectodermal elements of the paraphysis cerebri, or they may be derived from the migration of endodermal elements into the velum interpositum during early CNS development [3,4]. In favour of the latter, recent immunohistochemical analysis has revealed the presence of several different cellular types in the cyst membrane, including ciliated and non-ciliated, basal, goblet, and squamous cells [5]. The cyst contains mucoid and gelatinous material, which stain positive for Periodic Acid Schiff (PAS) and Alcian blue.

The true incidence of colloid cysts in the population is complicated by the distinction between asymptomatic and symptomatic lesions. In those undergoing MR imaging, 0/1000 and 1/3672 scans revealed incidental colloid cysts [6,7]; autopsy studies have variably shown colloid cysts in approximately 1 in 1000 autopsies [8,9]. De Witt Hamer reported an estimated incidence of *symptomatic* colloid cysts in the Dutch population of $1/10^6$ person-years [10], and Hernesniemi reported $3/10^6$ person-years in Finland [11].

> ✪ **Learning point** Colloid cyst histology
>
> Recent immunohistochemistry studies have challenged the notion of a neuroepithelial origin of colloid cysts. Migration of endodermal elements during early development, and either slow or delayed growth in the roof of the third ventricle are likely to be factors in their aetiology.

Colloid cysts can present in a variety of ways. In a review of thirteen case series of colloid cysts, Hellwig reported that the commonest symptoms were: headache (76%), followed by vomiting (24%), visual failure (21%), ataxia (12%), and memory deficit (10%) [12].

Imaging characteristics are classically of a hyperdense lesion in the roof of the third ventricle, with or without hydrocephalus, but MR allows further characterization of the cyst contents (typically hyperintense on T2-weighted and hypointense on T1-weighted imaging). This may be important if stereotactic aspiration of the cyst is the favoured option of management, since it is likely that the MR appearance will correlate with the viscosity of the cyst contents.

There are numerous case reports detailing family histories of colloid cysts. For example, Nader-Sepahi reported a mother and two daughters presenting with colloid cysts [13]; Joshi reported two sisters with confirmed colloid cysts and two other family members who died suddenly (causes unconfirmed) [14]; Akins reported a father and son with colloid cysts [15]. In 2004, Partington reviewed the literature of familial occurrence of colloid cyst, and postulated a possible autosomal dominant inheritance pattern albeit based on ten families [16].

Colloid cysts are associated with sudden death, but the strength of this association is controversial. The size of the cyst may be an important factor in this regard. Appuzzo stated that all cysts larger than 1cm in diameter should be surgically resected [17]. In two case series of autopsies of patients with sudden death attributable to colloid cysts, sizes ranged between 1.5–1.7cm [18] and 1–1.5cm [19]. Buttner in a review of 98 cases, reported a wide range of colloid cyst diameter in cases of sudden death, between 0.8 and >4cm [20].

The literature tells us that asymptomatic colloid cysts can be serially observed [21]. Symptomatic colloid cysts however have a high incidence (33%) of life-threatening progression [10].

Learning point Incidence of colloid cysts

The true incidence of colloid cysts is not known. A distinction should be drawn between asymptomatic and symptomatic lesions in this regard. Symptomatic colloid cyst incidence is approximately 1–3/10^6 person-years, and they account for 0.5–1% of all brain tumours.

Expert comment

Headache is usually a non-specific symptom, but progressive headache associated with visual obscurations and vomiting merits a scan even if there is no papilloedema on examination. Headache on waking is suggestive of raised ICP. The imaging is characteristic of a colloid cyst and these often present with intermittent raised ICP, headache, and on occasion respiratory arrest and sudden death. Although not normally familial, there have been reports of families where many siblings are affected (see LEARNING POINT: Family history).

Learning point Family history

There are multiple case reports of familial occurrences of colloid cyst. It is important to seek a family history. However, it is not clear how many first degree relatives need to be affected to justify screening the rest of the family. If a first degree relative of a patient with a known colloid cyst becomes symptomatic, it has been suggested that prompt scanning is appropriate.

Expert comment

Hydrocephalus does not always resolve after cyst resection. The first medical negligence damages in the UK to top 1 million pounds was to a student who had a colloid cyst resected and became acutely unwell, with raised ICP 1 week after surgery. For a variety of reasons this was not detected/treated promptly and the patient was left severely brain-injured as a result. Placement of a CSF access device at the end of the operation gives an easy method of relieving raised pressure in the post-operative period, and can be converted to a VP shunt if necessary.

Evidence base

There are two important papers in the literature addressing the natural history of colloid cysts. Both are retrospective case series and therefore represent NHS level C evidence.

Pollock et al. observed 68 patients with **asymptomatic** colloid cysts over a mean period of 79 months; the mean age was 57 years, and mean cyst size 8mm (8–14mm). Interestingly, 19 (28%) of these 'asymptomatic' patients initially presented with headache, but this symptom was thought to be unrelated to the cyst on further neurological assessment. There were no sudden deaths over the time frame, with one patient developing hydrocephalus, and one patient demonstrating cyst enlargement on serial imaging. All in all, 8% became symptomatic over a maximum of 10 years follow-up. The

(continued)

conclusion Pollock drew from this study was that patients in whom asymptomatic cysts are diagnosed can be cared for safely with observation and serial neuroimaging [21].

De Witt Hamer et al. retrospectively analysed 78 patients with **symptomatic** colloid cysts over 4 years. They found that 25 (32%) acutely deteriorated over that period of time, including four (12%) sudden deaths. A shorter duration (crescendo symptoms) and hydrocephalus were two risk factors for acute deterioration. The conclusion of this case series was that neurosurgical intervention was strongly advocated in those patients with symptomatic colloid cysts [22].

The management of colloid cysts is still keenly debated. Bilateral ventriculoperitoneal shunting historically was largely reserved for patients who were poor candidates for craniotomy. Stereotactic aspiration unfortunately has a high recurrence rate [22], and is limited by variable 'colloid' viscosity, sometimes precluding aspiration.

There are three major neurosurgical approaches to colloid cyst resection—transcortical trans/intra-ventricular, interhemispheric transcallosal, and the transcortical endoscopic or endoscope-assisted.

The transcallosal approach avoids the recognized complication of post-operative epilepsy associated with the transcortical approach. However, the transcallosal approach risks venous infarction, pericallosal artery injury, forniceal damage causing memory deficit (obviated by the modified far lateral approach [23]), and disconnection syndrome.

The use of endoscopes has allowed a minimal access approach to cyst management. However, cyst remnant is common after endoscopic surgery. Comparative studies are starting to be published comparing one modality of management to another. Horn et al. retrospectively compared twenty-eight patients treated endoscopically with twenty-seven undergoing transcallosal surgery. The associated hydrocephalus incidence was similar in both groups pre-operatively. Although the infection rate was greater in the transcallosal group (19%) compared with the endoscopic route (0%), and mean hospital stay was greater in the transcallosal group by 1 day, there was a 47% incidence of residual cyst in the endoscopic group compared with only 6% in the transcallosal [24].

> ➕ **Clinical tip** Common complications after colloid cyst resection
>
> The transcortical intraventricular approach can be complicated by seizure development, and CSF leakage. The interhemispheric transcallosal approach risks cortical venous infarction, contralateral leg weakness and the development of disconnection syndrome (although this is minimized by restricting the callosotomy to 1cm). The endoscopic approach has a high rate of cyst remnant, memory loss due to forniceal damage sustained during endoscope leverage, and has a steep learning curve for many operators.

> ➕ **Clinical tip** Surgical approaches to colloid cysts
>
> As a general rule, stereotactic aspiration of colloid cysts and bilateral VP shunt insertion are considered to be second-line management options. The choice between an interhemispheric transcallosal approach and a transcortical intraventricular approach to cyst resection is, in large part, based on the presence of hydrocephalus (favouring the latter). This is particularly the case if the endoscopic transcortical approach is being considered.

> ❝ **Expert comment**
>
> The emergency management of hydrocephalus due to a colloid cyst is often placement of bilateral external ventricular drains, and on occasion bilateral VP shunts. This approach collapses the ventricles and makes a transfrontal, transventricular approach more difficult.

> ⊙ **Learning point** Management of cyst remnant
>
> Particularly with the endoscopic approach, incomplete cyst wall resection results in a remnant that can be observed over time. Actual symptomatic recurrence of cysts from wall remnants is between 5 and 10%, and imaging characteristics often differ from the original colloid cysts on follow-up.

A final word from the expert

Microneurosurgery has revolutionized the management of this sometimes life-threatening cyst located in the deepest part of the brain. The neurosurgeon must reflect on his/her own practice and determine whether outcomes are better with one or other of the approaches described and with/without an endoscope. Hydrocephalus of the lateral ventricles in the absence of fourth ventricular dilatation mandates further imaging of the third ventricle. The relationship between the size of a colloid cyst, and development of symptoms and requirement for surgical intervention is not clearly defined in the literature.

References

1. Frisen L Swelling of the optic nerve head: a staging scheme Journal of Neurology, Neurosurgery and Psychiatry 1982; 45: 13–18.
2. Wallmann H. Eine colloidcyste im dritten Hirnventrikel und ein Lipom im plexus Choroides. Virchows Archiv Pathology and Anatomy 1858; 14: 385.
3. Nagaraju S1, O'Donovan DG, Cross J, et al. Colloid cyst of the third cerebral ventricle with an embryological remnant consistent with paraphysis cerebri in an adult human. Clinical Neuropathology 2010; 29 (3): 121–6.
4. Ho KL, Garcia JH. Colloid cysts of the third ventricle: ultrastructural features are compatible with endodermal derivation. Acta Neuropathologica 1992; 83 (6): 605–12.
5. Parwani AV, Fatani IY, Burger PC, et al. Colloid cyst of the third ventricle: cytomorphologic features on stereotactic fine-needle aspiration. Diagnostic Cytopathology 2002; 27 (1): 27–31.
6. Katzman GL, Dagher AP, Patronas NJ. Incidental findings on brain magnetic resonance imaging from 1000 asymptomatic volunteers. Journal of the American Medical Association 1999; 282: 36–9.
7. Yue NC1, Longstreth WT Jr, Elster AD, et al. Clinically serious abnormalities found incidentally at MR imaging of the brain: data from the Cardiovascular Health Study Radiology 1997; 202: 41–6.
8. Keiding D, Gregersen M, Charles AV. Intracranial tumors and angiomatous malformations in autopsy material of a medicolegal service. Ugeskrift for Laeger 1987; 149: 3002–15.
9. DiMaio SM, DiMaio VJ, Kirkpatrick JB. Sudden, unexpected deaths due to primary intracranial neoplasms. American Journal of Forensic Medical Pathology 1980; 1: 29–45.
10. de Witt Hamer PC, Verstegen MJ, De Haan RJ, et al. High risk of acute deterioration in patients harboring symptomatic colloid cysts of the third ventricle. Journal of Neurosurgery 2002; 96: 1041–5.
11. Hernesniemi J, Leivo S. Management outcome in third ventricular colloid cysts in a defined population: a series of 40 patients treated mainly by transcallosal microsurgery. Surgical Neurology 1996; 45: 2–14.
12. Hellwig D, Bauer BL, Schulte M, et al. Neuroendoscopic treatment for colloid cysts of the third ventricle: the experience of a decade. Neurosurgery 2003; 52 (3): 525–33.
13. Nader-Sepahi A, Hamlyn PJ. Familial colloid cysts of the third ventricle: case report Neurosurgery 2000; 46 (3): 751–3.
14. Joshi SM, Gnanalingham KK, Mohaghegh P, et al. A case of familial third ventricular colloid cyst. Emergency Medicine Journal 2005; 22 (12): 909–10.
15. Akins PT, Roberts R, Coxe WS, et al. Familial colloid cyst of the third ventricle: case report and review of associated conditions. Neurosurgery 1996; 38 (2): 392–5.
16. Partington MW, Bookalil AJ. Familial colloid cysts of the third ventricle. Clinical Genetics 2004; 66 (5): 473–5.
17. Apuzzo MLJ. Surgery of the third ventricle 2nd edn. Baltimore: Williams & Wilkins, 1998.
18. Brun A, Egund N. The pathogenesis of cerebral symptoms in colloid cysts of the third ventricle: a clinical and pathoanatomical study. Acta Neurologica Scandinavica 1973; 49 (4): 525–35.
19. Ryder JW, Kleinschmidt-DeMasters BK, Keller TS. Sudden deterioration and death in patients with benign tumors of the third ventricle area. Journal of Neurosurgery 1986; 64 (2): 216–23.
20. Büttner A, Winkler PA, Eisenmenger W, et al. Colloid cysts of the third ventricle with fatal outcome: a report of two cases and review of the literature. International Journal of Legal Medicine 1997; 110: 260–6.
21. Mathiesen T, Grane P, Lindquist C, et al. High recurrence rate following aspiration of colloid cysts in the third ventricle. Journal of Neurosurgery 1993; 78: 748–52.

22. Hernesniemi J, Romani R, Dashti R, et al. Microsurgical treatment of third ventricular colloid cysts by interhemispheric far lateral transcallosal approach—experience of 134 patients. Surgical Neurology 2008; 69: 447–56.

23. Pollock BE, Huston J 3rd. Natural history of asymptomatic colloid cysts of the third ventricle. Journal of Neurosurgery 1999; 91: 364–9.

24. Horn EM, Feiz-Erfan I, Bristol RE, et al. Treatment options for third ventricular colloid cysts: comparison of open microsurgical versus endoscopic resection. Neurosurgery 2007; 60 (4): 613–20.

9 Bilateral vestibular schwannomas: the challenge of neurofibromatosis type 2

Patrick Grover

✪ Expert commentary Robert Bradford

Case history

A 17-year-old female presented to her GP with a 1-year history of left-sided hearing loss, worsening balance, generalized headaches, and numbness affecting the left side of her face and tongue. She had previously been treated for left-sided otitis media and externa, and had undergone ear syringing for wax. Her previous medical history included meningitis as a child, but she had suffered no permanent neurological deficits. She had no family or social history of note.

On examination she had multiple café au lait spots over her abdomen and nodular fleshy polyps on her elbows, knees, and shins. She had bilateral sensorineural hearing deficits worst on the left side. Light touch and pin prick sensations were reduced on the left side of her face in the V2 and V3 dermatomes. Corneal reflex was absent in the left eye. There was uvular deviation to the left and tongue deviation to the left with right-sided wasting, consistent with glossopharyngeal and hypoglossal cranial nerve deficits. There was no facial nerve dysfunction. Cerebellar examination elicited slight left-sided dysmetria.

MRI demonstrated bilateral homogenously enhancing cerebellopontine angle mass lesions expanding the internal acoustic meati (Figure 9.1). The left-sided lesion measured 37 × 27 × 25mm and caused significant compression of the pons and medulla. The right-sided lesion was smaller at 23 × 14 × 11mm. Two further small extra-axial enhancing lesions were present in the right olfactory groove and abutting the right petrous ridge. There was no associated hydrocephalus. Audiometry confirmed bilateral sensorineural hearing loss particularly on the left side.

These findings were consistent with bilateral vestibular schwannoma and additional supratentorial meningiomata, with an underlying diagnosis of NF2. The patient's symptoms and signs were predominantly localized to the larger left cerebellopontine angle lesion, which was debulked through a left retrosigmoid craniotomy and sub-occipital approach. The patient was started on dexamethasone (4mg qds po/iv). Post-operatively, the patient experienced hearing loss in her left ear, but no additional cranial nerve dysfunction. She subsequently developed hydrocephalus, for which a ventriculo-peritoneal shunt was inserted, and recovered well thereafter.

The gross pathological appearance of the resected fragments was of tan/grey pieces of tissue with a granular appearance. Histology showed multiple interlacing bundles of spindle cells with no atypical features, characteristic of a WHO Grade I schwannoma (Table 9.1).

> **✪ Learning point** Diagnostic criteria for neurofibromatosis type 2
>
> The Manchester criteria are the most widely used criteria for defining neurofibromatosis [1]. They describe neurofibromatosis type 2 (NF2) associated lesions as meningioma, glioma, schwannoma, neurofibroma, or posterior subcapsular lenticular opacities. Diagnosis requires one of the following:
>
> - Bilateral vestibular schwannomas
> - A first-degree relative with NF2 and either a unilateral vestibular schwannoma or two NF2 associated lesions.
> - Unilateral acoustic neuroma and two NF2 associated lesions.
> - Multiple meningiomas and either a unilateral acoustic neuroma or two NF2 associated lesions.

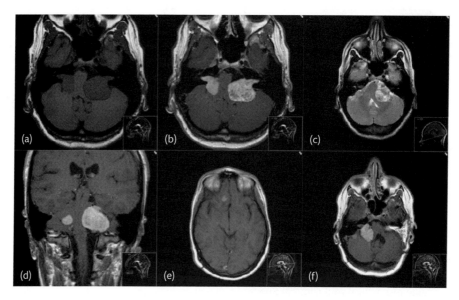

Figure 9.1 MRI images demonstrating pre- and post-surgical appearance of bilateral vestibular schwannomas and additional intracranial meningiomas. (a) T1-weighted axial MRI. (b) T1-weighted with gadolinium. (c) T2-weighted. (d) Sagittal T1-weighted with gadolinium. (e) T1-weighted with gadolinium demonstrating olfactory groove meningioma. (f) T1-weighted with gadolinium after two surgical resections of the left tumour.

Her 6-month follow-up MRI unfortunately revealed progressive growth of the left-sided tumour and the patient underwent further planned subtotal excision via a translabyrinthine approach (Figure 9.1). Post-operative MRI scans at 3 and 11 months showed stable appearances of the remaining right-sided tumour and small left-sided residual. The patient has not experienced any further progression of her symptoms and has retained hearing in her right ear with moderate loss to 55 dB at 2000Hz and 30–40dB at high frequencies (Figure 9.2). She has no hearing in the left ear. The patient's family are currently undergoing genetic testing, although no other member has clinical symptoms or signs of neurofibromatosis.

Table 9.1 Histopathological classification of central and peripheral nerve sheath tumours based on the 2007 World Health Organization (WHO) classification [30].

Subtypes	Histological variants	Description
Schwannoma (neurilemoma, neurinoma)	Cellular, plexiform, melanotic	Encapsulated nerve sheath tumour composed of well-differentiated neoplastic Schwann cells
Neurofibroma	Plexiform	Unencapsulated fusiform nerve sheath tumour composed of a mix of neoplastic Schwann cells, perineural cells, and fibroblasts in a collagen matrix
Perineuroma	Perineuroma, malignant perineuroma	Tumours of perineural cells, which form either intraneurally encasing the nerve or within soft tissue
Malignant peripheral nerve sheath tumour (MPNST)	Epitheloid, melanotic, MPNST with glandular differentiation, MPNST with mesenchymal differentiation	Malignant and invasive peripheral nerve sheath tumour composed of spindle cells. Hypercellular with high mitotic activity, hyperchromatic nuclei and necroses

Perry A LD, Scheithauer BW, Budka H, von Diemling A. World Health Organization Classification of Tumours of the Central Nervous System, ed 4. Lyon: IARC, 2007.

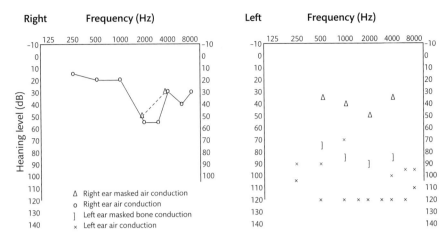

Figure 9.2 Post-surgical audiometry demonstrating bilateral sensorineural hearing loss with no useful hearing on the left side.

Discussion

Vestibular schwannomas are benign tumours that are said to originate predominantly from the superior vestibular nerve. Their incidence is estimated to be between two and twenty cases per million worldwide, comprising approximately 5–10% of intracranial tumours [2]. They arise in the cerebellopontine angle accounting for approximately 90% of mass lesions in this location [3]. Speculation that their incidence may be increased by mobile phone exposure has been the subject of several studies, most of which have found no association [4]. However, the recent multi-national INTERPHONE case-control study suggested an increased incidence of ipsilateral tumours after 10 years usage [5]. They compared 678 cases of vestibular schwannoma and 3553 controls, retrospectively, interviewing participants to determine mobile phone usage. There was no overall increase in the risk of developing vestibular schwannoma (OR 0.9, 95% CI 0.7–1.1), but the risk of developing a tumour on the same side of the head as reported phone usage was statistically greater after 10 years (OR 1.8, 95% CI 1.1–3.1).

Vestibular schwannomas arise from the neurolemmal sheath of the vestibular nerve at the junction between oligodendrocytes and Schwann cells known as the Obersteiner–Redlich zone, approximately 8–12mm from the brainstem. They are characterized by spindle cells arranged in tightly compact fascicles within Antoni type A areas, and loosely compacted in Antoni type B areas. Bilateral vestibular schwannomas are pathognomonic of NF2 and are caused by mutations of the *neurofibromin 2* gene found on chromosome 22q. This codes for tumour suppressor protein merlin, also known as schwannomin, which has roles in cellular proliferation and cell adherence [6]. Mutations in *neurofibromin 2* are also found in a significant proportion of sporadic vestibular schwannomas [7].

Nearly all patients present with unilateral hearing loss with or without tinnitus. Balance disturbance affects around two-thirds of patients and headaches are similarly common. Facial numbness due to trigeminal nerve involvement can be a feature in up to one-third, whereas symptoms relating to the other surrounding cranial nerves are uncommon. On examination, a sensorineural hearing deficit is

> ✪ **Learning point** Genetics of neurofibromatosis type 2
>
> NF2 is autosomal dominant with high penetrance in inherited cases leading to clinical manifestations by the age of 60 in almost all affected individuals [8]. However, more than 50% of cases are sporadic and, of these, approximately one-third are mosaic—only a proportion of cells carry the mutation, which occurs after conception [8]. These patients will have a milder clinical course and a less than 50% chance of passing the mutation to their offspring.

❝ Expert comment The presentation of neurofibromatosis type 2

In adulthood, NF2 most commonly presents with symptoms and signs of vestibular schwannoma, particularly unilateral hearing loss. A smaller proportion are diagnosed from alternative lesions, such as intracranial meningiomas causing seizures and headaches, ocular tumours leading to visual loss, spinal masses resulting in limb weakness and sensory disturbance, and cutaneous stigmata. More severe cases present in the paediatric population, where symptoms and signs from these alternative lesions are more prevalent [11].

almost universal. Nystagmus, facial hypoaesthesia and an abnormal corneal reflex are each elicited in approximately one-third of patients. Facial weakness and oculo-motor nerve palsy may be detected infrequently. Large tumours (>3cm) can present with symptoms and signs of brainstem compression, lower cranial nerve damage, ataxia, or raised intracranial pressure due to obstruction of the fourth ventricle caus-ing non-communicating hydrocephalus [9,10].

✚ Clinical tip Cranial nerve examination in vestibular schwannoma

The differential diagnosis of a patient with unilateral hearing and balance loss remains wide and a thorough cranial nerve examination is crucial. Although intimately associated with the VIIIth cranial nerve (Figure 9.3), the VIIth nerve is much less often clinically affected by compression. Symptoms and signs of trigeminal nerve involvement are slightly more common although still seen in less than 20% of cases [10]. Loss of the corneal reflex is a particularly useful sign as it often precedes facial hypoaesthesia [9].

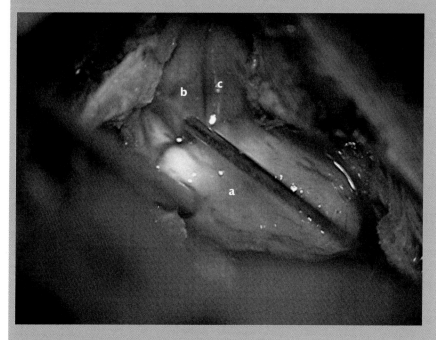

Figure 9.3 Vestibular schwannoma and relations to cranial nerves. a, vestibular schwannoma; b, facial nerve (VII); c, vestibulocochlear nerve (VIII).

The investigation of choice in patients clinically suspected of vestibular schwan-noma is MRI [12,13]. Our recommendation is that any patient with unilateral sensori-neural hearing loss should have an MRI scan [13]. The spatial resolution of MRI is now such that the sensitivity of non-contrasted thin-slice T2- and T2*-weighted imaging approaches 100% for cerebellopontine angle lesions with a specificity of between 90 and 100% [12,14]. Contrasted scans only improve sensitivity if dedicated internal acoustic meatus (IAM) views are not undertaken and are usually unnecessary.

Abnormalities of the auditory brainstem response waveform are reliably found in tumours greater than 1cm in size, but this test is not specific and is now rarely per-formed as MRI has become more widely available [15]. CT with contrast will miss up to 10% of cases, but may be useful to demonstrate bony anatomy. Audiometry is of value in serial monitoring of hearing but its use as a diagnostic tool is limited to the detection of hearing loss in advance of scanning. Speech discrimination is typically disproportionately impaired relative to pure tone threshold.

> ✪ **Learning point**
>
> The American Academy of Otolaryngology-Head and Neck Surgery (AAO-HNS) hearing classification is the most widely used in vestibular schwannoma assessment (see Table 9.2) [16]
>
> **Table 9.2** The American Academy of Otolaryngology-Head and Neck Surgery (AAO-HNS) hearing classification
>
> | Class | Pure tone threshold (dB) | Speech discrimination (%) |
> | --- | --- | --- |
> | A | ≤30 | ≥70 |
> | B | 30.1–50 | ≥50 |
> | C | >50 | ≥50 |
> | D | Any level | <50 |

Vestibular schwannomas may be managed conservatively, surgically or with radiotherapy. Combined modality treatment has also been successfully reported, e.g. sub-total debulking followed by gamma knife therapy for large vestibular schwannomas [17]. Smouha et al. (2005) carried out a meta-analysis of the conservative management of 1345 cases in twenty-one studies, with a mean follow-up of 3.2 years [18]. Mean growth rate was 1.9mm/year with 43% of cases progressing, and 57% not growing or regressing. Fifty-one percent of the 347 patients in whom data was available lost hearing. It is important to remember this represents a small selected cohort of patients not felt suitable for immediate intervention. For example, of 432 patients referred with vestibular schwannomas to the Northwestern otolaryngology unit in Chicago, USA, fifty-three were initially managed conservatively [19]. These patients tend to be older (mean age = 62) with smaller tumours (mean size = 11.8mm) [18]. It is also important to note that these tumours may show non-linear growth, with enlargement after a period (which may be many years) with no apparent growth.

Selecting which patients are suitable for conservative management is difficult due to a lack of factors predictive of clinical progression. Twenty percent of patients in the Smouha et al. meta-analysis failed conservative management, and progressed to surgery or radiotherapy. Mean growth rate at 1 year has been shown to be predictive of the eventual need for treatment in conservatively managed patients but not routinely so [20,21].

> 🎓 **Expert comment** Suitability for conservative management
>
> A suitable patient is one who makes a fully-informed decision, based on balancing the risks and benefits in collaboration with their surgeon. Patients with small masses and preserved hearing may wish to forgo the risk of losing their hearing in the short-term, accepting a greater risk of hearing loss and other complications in the future. Older patients and those with multiple comorbidities have a higher risk of peri-operative complications, which might outweigh the potential benefits of surgery.

Tumours may be approached surgically via three approaches. The two most commonly used are retrosigmoid transmeatal and translabyrinthine, with the middle cranial fossa approach less prevalent. The retrosigmoid transmeatal approach

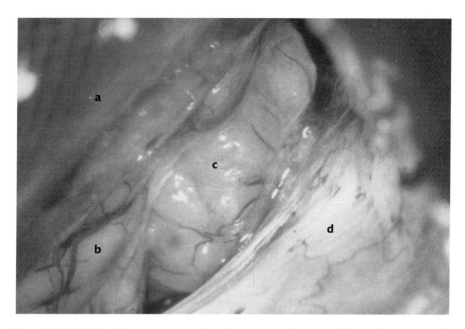

Figure 9.4 Vestibular schwannoma as seen through a retrosigmoid transmeatal approach. a, retractor; b, cerebellum; c, vestibular schwannoma; d temporal bone.

❝ Expert comment

Indications for intervention in vestibular schwannoma in NF2 used in our practice include tumours that are:

- Greater than 3cm.
- 2–3cm if enlarging on serial imaging.
- 1–2cm if growing, with poor hearing. In those with good hearing, hearing preservation surgery may be undertaken with cochlear nerve implant if required

❝ Expert comment
Cerebrospinal fluid leakage

CSF leakage is a common and troublesome complication of vestibular schwannoma surgery causing significant morbidity. Rates tend to be highest with the translabyrinthine approach. The incidence can be minimized with meticulous dural closure (not possible with translabyrinthine surgery), intra-operative fat and fascia grafting, use of fibrin glue, and post-operative lumbar CSF drainage.

enables access to almost all tumours with the possibility of hearing preservation (Figure 9.4) [22]. However, cerebellar retraction is required and the facial nerve is encountered late, resulting in higher rates of facial nerve palsy.

The translabyrinthine approach sacrifices vestibular and cochlear function on that side, but has the advantage of being a predominently extracranial approach with early identification of the facial nerve. Preservation rates of greater than 90% for small tumours and 50% for large tumours may be expected with this technique [23]. The middle cranial fossa approach is largely extradural and enables hearing preservation also, but is limited to small intracanalicular tumours, and carries a high risk of damage to the geniculate ganglion and facial nerve palsy [24]. It is important to recognize that these rates are case series from experienced centres representing exceptional outcomes. Rates of serviceable hearing preservation after surgery, for example, are not typically as high as quoted in the literature. Furthermore, all procedures carry a risk of CSF leakage in between 10 and 20% of cases, and a small risk of mortality (<1%).

Stereotactic radiosurgery and fractionated radiotherapy are increasingly used in the management of small vestibular schwannomas. A non-randomized prospective study of eighty-two patients treated at the Mayo clinic, Minnesota, USA, compared gamma knife stereotactic radiosurgery in forty-two patients, with microsurgery carried out on thirty-six patients for tumours of similar size and clinical profile [25]. At a mean of 42 months follow-up, facial nerve function was preserved in 96% of the gamma knife group and 75% of the surgical group, while useful hearing was maintained in 63% of gamma knife patients compared with only 5% of the surgical cohort. Operated patients also had significantly worse physical functioning, and pain at 3- and 12-month follow-up.

These data demonstrate a significantly better side effect profile for stereotactic radiosurgery, but it should be noted that evidence on long-term tumour control is lacking as the gamma knife has been in use in its current form only since 1985, with progressive dose reduction over the past 20 years. Furthermore, there is concern regarding the development of radiation-induced tumours or malignant transformation, which again may only be uncovered after a long follow-up period. At present, the risk appears to be in the region of 1:5000–1:10,000 for sporadic tumours, but it is probably much greater for NF2 tumours, which are inherently less stable. Multiple modalities of radiotherapy administration have shown efficacy in acoustic neuroma including Linear Accelerator (LINAC) radiosurgery [26] and Cyberknife® [27], with the longest follow-up for gamma knife single fraction treatment. Staged or fractionated protocols apply lower radiation doses multiple times and may result in reduced rates of damage to surrounding structures [28]. From our 12 years' experience of fractionated radiotherapy, we quote control rates of greater than 90%, with a 3% risk of cranial nerve damage and 50% risk of loss of useful hearing.

A final word from the expert

Treatment of these tumours will increasingly depend on less invasive modalities including focused radiation techniques and molecular chemotherapeutics. Radiosurgery is significantly less effective in NF2-associated schwannomas and this represents a particular challenge in management. Clinical trials of bevacizumab (a VEGF inhibitor), and lapatinib (a tyrosine kinase inhibitor) in NF2 are ongoing [29].

Acknowledgements

The authors wish to thank Professor Shakeel Saeed who proof-read the article and contributed to the expert commentary.

References

1. Evans DG, Baser ME, O'Reilly B, et al. Management of the patient and family with neurofibromatosis 2: a consensus conference statement. British Journal of Neurosurgery 2005; 19 (1): 5–12.
2. Tos M, Stangerup SE, Caye-Thomasen P, et al. What is the real incidence of vestibular schwannoma? Archives of Otolaryngology—Head and Neck Surgery 2004; 130 (2): 216–20.
3. Brackmann DE, Bartels LJ. Rare tumors of the cerebellopontine angle. Otolaryngology—Head and Neck Surgery 1980; 88 (5): 555–9.
4. Han YY, Kano H, Davis DL, et al. Cell phone use and acoustic neuroma: the need for standardized questionnaires and access to industry data. Surgical Neurology 2009; 72 (3): 216–22 ; discussion 222.
5. INTERPHONE Study Group. Acoustic neuroma risk in relation to mobile telephone use: results of the INTERPHONE international case-control study. Cancer Epidemiology 2011; 35 (5): 453–64.
6. Sughrue ME, Yeung AH, Rutkowski MJ, et al. Molecular biology of familial and sporadic vestibular schwannomas: implications for novel therapeutics. Journal of Neurosurgery 2011; 114 (2): 359–66.

7. Irving RM, Moffat DA, Hardy DG, et al. Somatic NF2 gene mutations in familial and non-familial vestibular schwannoma. Human Molecular Genetics 1994; 3 (2): 347–50.

8. Evans DG, Sainio M, Baser ME. Neurofibromatosis type 2. Journal of Medical Genetics 2000; 37 (12): 897–904.

9. Harner SG, Laws ER, Jr. Clinical findings in patients with acoustic neurinoma. Mayo Clinic Proceedings 1983; 58 (11): 721–8.

10. Matthies C, Samii M. Management of 1000 vestibular schwannomas (acoustic neuromas): clinical presentation. Neurosurgery 1997; 40 (1): 1–9; discussion 9–10.

11. Evans DG, Birch JM, Ramsden RT. Paediatric presentation of type 2 neurofibromatosis. Archives of Diseases of Childhood 1999; 81 (6): 496–9.

12. Fortnum H, O'Neill C, Taylor R, et al. The role of magnetic resonance imaging in the identification of suspected acoustic neuroma: a systematic review of clinical and cost effectiveness and natural history. Health Technology Assessment 2009; 13 (18): iii–iv, ix–xi, 1–154.

13. Wright A, Bradford R. Management of acoustic neuroma. British Medical Journal 1995; 311 (7013): 1141–4.

14. Soulie D, Cordoliani YS, Vignaud J, et al. MR imaging of acoustic neuroma with high resolution fast spin echo T2-weighted sequence. European Journal of Radiology 1997; 24 (1): 61–5.

15. Schmidt RJ, Sataloff RT, Newman J, et al. The sensitivity of auditory brainstem response testing for the diagnosis of acoustic neuromas. Archives of Otolaryngology—Head and Neck Surgery 2001; 127 (1): 19–22.

16. Monsell EM. New and revised reporting guidelines from the Committee on Hearing and Equilibrium. American Academy of Otolaryngology-Head and Neck Surgery Foundation, Inc. Otolaryngology—Head and Neck Surgery 1995; 113 (3): 176–8.

17. van de Langenberg R, Hanssens PE, Verheul JB, et al. Management of large vestibular schwannoma. Part II. Primary gamma knife surgery: radiological and clinical aspects. Journal of Neurosurgery 2011; 115 (5): 885–93.

18. Smouha EE, Yoo M, Mohr K, et al. Conservative management of acoustic neuroma: a meta-analysis and proposed treatment algorithm. Laryngoscope 2005; 115 (3): 450–4.

19. Wiet RJ, Zappia JJ, Hecht CS, et al. Conservative management of patients with small acoustic tumors. Laryngoscope 1995; 105 (8 Pt 1): 795–800.

20. Deen HG, Ebersold MJ, Harner SG, et al. Conservative management of acoustic neuroma: an outcome study. Neurosurgery 1996; 39 (2): 260–4; discussion 264–6.

21. Sughrue ME, Kane AJ, Kaur R, et al. A prospective study of hearing preservation in untreated vestibular schwannomas. Journal of Neurosurgery 2011; 114 (2): 381–5.

22. Gormley WB, Sekhar LN, Wright DC, et al. Acoustic neuromas: results of current surgical management. Neurosurgery 1997; 41 (1): 50–8; discussion 58–60.

23. Sterkers JM, Morrison GA, Sterkers O, et al. Preservation of facial, cochlear, and other nerve functions in acoustic neuroma treatment. Otolaryngology—Head and Neck Surgery 1994; 110 (2): 146–55.

24. Shelton C, Brackmann DE, House WF, et al. Middle fossa acoustic tumor surgery: results in 106 cases. Laryngoscope 1989; 99 (4): 405–8.

25. Pollock BE, Driscoll CL, Foote RL, et al. Patient outcomes after vestibular schwannoma management: a prospective comparison of microsurgical resection and stereotactic radiosurgery. Neurosurgery 2006; 59 (1): 77–85.

26. Friedman WA. Linear accelerator radiosurgery for vestibular schwannomas. Progress in Neurological Surgery 2008; 21: 228–37.

27. Chang SD, Gibbs IC, Sakamoto GT, et al. Staged stereotactic irradiation for acoustic neuroma. Neurosurgery 2005; 56 (6): 1254–61 ; discussion 1261–3.

28. Williams JA. Fractionated stereotactic radiotherapy for acoustic neuromas. International Journal of Radiation Oncology • Biology • Physics 2002; 54 (2): 500–4.

29. Chang, S.D., et al. Staged stereotactic irradiation for acoustic neuroma. Neurosurgery, 2005. 56 (6): 1254–61 ; discussion 1261–3.

30. Perry A LD, Scheithauer BW, Budka H, et al. World Health Organization Classification of Tumours of the Central Nervous System, 4th edn. Lyon: IARC, 2007.

Multimodality monitoring in severe traumatic brain injury

Adel Helmy

⊕ Expert commentary Peter J. Hutchinson

Case history

A 23-year-old, right-handed female presented to the A&E department following a road traffic accident. The patient was a single restrained occupant and collateral history suggested that, following loss of control of the vehicle, the driver collided with a tree at 60–70mph. There was significant intrusion into the vehicle on the passenger side resulting in a 1-hour extrication time. Medical first responders noted a GCS on scene of E1 V1 M4 (6/15) and that both pupils were small (3mm) and reactive to light. Following extrication, the patient was intubated and ventilated, and airlifted to the nearest trauma centre.

> **✪ Learning point** Glasgow Coma Score
>
> The GCS was developed as a tool for the objective assessment of coma by Teasdale and Jennet in the 1970s [1]. The GCS has three distinct components, which should be reported individually, namely eye-opening (1–4), verbal (1–5), and motor (1–6) response. The best response is always used and provides a measure of global responsiveness. While the GCS has been criticized as having poor inter-observer validity in the non-expert assessor [2], it remains an important tool for both stratification of severity and prognostication following traumatic brain injury (TBI) [3].

The patient was managed in line with Advanced Trauma and Life Support (ATLS) protocols. Secondary survey did not note any further extracranial injuries. On arrival in A&E 90 minutes after injury, the patient had adequate ventilation ($PO_2 = 17$kPa, $PCO_2 = 4.7$kPa) and was haemodynamically stable, with a pulse rate of 85 and a blood pressure of 130/85mmHg. However, on reassessment, her pupils were found to be bilaterally fixed and dilated.

> **✪ Learning point** Hyperventilation following traumatic brain injury
>
> Therapeutic hyperventilation can be used in the intensive care setting to reduce ICP. CO_2 is an important determinant of vascular tone. Hyperventilation results in relative vasoconstriction, reduction in arterial blood volume, and a consequent reduction in ICP. However, vasoconstriction reduces cerebral blood flow and there is a trade-off between the reduction in ICP and the risk of ischaemia [4]. For this reason, outside the setting of the neurointensive care unit and appropriate monitoring of oxygenation (such as brain tissue oxygen or jugular venous oximetry) it is not recommended [5]. Nevertheless, PCO_2 should be kept in the low normal range (4.5–5.0 kPa) in those with suspected raised ICP.

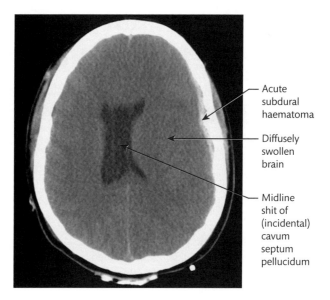

Acute
subdural
haematoma

Diffusely
swollen
brain

Midline
shit of
(incidental)
cavum
septum
pellucidum

Figure 10.1 A brain window CT scan demonstrates a thin left-sided acute subdural haematoma and diffuse brain swelling.

The patient was catheterized and administered 200mL of 20% mannitol intravenously. She was transferred to the CT scanner. Figure 10.1 shows a representative axial slice on CT scan of the brain. This demonstrated a thin acute left subdural haematoma, brain swelling, but no evidence of vault or base of skull fracture. No other extracranial or spinal injuries were identified.

> **🗨 Expert comment** Base of skull fracture
>
> Base of skull fractures can provide circumstantial evidence for the magnitude of force applied to the skull. They are sometimes missed and can be associated with several complications. CSF leak can mitigate rises in ICP by reducing intracranial CSF volume; however, they are associated with an increase in risk of meningitis. Prophylactic antibiotics do not play a role, but recent NICE guidelines recommend the administration of pneumoccal vaccine (pneumovax) in all patient [6]. Most CSF leaks will resolve spontaneously over a few days without the need for operative intervention.
>
> There is an increasing recognition of vascular injury to the intrapetrous carotid in base of skull fractures that traverse the carotid canal (as well as vertebral artery injury in fractures that traverse the relevant transverse foraminae) and we now recommend CT angiography in these cases. While anticoagulation may prove high risk in patients with severe TBI, endovascular interventions may still be an option if an intimal dissection is identified.

CT scan of C-spine, chest, abdomen, and pelvis did not demonstrate any other injury. The patient was immediately transferred to the theatre where a left-sided craniotomy and evacuation of subdural haematoma was carried out. The brain appeared swollen at the time of craniotomy and the bone flap was therefore not replaced. ICP, brain tissue oxygen, and microdialysis (to monitor brain chemistry) monitors were inserted in the right frontal lobe anterior to the coronal suture and the patient was returned to the intensive care unit.

The initial ICP was 18mmHg, but over the following 6 hours this gradually rose to 20–25mmHg requiring an escalation in ICP control measures, including moderate hypothermia to 35°C. Cerebral perfusion pressure (CPP) was maintained within the

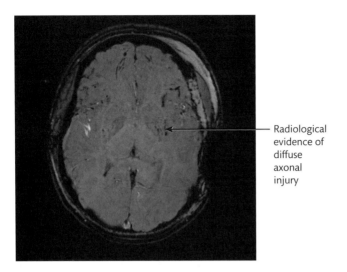
Radiological
evidence of
diffuse
axonal
injury

Figure 10.2 Certain MR sequences (gradient-echo, susceptibility-weighted images) are particularly sensitive to blood product and can be used to identify small petechial haemorrhages not apparent on CT or conventional MRI. The widespread dots of low signal on this image are indicative of a diffuse brain injury, which is often interpreted as diffuse axonal injury. Strictly speaking, diffuse axonal injury is a post-mortem histological diagnosis with evidence of axonal retraction balls.

target range of 60–65mmHg. An MRI scan (susceptibility-weighted image) taken 24 hours post-operatively is shown in Figure 10.2.

At approximately 60 hours following craniectomy there was a sharp increase in lactate/pyruvate (L/P) ratio above 25, despite adequately controlled ICP (Figure 10.3). L/P ratio is a measure of cellular redox state and reflects the degree of anaerobic metabolism occurring within a tissue: a threshold of more than 25 is used to identify cerebral ischaemia [7]. A repeat CT scan did not reveal any further intracranial lesions, but as the brain tissue oxygen demonstrated a co-existent drop (not shown), a decision was made not to de-escalate ICP control measures.

At approximately 70 hours following craniotomy there was a sharp increase in ICP to above 40mmHg requiring further escalation of ICP control measures, including cooling to 33°C, more aggressive hyperventilation to a CO_2 of 4kPa and repeated boluses of 5% hypertonic saline until the serum Na^+ reached 160mmol/L and the serum osmolarity reached 320mmol/L. During aggressive hyperventilation, the brain tissue oxygen tension was not permitted to drop below 15mmHg. As ICP was difficult to control an EVD was inserted at this time (Figure 10.4) as a further measure. Figure 10.5 shows the output from ICM+ demonstrating the Pulse Reactivity Index (PRx) for the patient in question. Figure 10.6 shows a plot of the PRx in relation to 5mmHg CPP bins.

> ✪ **Learning point** Pulse Reactivity Index
>
> PRx is the moving correlation coefficient between mean arterial pressure (MAP) and ICP that varies from −1 to +1. The normal autoregulatory response maintains constant cerebral blood flow in the face of variations in MAP. This is achieved by vasoconstriction in the cerebral vasculature in response to an increase in MAP. This vasoconstriction would normally reduce ICP, and in this way MAP and ICP should be inversely correlated. In this way, in the normal brain PRx should be negative. Following TBI, autoregulation can be impaired or absent such that increasing MAP causes a passive distension of the cerebral vessels, an increase in arterial blood volume and an increase in ICP. In this case, PRx will be increasingly positive [8].

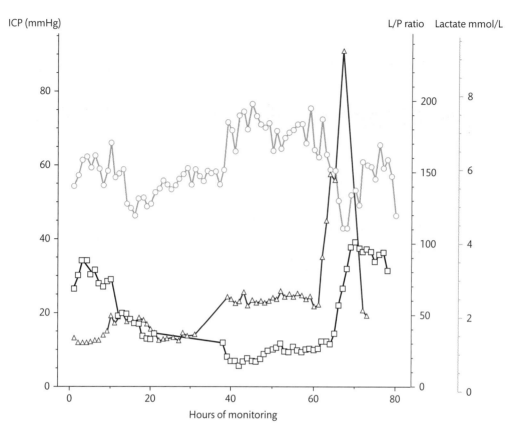

Figure 10.3 ICP (left hand axis) and L/P (right hand blue axis) ratio are plotted over time since commencement of monitoring. The L/P ratio jumps from around 20–25 to 60–80 around 60 hours. This precedes an ICP spike to a plateau of 40mmHg at around 70 hours.

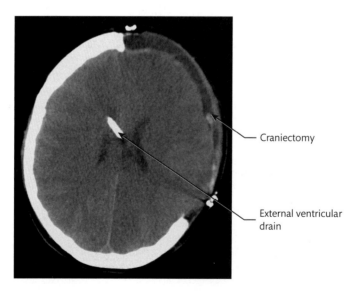

Figure 10.4 Axial CT scan demonstrates the left-sided craniectomy and an external ventricular drain from the right frontal approach.

With thanks to Dr Karol Budohoski and Dr Marek Czosynka for providing these images.

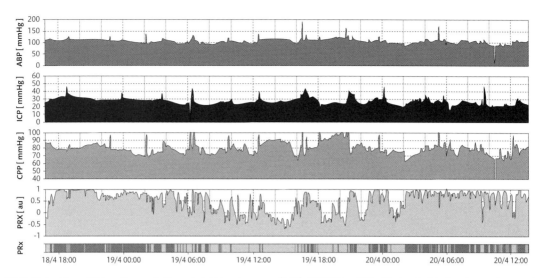

Figure 10.5 Output from ICM+ software plotting arterial blood pressure (ABP), ICP, CPP, and PRx. PRx is calculated as the moving correlation coefficient between ABP and ICP.

With thanks to Dr Karol Budohoski and Dr Marek Czosynka for providing these images.

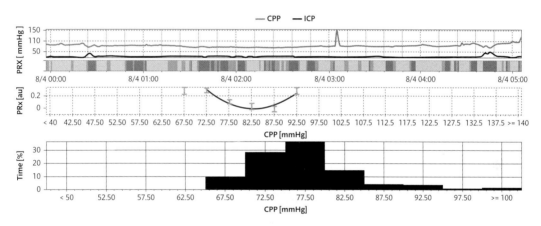

Figure 10.6 Output from ICM+ software. PRx is plotted in the top panel. In the middle panel, the mean PRx value has been plotted against the CPP. A clear nadir is seen at 82.5–87.5mmHg indicating that at this value of CPP, PRx is minimized, and at this level of CPP the cerebral vasculature is autoregulating most effectively. Some authors have suggested that this is the optimal CPP to ensure adequate delivery of metabolic substrates to the injured brain. The lower panel shows the percentage of time the patient has spent at each CPP value.

> **❝ Expert comment** Optimizing cerebral perfusion pressure
>
> The Brain Trauma Foundation have provided guidelines on CPP targets—current guidelines suggest a range of 50–70mmHg. PRx may provide a method for individualizing CPP targets in two ways. First, if the PRx is negative and ICP is difficult to control increasing MAP can be used as a method of controlling ICP. Secondly, some authors have suggested that by targeting a CPP in which PRx can be shown to be negative may be beneficial as it provides a sufficient perfusion pressure, such that the brain can regulate its own needs physiologically.

A higher CPP target was adopted in this patient (75mmHg) resulting in improved control of ICP to below 20mmHg. After a further period of 24 hours, ICP began to fall consistently to the range of 15–20mmHg. A trial of raising CO_2 to 4.5kPa from

4kPa was attempted. This resulted in a rapid increase in ICP to 30mmHg and, there-fore, PCO_2 was returned to 4kPa for a further 24 hours. A repeat trial of raised CO_2 was carried out at this point, which was well tolerated. This allowed further de-escalation with gradual re-warming to 35°C then 37°C.

> **⊕ Clinical tip** De-escalation of intracranial pressure control
>
> Patients with raised ICP often have poor intracranial compliance, i.e. small changes in intracranial volume lead to large changes in ICP. When reducing ICP control measures a CO_2 challenge is a useful method for gauging intracranial compliance and whether a patient will tolerate such de-escalation. As CO_2 can be manipulated quickly and easily by alteration of minute volume it is preferable to de-escalation of other ICP control measures, such as rewarming from hypothermia. Rewarming can take several hours and if ICP were to rise, it can take several hours to re-institute. This can lead to poor ICP control for several hours, and potentially further secondary injury.

Over the following 48 hours, all ICP control measures were reversed. On stopping sedation, the patient achieved a GCS: E2, V: intubated; M5. The patient underwent tracheostomy and continued to improve over the following 2 weeks to a GCS: E4 V: tracheostomy; M6. A repeat CT scan (Figure 10.7) at this time showed a large sub-dural hygroma on the non-operated side. As the flap was soft and the patient was clinically improving, a decision was made to proceed to early cranioplasty and burr hole drainage of the hygroma. Figure 10.8 shows a CT scan 3 days post-cranioplasty showing resolution of the subdural hygroma.

The patient remains in a poor clinical state 6 months following injury with a Glasgow Outcome Score of 3 (severe disability). The patient has been referred for neuro-rehabilitation.

1. Presenting CT scan (brain window and bone window).
2. MRI scan (susceptibility-weighted image/gradient echo).
3. LP ratio and ICP.

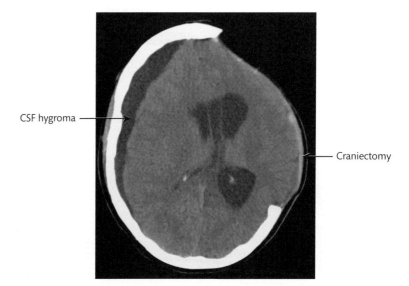

Figure 10.7 Axial CT scan demonstrating CSF hygroma contralateral to the side of decompressive craniectomy.

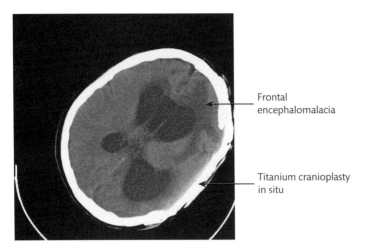

Frontal
encephalomalacia

Titanium cranioplasty
in situ

Figure 10.8 Axial CT scan following cranioplasty insertion. Although the subdural hygroma has resolved, the ventricles have now dilated. This is likely to be secondary to brain atrophy. Areas of low density, most marked in the right frontal lobe, indicate encephalomalacia.

4. CT scan with EVD in situ.
5. PRx trace from ICM+.
6. CPP optimal from ICM+.
7. CT scan with subdural hygroma.
8. CT scan post-cranioplasty.

Discussion

TBI is the commonest cause of death in those under 40 years of age in the UK. Although there is a long-term declining trend in severe TBI, largely related to the widespread introduction of road safety measures, such as seatbelts and cycle helmets, it still exacts a heavy economic and social toll. The management of severe TBI can provide many challenges, both to the neurosurgeon and to the neuro-intensivist. Great strides have been made by developing protocol treatment regimens for the intensive care management of ICP [9], which have led to improvements in patient outcome when compared with historical controls [10]. However, no Class 1 evidence exists for the use of ICP monitoring. In the developed world it is unlikely that there will ever be the ethical basis to run a trial in severe TBI, randomizing between ICP-driven therapy and management without ICP measurement. ICP measurement is recommended (based on the Brain Trauma Foundation Guidelines) in TBI patients presenting in coma (GCS ≤ 8), those with significant intracranial pathology on CT scan that are likely to deteriorate, and in some patients in which prolonged sedation and paralysis are required for extracranial injuries that would preclude clinical neurological monitoring.

> **❝ Expert comment** Prognostic models
>
> Two large clinical databases have been used to provide multivariate prediction models for outcome following TBI: CRASH-3 and IMPACT [11]. These models use admission characteristics to predict mortality and unfavourable outcome. This is potentially of key importance in risk stratification in
>
> (continued)

clinical trials however these prognostic models must be used with caution in the clinical setting for several reasons [12]. Most importantly, prognostic models use population data to generate population statistics, but these cannot be accurately applied to a given patient. Furthermore, only admission characteristics are used within the models. This does not take into account either the clinical progress of the patient or the impact of the interventions during their clinical management. In practice, the clinical progress of a patient is used to make decisions about whether continued intervention is futile, rather than prognostic modelling of this sort.

The use of craniectomy in TBI has long been recognized as a method for reducing ICP [13]. The questions around its use centre on whether the reduction in ICP and potentially in mortality salvage patients with devastating injuries. The recently published DECRA study [14] addressed the question of whether early craniectomy could improve patient outcome by rapidly controlling ICP and preventing some of the pathophysiological consequences of raised ICP. The study randomized 155 patients to either decompressive craniectomy or medical management if they had a spike of ICP in the first 72 hours following admission. It demonstrated that there was an increased risk of unfavourable outcome in the decompressive craniectomy group (craniectomy group 70%; standard care group 42%; odds ratio 2.21) and a similar rate of mortality (19% craniectomy group, 18% medical care group). Several issues have been raised with this important study, including:

- Early randomization of patients with relatively modest ICP (15 minutes of ICP > 20mmHg).
- Imbalances between the two study groups, for example, many more patients in the decompressive craniectomy group had fixed dilated pupils (27% in decompressive craniectomy group and 12% in medical group).
- Only a tiny proportion of patients eligible for the trial (155 patients recruited from 3478 eligible) were randomized.

Nevertheless, this study highlights the fact that craniectomy should not be used in every patient, as it may not benefit all survivors of TBI.

In this particular case, the bone flap was not returned because of brain swelling and the perceived risk of further swelling, based on the mechanism of injury. The use of craniectomy after evacuation of a mass lesion is a contentious issue in its own right and one for which no clear evidence base exists.

❝ Expert comment Dangers and uses of decompressive craniectomy

Craniectomy has several potential risks that may ameliorate some of the benefits of its effect on ICP. It can result in several problems, such as abnormalities in CSF dynamics (as seen in this case study) and a greater risk of developing kinking of the cortical veins at the margins of craniectomy [15], the syndrome of the trephined and the need for a delayed procedure (cranioplasty) to restore the skull contour. There is a risk that some patients undergoing decompressive craniectomy do not require the procedure and could be managed with medical therapy. This may have diluted out the benefits of this procedure in the DECRA study group. It is unfortunate that the randomization in this study led to so many more patients with bilateral fixed, dilated pupils in one arm of the study, which also makes the study difficult to interpret.

The Randomized Evaluation of Surgery with Craniectomy for Uncontrollable Elevation of Intra-Cranial Pressure (RESCUEicp) study (www.rescueicp.com) specifically randomized patients that have ICP refractory to medical therapy to decompressive craniectomy or further medical therapy (including barbiturate coma). This study is still recruiting and will specifically address whether decompressive craniectomy is of benefit in those patients in whom ICP is difficult to control.

> **⊕ Clinical tip** Craniectomy
>
> Craniectomy can be carried out in several ways including unilateral (fronto-temporoparietal), bilateral fronto-temporoparieta leaving a bridge of bone over the sagittal sinus ('bucket-handle'), and bifrontal. Unilateral craniectomies are recommended where there is a clear mass lesion or midline shift, while bifrontal craniectomies are recommended for diffuse brain swelling. Whatever method is used, the size of the craniectomy relates directly to the increase in intracranial volume achieved, and the risk of brain herniation causing kinking of cortical vessels and damage to the herniating brain edges. For this reason, a wide craniectomy (>12cm in diameter) is of benefit. Opening of the dura facilitates further brain expansion as does transfixing and dividing the anterior aspect of the sagittal sinus in bifrontal decompression. A layer of Surgicel® (Ethicon, Johnson and Johnson, USA) or thin dural substitute over the exposed brain creates a further layer that facilitates dissection of the scalp at the time of subsequent cranioplasty.

MRI imaging is not used routinely in the management of cerebral trauma, but it can be used to demonstrate diffuse injuries, believed to radiologically correlate with regions of diffuse axonal injury (DAI) that are not visible on CT imaging. The most sensitive MRI sequences for diffuse brain injury are those that exaggerate the signal that arises from blood products, such as gradient-echo and susceptibility-weighted imaging.

As well as the use of ICP monitoring, advanced monitoring techniques include brain tissue oxygenation and microdialysis monitoring. Using brain tissue oxygen probes, a value of 15mmHg regional PbO_2 has been suggested as a threshold for cerebral ischaemia. Microdialysis is a technique for sampling the brain extracellular space by passing a flexible probe, lined with a semi-permeable membrane into the brain substance, which is constantly perfused with a physiological solution. Substances within the brain, such as glucose, lactate, and pyruvate, can diffuse into the catheter, and be recovered and measured at the bedside in the perfusing fluid. The ratio between L/P is used as a marker of aerobic versus anaerobic metabolism and a threshold of 25 is used to suggest anaerobic metabolism [7].

In both monitoring techniques, observational studies have demonstrated that derangements of brain tissue oxygenation [16] and microdialysis parameters [7] correlate to TBI outcome, even in a multivariate analysis. However, it is not clear which interventions are best suited to manipulate these parameters and whether targeting them will lead to improvements in outcome. Furthermore, as these are focal monitors, there is an on-going debate as to how data from these monitors should be used to guide therapy for the brain as a whole. In this case, there was a clear derangement in L/P ratio that preceded a dramatic ICP spike and provided an early warning of impending swelling.

> **❝ Expert comment** Advanced monitoring techniques
>
> While these monitors are used in many units, specialist expertise is required to integrate the information from these monitors and individualize a given patient's ICP and CPP targets. The data derived from these monitors must be interpreted in the context of the patient's clinical state, as well as the position of the monitors on neuroimaging and are currently undergoing further evaluation to determine their clinical role on an individual patient intention-to-treat basis. Several other monitors exist, such as cerebral blood flow monitors and near infra-red spectroscopy. The utility of these monitors is an area of active clinical research.

Following craniectomy, CSF dynamics can change and lead to ventriculomegaly or subdural hygromas (either over the convexity or in the interhemispheric fissure). Whether these changes on CT scan represent hydrocephalus and impact on patient recovery or are a passive epiphenomenon of the change in ICP dynamics is not clear. In this case, early cranioplasty led to a partial resolution of the hygroma and the patient remains shunt free.

In this case, the patient did not have prophylactic anti-epileptic medication as there is a recognition that this does not ameliorate the long-term risk of epilepsy [17]. However, following head injury, patients are at risk of post-traumatic seizures, which can have potentially profound implications for quality of life and socioeconomic status. This applies both to patients who actually suffer from seizures, but also those deemed at risk of seizures, whose activities, e.g. driving and employment, are restricted as a result of this risk. Identifying which patients are likely to go on to develop seizures remains one of the most vexing areas of TBI management. Jennett et al. [18] in his seminal studies identified risk factors for late post-traumatic seizures, including depressed skull fractures, intracranial haematomas, early seizures (within 1 week), and patients with post-traumatic epilepsy (PTA) of more than 24 hours. Annegers et al. [19] have defined the risk of seizure according to the severity of injury with patients in the severe category given a 10% risk at 5 years post-injury. More recently, Christensen et al. [20] have shown that the risk is increased even 10 years after injury. These studies help in terms of the population risk, but it is not currently possible to accurately predict the risk for an individual patient. This is important for the ability to return to driving in the UK, particularly for bus and truck licence holders, where the risk must be deemed to be less than 2% per annum.

A final word from the expert

Maintaining the perfusion of oxygenated blood through a swollen brain is likely to decrease the morbidity and mortality associated with TBI. The aim of multi-modality cerebral monitoring is to quantify intracranial parameters believed to be upset after TBI, and guide treatment in the operating room and on the intensive care unit in order to decrease secondary brain injury. Craniectomy helps to decrease ICP, but further studies are awaited to determine how it alters long-term outcome after TBI. The overall aim would be to minimize the long-term disability and dependency of the commonly young population of severe TBI sufferers.

References

1. Teasdale G, Jennett B. Assessment of coma and impaired consciousness. A practical scale. Lancet 1974; 2: 81–4.
2. Crossman J, Bankes M, Bhan A, Crockard HA. The Glasgow Coma Score: reliable evidence? Injury 1998; 29: 435–7.
3. MRC CRASH Trial Collaborators. Predicting outcome after traumatic brain injury: practical prognostic models based on large cohort of international patients. British Medical Journal 2008; 336: 425–9.

4. Coles JP, Fryer TD, Coleman MR, et al. Hyperventilation following head injury: effect on ischemic burden and cerebral oxidative metabolism. Critical Care Medicine 2007; 35: 568–78.

5. Bratton SL, Chestnut RM, Ghajar J, et al. Guidelines for the management of severe traumatic brain injury. XIV. Hyperventilation. Journal of Neurotrauma 2007; 24 (Suppl. 1): S87–90.

6. NationalInstitute for Health and Clinical Excellence, Head injury: Triage, assessment, investigation and early management of head injury in infants, children and adults. NICE guideline CG56, 2007. Available at: http://www.nice.org.uk/guidance/cg56

7. Timofeev I, Carpenter KL, Nortje J, et al. Cerebral extracellular chemistry and outcome following traumatic brain injury: a microdialysis study of 223 patients. Brain 2011; 134: 484–94.

8. Sorrentino E., Diedler J., Kaprowicz M., et al. Critical thresholds for cerebrovascular reactivity after traumatic brain injury. Neurocritical Care 2012; 16: 258–66.

9. Helmy A, Vizcaychipi M, Gupta AK. Traumatic brain injury: intensive care management. British Journal of Anaesthesia 2007; 99: 32–42.

10. Patel HC, Bouamra O, Woodford M, et al. Trends in head injury outcome from 1989 to 2003 and the effect of neurosurgical care: an observational study. Lancet 2005; 366: 1538–44.

11. Steyerberg EW, Mushkudiani N, Perel P, Butcher I, et al. Predicting outcome after traumatic brain injury: development and international validation of prognostic scores based on admission characteristics. PLoS Medicine 2008; 5: e165; discussion e165.

12. Helmy A, Timofeev I, Palmer CR, et al. Hierarchical log linear analysis of admission blood parameters and clinical outcome following traumatic brain injury. Acta Neurochirurgia (Wien) 2010; 152: 953–7.

13. Kocher T. Hirnerschütterung, hirndruck und chirurgische eingriffe bei hirnkrankheiten. In: H Nothnagel (ed.) Specielle pathologie und therapie, Vol. 9 (pp. 1–457). Vienna: Hölder, 1901.

14. Cooper DJ, Rosenfeld JV, Murray L, et al. Decompressive craniectomy in diffuse traumatic brain injury. New England Journal of Medicine 2011; 364: 1493–502.

15. Stiver SI. Complications of decompressive craniectomy for traumatic brain injury. Neurosurgery Focu S 2009; 26: E7.

16. van den Brink WA, van Santbrink H, Steyerberg EW, et al. Brain oxygen tension in severe head injury. Neurosurgery 2000; 46: 868–76; discussion 876–8.

17. Temkin NR, Dikmen SS, Anderson GD, et al. Valproate therapy for prevention of post-traumatic seizures: a randomized trial. Journal of Neurosurgery 1999; 91: 593–600.

18. Jennett B, Teather D, Bennie S. Epilepsy after head injury. Residual risk after varying fit-free intervals since injury. Lancet 1973; 2: 652–3.

19. Annegers JF, Hauser WA, Coan SP, et al. A population-based study of seizures after traumatic brain injuries. New England Journal of Medicine 1998; 338: 20–24.

20. Christensen J, Pedersen MG, Pedersen CB, et al. Long-term risk of epilepsy after traumatic brain injury in children and young adults: a population-based cohort study. Lancet 2009; 373: 1105–10.

11 Intracranial abscess

Ciaran Scott Hill

Expert commentary George Samandouras

Case history

A 20-year-old right-handed man presented to the Emergency department with a 4-week history of right-sided earache associated with a foul smelling purulent discharge. He had suffered from intermittent ear discharge since childhood, but he had been well for the previous year. The current episode had been treated with a 1-week course of antibiotics by the general practitioner without any effect. The patient then developed general malaise, positional headaches, and was now describing intermittent horizontal vertigo, the sensation of movement as if the environment were spinning. There were no meningitis symptoms. He had no headache, neck stiffness, or photophobia. His past medical history was otherwise unremarkable.

On examination, there was an erythematous, boggy swelling over the right mastoid process. The right external auditory meatus was completely occluded by pus and the pinna was pushed anteriorly.

The patient was admitted under the ear, nose, and throat surgeons who requested routine laboratory investigations and a microbiology swab that was sent for microscopy, culture, and sensitivity. A CT scan was performed and the CT images are shown in Figure 11.1.

A diagnosis of mastoiditis was made and the patient was placed on the emergency theatre list for an exploratory mastoidectomy. However, the next day the patient was noted to have developed a mild right-sided hemiparesis and was referred to neurosurgery. Review of the CT scans (Figure 11.2) with brain windows demonstrated a hypodensity of the right cerebellum in association with subtle triventricular hydrocephalus and displacement of the IVth ventricle.

It was felt these images were consistent with cerebritis and a T1, T2 and T2 FLAIR MR scan was requested (Figure 11.3). Additionally, a T1 scan with contrast (Figure 11.4), diffusion-weighted imaging (Figure 11.5) and magnetic resonance venography (MRV) was performed (Figure 11.6).

> **⚬ Expert comment**
>
> The classic clinical triad of headache, high temperature, and focal neurological deficit occurs in <50% of cases. When no obvious source of infection is identified an extensive septic work up is mandatory.

> **⚬ Expert comment**
>
> The role of steroids remains controversial in the literature, with some studies supporting their use, while others advocate against them.
>
> Cerebral oedema is a major cause of morbidity and mortality in patients with brain abscess. When the patient is on a targeted antibiotic treatment, administration of dexamethasone, in the presence of oedema on imaging, is often an essential part of the patient's management. Long-term use should be discouraged.
>
> Rapidly deteriorating patients referred from district general hospitals requiring urgent treatment can have, prior to transfer, administration of broad spectrum antibiotics and dexamethasone after obtaining blood cultures.

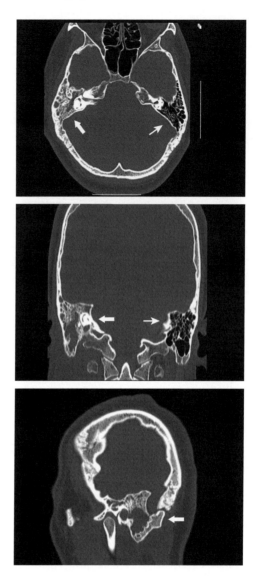

Figure 11.1 CT scan with bone windows demonstrates a right-sided opacification of the mastoid air cells with bony expansion in the inferior aspect and bony sclerosis superiorly (white block arrows). The left mastoid process is well aerated and normal in appearance (white line arrows).

❝ Expert comment

Cortical thrombophlebitis is a major cause of cortical neurological deficits in patients with white matter brain abscesses. This may be the result of occlusion of specific veins, such as the vein of Labbé or a diffuse process involving cortical territory. Involvement of deep venous systems, although not as common can occur.

The imaging studies demonstrated cerebellar and right mastoid abscesses in keeping with an otogenic origin. The MRV showed patent sinuses and large veins, with no signs of lateral sinus thrombosis (Figure 11.6). Cultures obtained from the ear canal swab grew **Group A beta haemolytic streptococci** and *Pseudomonas* and the patient was started on intravenous ceftriaxone, 2g bd, and clindamycin, 600mg qds.

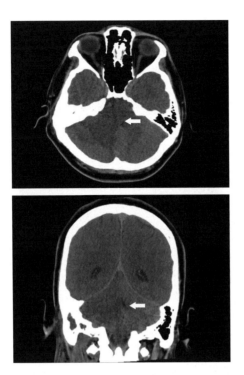

Figure 11.2 Non-enhanced CT scan with brain windows show an ill-defined right cerebellar hypodensity (white block arrows).

⭐ **Learning point** Stages of brain abscess formation

Stages of brain abscess formation as defined by Britt et al. (pathological) and Osborn et al. (radiological) (see Table 11.1) [1,2].

Table 11.1 Stages of brain abscess

Stage	Day	Microscopic features	MRI T1	MRI T1 + contrast
Early cerebritis	0–3	Acute inflammatory reaction with polymorphonuclear leukocytes. Fibroblasts appear and angiogenesis begins.	Poorly-defined hypo/isointense lesion	Patchy enhancement
Late cerebritis	4–9	Necrosis. Macrophage recruitment. Neovascularization and associated vasogenic oedema. Fibroblastic collagen deposition.	Hypointense centre and iso/hyperintense rim	Intense irregular rim enhancement
Early capsule	10–13	Progressive central necrosis and collagen deposition in capsule. Peripheral gliosis.	Centre becomes more hyperintense than CSF and rim more hyperintense than white matter	Well-defined, thin-walled capsule
Late capsule	14+	Reduction in inflammatory cells. Multiple layers of collegen capsule form surrounded by increasing numbers of reactive astrocytes.	Capsule thickens and cavity may collapse	Thick capsule with possible cavity collapse. Capsule is thicker on cortical side and thinner on ventricle side.

Samandouras G. *The Neurosurgeon's Handbook*. 2011. Oxford University Press.

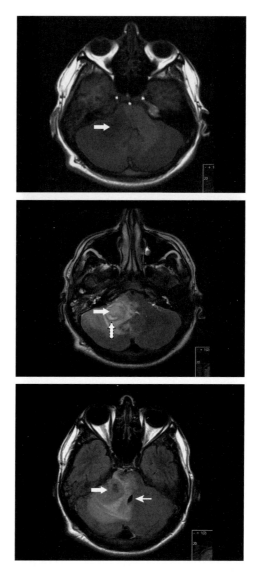

Figure 11.3 MR T1, T2, and T2 FLAIR images, top to bottom, demonstrate a lesion near the right cerebellopontine angle (CPA) involving the right cerebellar peduncle and abutting the brainstem (white block arrow). The perifocal oedema affects the cerebellum, particularly the vermis, the pons, and midbrain (white line arrows). The classical T2 hypointense rim caused by the susceptibility artefacts of a maturing abscess is demonstrated (dotted arrow).

In this case the radiological features and clinical timeline are consistent with the late capsule phase.

> **⊕ Clinical tip**
> Cases referred to neurosurgeons are often at the late abscess stage. When a cerebritis stage abscess is suspected, microbiologists often request CSF analysis. This should be discouraged, as it is not only dangerous in the presence of mass effect, but provides low diagnostic yield. CSF findings when obtained, typically show normal glucose, raised protein, and raised WCC (1–1000/mm^3) with lymphocytes predominating.

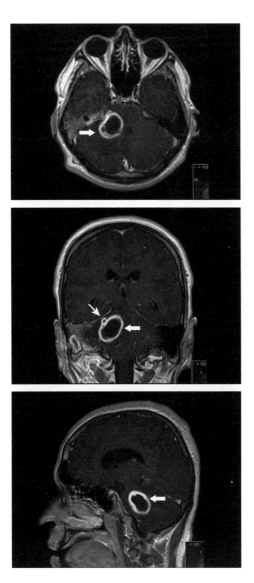

Figure 11.4 MR T1 after gadolinium administration show a smooth, well-demarcated right cerebellar ring-enhancing 3 × 3 × 2.5cm lesion with a thin wall (white block arrow). The hypointense surrounding area is consistent with oedema. On the coronal views (middle) a second ring enhancing 'daughter' lesion is seen in contact with the lesion superiorly (white line arrow). There is also ring-enhancement (1.8 × 1.5cm) in the right mastoid. There is moderate enhancement of the right cerebellar tentorium.

The patient was taken to theatre urgently for aspiration of the abscess. In the lateral position and without image-guided neuronavigation, a Dandy cannula was inserted aiming just lateral to the right CP angle. Pus was aspirated at the first attempt, but at the second attempt frank blood was aspirated. The resulting haemorrhage was difficult to control and, therefore, it was decided to convert the burr hole to a small posterior fossa craniectomy. The haemorrhage was finally controlled and it was felt by the operating surgeon that he could uneventfully remove the capsule that was prominent in the operative field. After dissection, the abscess capsule was excised. The post-operative CT is shown in Figure 11.7.

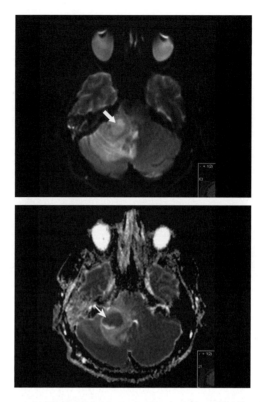

Figure 11.5 Diffusion-weighted MRI shows a high signal lesion in the right CPA with restricted diffusion (white block arrow). This is confirmed with the ADC map below that shows a central region of low signal (white line arrow).

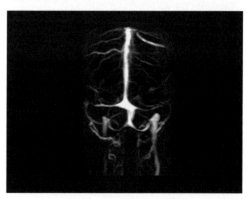

Figure 11.6 MRV. There is no evidence of thrombosis. The transverse sinuses bilaterally are gracile and hypoplastic, but the sigmoid sinuses are of normal calibre. There is incidental anatomical variation as the superior sagittal sinus divides caudally into two branches that drain to the internal jugular veins.

Post-operatively he was unable to abduct his right eye, but other movements were unaffected. There was also a complete loss of right-sided facial cutaneous sensation in V1–V3 distribution and an associated palsy of the muscles of mastication. He was noted to have developed a right-sided House–Brackmann Grade 5 lower motor neurone facial paresis. These findings were consistent with lesions of the abducens, trigeminal, and facial nerves.

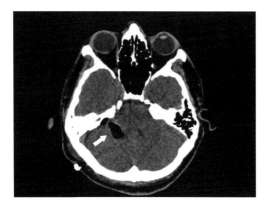

Figure 11.7 Enhanced axial CT shows complete capsule excision and a small amount of intra-operative air.

> **❝ Expert comment**
>
> This case demonstrates that free-hand aspiration has a limited role in the management of cerebral abscess, even in large or very superficial lesions.
>
> Image guidance systems, either frameless or frame based are very useful in achieving target acquisition and optimum aspiration of the centre of the volumetric space allowing maximum removal of the infective material and planning of a minimally invasive trajectory.
>
> An additional benefit of image guidance systems is the stabilization of a fixed trajectory. Hand-held probes, even with minute hand movements, inadvertently and unnecessarily widen the tract disturbing or damaging neural tissue at the walls of the tract.
>
> The decision to excise the abscess capsule should be planned, especially when the capsule is adjacent to eloquent areas, and is usually indicated when, despite repeated aspirations and targeted antibiotic treatment, there is no radiological resolution and no clinical improvement of the patient.
>
> The capsule of the abscess is adherent and tough and is not similar to the soft capsule of a metastatic lesion or of a circumscribed meningioma.
>
> Even removal of the capsule does not guarantee eradication of the abscess as recurrences have been observed after complete abscess capsule removal.

Although not a common practice, the stereotactic insertion of an Ommoya reservoir to allow repeated aspiration and antibiotic infiltration has been described [3].

> **✪ Learning point** House–Brackmann classification
>
> The original House–Brackmann classification of facial nerve weakness is shown in Table 11.2 [4].
>
> **Table 11.2 House–Brackmann classification**
>
> | Grade | Description of facial weakness | Score | Percentage motor function |
> |---|---|---|---|
> | 1 | None | 8/8 | 100 |
> | 2 | Slight | 7/8 | 76–99 |
> | 3 | Moderate with full eye closure | 5–6/8 | 51–75 |
> | 4 | Moderate with incomplete eye closure | 3–4/8 | 26–50 |
> | 5 | Severe | 1–2/8 | 1–25 |
> | 6 | Complete | 0/8 | 0 |
>
> (continued)

The overall score is calculated by measuring the movement of the mid-portion of the superior aspect of the eyebrow in a superior direction and the movement of the angle of the mouth laterally. The eye is scored from 0 to 4 with one point given for each 0.25cm of cephalic movement. The mouth is also scored out of 4 with 1 point given for each 0.25cm of lateral movement. The maximum score is 8. This does not consider the sensory or parasympathetic innervation of the facial nerve. A graphical version was produced by Lazarini et al., this is simple to use and offers the advantage of speed over the tabulated scale [5].

Two days later he underwent a mastoidectomy and tympanoplasty. A pneumatized mastoid cavity full of granulation tissue was drilled to healthy bone. The facial nerve was decompressed by opening its bony canal. Within 2 weeks, his cranial neuropathies had improved with only mild weakness of mastication, normal facial sensation, minimal diplopia, and a House–Brackman Grade 3 facial weakness remaining. The intra-operative pus samples were sterile and a peripherally inserted central catheter (PICC) line was inserted so the patient could receive 6 weeks of intravenous antibiotics.

Discussion

The earliest successful series of posterior fossa intracranial operations were those of the Sir William Macewen over 100 years ago. The original technique involved blind drainage of a cerebellar abscess through a trephined opening in the temporal mastoid bone [6,7]. Macewen was also perhaps the first surgeon to champion the use of the electric burr, a tool that in combination with the operating microscope and suction irrigation would allow surgeons to unlock the complexities of the skull base. Mastoidectomies were popularized by the German otologist Hermann Schwartze and modified to achieve their current form under William F. House [8].

Chronic suppurative otitis media is a longstanding infective disease of the middle ear. It is usually easily treated in the early stages with antibiotics, with or without myringotomy. If treatment is delayed or ineffective the complications can be severe. Most intracranial complications develop in patients with a chronically discharging ear. The complications that are the primary concern to neurosurgeons are extra-axial (such as subdural empyema) or intra-axial (such as brain abscess). A brain abscess is a focal suppurative process that involves the brain parenchyma. At least 50% of all adults brain abscesses are thought to be otogenic in origin [9]. The possible causes of brain abscesses are outlined in Table 11.3.

Table 11.3 Aetiology of brain abscess from The Neurosurgeon's Handbook by G. Samandouras (reproduced with permission).

Primary infection	Micro–organisms
Frontal sinus	**Aerobic and anaerobic streptococci** *Strep milleri, Bacteroides* species, *Haemophilus* species, *Enterobacteriaceae, Staph. aureus*
Middle ear/mastoid bone	**Aerobic and anaerobic streptococci** *Bacteroides fragilis, Enterobacteriaceae, Pseudomonas aeruginosa*
Haematogenous spread	Polymicrobial *Bacteroides* species, *Streptococcus* species
Penetrating trauma	*Staph. aureus, Clostridium* species, *Bacillus* species, *Enterobacteriaceae*

🕂 Clinical tip

Temporal lobe abscesses secondary to middle ear infection are best managed operatively in conjunction with the ear, nose, and throat (ENT) surgeon. Petrosectomy or mastoidectomy are often necessary and, ideally, when indicated, should be performed at the same operative session as the abscess drainage.

Spread of contiguous infection from an otogenic source to the brain is thought to be a key cause of cerebellar abscesses and has been found in up to 93% of cases [10]. Intracranial entry can occur by a number of pathways.

The management of brain abscesses from an otogenic origin is controversial. Otological infections that spread to the brain lie at the interface of neurosurgery, ENT, and microbiology. Treatments include pure pharmacological management, single or repeat aspirations, capsule excision, and extensive ENT procedures.

✔ Evidence base

Staged operative approach

The classical approach to intracranial complications of chronic suppurative otitis media is first to treat the intracranial disease (with either aspiration or capsule excision) and then remove the offending source via mastoidectomy at a later date. This was described by Joe Pennybacker in 1948 who reported eighteen cases of otogenic cerebellar abscesses. Interestingly, he notes that only two of the nine survived in the pre-antibiotic era, whereas after penicillin was introduced eight out of nine survived, underlining the importance of antimicrobial therapy [13] (Class IV evidence). In 1981, Shu-Yuan Yang reported 400 cases of brain abscess (115 cerebellar) treated over 20 years in China without the aid of CT imaging. They found no difference in mortality between simple aspiration or capsule excision (Class IV evidence). In 2011, a review of 973 brain abscesses (38.6% otorhinogenic) over a 20-year period in Durban, South Africa recommended abscess drainage and separate eradication of infection source. This study was limited by its lack of direct comparison with other strategies [14]. A review of the literature pertaining to aspiration versus capsule excision over a 78-year period by Ratnaike et al. favoured aspiration because of a 6.6% mortality rate versus 12.7% in the capsule excision group [15]. However, the validity of this final conclusion is questionable because abscesses location, aetiology or adjuvant therapy was not addressed. A modern consensus document on treatment of bacterial brain abscesses states that the type of surgical approach does not appear to be critical in determining outcome but that the speed of the therapeutic operation, including surgery, appear to be the more decisive factors for the final outcome [16] (Class V evidence).

Combined approach (neurosurgery and ENT surgeons)

The location of cerebral abscesses that originate in the ear is remarkably constant. In twenty-six cases of otogenic abscesses that were treated over 15 years all were found immediately adjacent to the petrous temporal bone. In the pre-CT era, this consistency of location allowed blind drainage. More recently, it has facilitated a concurrent approach to the abscess and mastoid infection through a single incision [17]. Morwani & Jayashankar propose a single stage, transmastoid approach as a safe treatment modality for otogenic intracranial abscesses [18] (Class IV evidence). They retrospectively reviewed sixty-one patients who had undergone transmastoid abscess drainage and concurrent tympanomastoidectomy (canal wall up or down depending on pathology). Follow-up was for a minimum of 24 months. Their mortality was 3%, there was a 6% complication rate (CSF leak or meningitis), and a 3% abscess recurrence rate. They conclude that this is a safe and effective treatment strategy. This view is also supported by the work of Singh and Maharaj who found lower mortality (13% versus 36%) when procedures were combined or performed within 12 hours of each other [19] (Class IV evidence). Kurien et al. also adopted concurrent craniotomy and mastoidectomy, and in their report of thirty-six patients found this to be a safe procedure [20] (Class IV evidence). It has been suggested that early surgical intervention is important to achieve a good outcome and transtemporal drainage of the abscess allows eradication of the primary mastoid disease at the same time as treating the intracranial complications [11,21].

Non-surgical management

Wanna et al. have suggested that an initial non-surgical approach to otogenic intracranial abscess with 6 weeks of broad-spectrum antibiotics (vancomycin, ceftriaxone, and metronidazole) and a shorter intravenous steroid course is safe and effective (Class IV evidence) [12]. They reserve surgical

(continued)

> ✪ **Learning point** Routes of intracranial infection from the middle ear
>
> - Direct spread through a bone defect in the tegmen tympani (the very thin layer of temporal bone that separates the tympanic cavity from the middle cranial fossa) or via Trautmann's triangle (demarcated by the angle between the sigmoid sinus, the superior petrosal sinus and the osseous labyrinth).
> - A retrograde thrombophelbitis of the emissary veins may allow communication through the skull into the venous sinuses and then to the brain parenchyma [11,12].

intervention for patients with an abscess that is expanding with mass effect, despite therapy, or shows a poor response to treatment. They also state that neurosurgical intervention is indicated if the abscess looks likely to rupture into the ventricles as this is a recognized poor prognostic marker, with up to 80% mortality. Interval mastoidectomy is performed once the intracranial disease is stable unless neurosurgical intervention is needed, in which case it is performed as a combined procedure wherever possible. It has been suggested that perhaps mastoidectomy can also be avoided in these patients. In separate studies, Kenna et al. and Dagan et al. treated mastoiditis with daily aural toilet and intravenous antibiotics [22,23]. This approach has not been widely adopted and Wanna et al. urge caution, given the severe potential complications of mastoiditis, including sinus thrombosis and further abscess development. The results of Wanna et al. in ten consecutive patients with intracranial complications from chronic supperative otitis media (four temporal abscesses, one cerebellar abscess, four sagittal sinus thrombosis, and one subdural empyema) showed 0% mortality and no recurrence. Mean hospital stay was 6.4 days. Although firm evidence is lacking, it has been suggested that medical treatment alone may be more successful if it is begun during the cerebritis stage, if the lesion is less than 2.5cm, if GCS is >12, and a specific organism is known (Class V evidence) [16,24]. Other authors have found higher mortality rates with Hsiao et al. reporting an overall case fatality rate of 48% in thirty-one cases of brain abscess that were managed non-operatively. They identified a low GCS as a key poor prognostic marker in these patients (Class IV evidence) [25].

The optimum antibiotic regimen has not been firmly established, but an 'Infection in Neurosurgery' working party review in 2000 suggested ampicillin, metronidazole, and ceftazidime (or gentamicin), as the first line empirical therapy (Class V evidence) [26].

A final word from the expert

To date, there has not been a blinded, randomized trial comparing the different treatment approaches to intracranial abscesses. Neither has there been any meta-analysis of the existing evidence. There remains clinical equipoise as to the most effective strategy for treating otogenic posterior fossa brain abscesses. However, in the presence of a large posterior fossa abscess at early- or late-stage capsule, stereotactic aspiration to obtain diagnosis and reduce the microbial load appears to be a reasonable initial approach within the context of multidisciplinary management.

References

1. Britt RH, Enzmann DR, Yeager AS. Neuropathological and computerized tomographic findings in experimental brain abscess. Journal of Neurosurgery 1981; 55(4): 590–603.
2. Osborn AG, Salzman KL, Barkovich AJ. Diagnostic imaging: brain. Salt Lake City: Amirsys, 2004.
3. Shen H, Huo Z, Liu L, et al. Stereotatic implantation of Ommaya reservoir in the management of brain abscesses. British Journal of Neurosurgery. 2011; 25(5): 1–5.
4. House JW, Brackmann DE. Facial nerve grading system. Otolaryngology—head and neck surgery 1985; 93(2): 146–7.
5. Lazarini P, Mitre E, Takatu E, et al. Graphic visual adaptation of House-Brackmann facial nerve grading for peripheral facial palsy. Clinical Otolaryngology 2006; 31(3): 192–7.
6. Canale DJ. William Macewen and the treatment of brain abscesses: revisited after one hundred years. Journal of Neurosurgery 1996; 84(1): 133–42.
7. Macewen SW. Pyogenic infective diseases of the brain and spinal cord. Basingstoke: Macmillan, 1893.

8. Sunder S, Jackler RK, Blevins NH. Virtuosity with the Mallet and Gouge: the brilliant triumph of the 'modern' mastoid operation. Otolaryngologic Clinics of North America. 2006; 39(6): 1191.

9. Syal R, Singh H, Duggal K. Otogenic brain abscess: management by otologist. Journal of Laryngology & Otology 2006; 120(10): 837–41.

10. Hsu CW, Lu CH, Chuang MJ, et al. Cerebellar bacterial brain abscess: report of eight cases. Acta Neurologica Taiwanica 2011; 20(1): 47–52.

11. Alaani A, Coulson C, McDermott AL, et al. Transtemporal approach to otogenic brain abscesses. Acta Otolaryngologica 2010; 130(11): 1214–19.

12. Wanna GB, Dharamsi LM, Moss JR, et al. Contemporary management of intracranial complications of otitis media. Otology & Neurotology 2010; 31(1): 111.

13. Pennybacker J. Cerebellar abscess: treatment by excision with the aid of antibiotics. Journal of Neurology, Neurosurgery, and Psychiatry 1948; 11(1): 1.

14. Nathoo N, Nadvi S.S., Narotam PK, & van Dellen JR. Brain abscess: management and outcome analysis of a computed tomography era experience with 973 patients. World neurosurgery. 2011; 75(5): 716–726.

15. Ratnaike TE, Das S, Gregson BA, et al. A review of brain abscess surgical treatment,78 years: aspiration versus excision. World Neurosurgery 2011; 76(5): 431–6.

16. Arlotti M, Grossi P, Pea F, et al. Consensus document on controversial issues for the treatment of infections of the central nervous system: bacterial brain abscesses. International Journal of Infectious Diseases 2010; 14: S79–92.

17. Penido NDO, Borin A, Iha LCN, et al. Intracranial complications of otitis media: 15 years of experience in 33 patients. Otolaryngology-Head and Neck Surgery. 2005; 132(1): 37–42.

18. Morwani K, Jayashankar N. Single stage, transmastoid approach for otogenic intracranial abscess. Journal of Laryngology and Otology 2009; 123(11): 1216.

19. Singh B, Maharaj TJ. Radical mastoidectomy: its place in otitic intracranial complications. The Journal of Laryngology & Otology 1993; 107(12): 1113–18.

20. Kurien M, Job A, Mathew J, et al. Otogenic intracranial abscess: concurrent craniotomy and mastoidectomy—changing trends in a developing country. Archives of Otolaryngology—Head and Neck Surgery 1998; 124(12): 1353.

21. Hippargekar P, Shinde A. Trans-mastoid needle aspiration for otogenic brain abscesses. Journal of Laryngology & Otology 2003; 117(5): 422–3.

22. Kenna MA, Bluestone CD, Reilly JS, et al. Medical management of chronic suppurative otitis media without cholesteatoma in children. Laryngoscope 1986; 96(2): 146–51.

23. Dagan R, Fliss DM, Einhorn M, et al. Outpatient management of chronic suppurative otitis media without cholesteatoma in children. Pediatric Infectious Disease Journal 1992; 11(7): 542–546.

24. Erdofüan E, Cansever T. Pyogenic brain abscess. Neurosurgery Focus 2008; 24(6): E2.

25. Hsiao SY, Chang WN, Lin WC, et al. The experiences of nonoperative treatment in patients with bacterial brain abscess. Clinical Microbiology and Infection 2011; 17(4): 615–20.

26. De Louvois EB, Bayston R, Lees PD, et al. The rational use of antibiotics in the treatment of brain abscess. British Journal of Neurosurgery 2000; 14(6): 525–30.

27. Kocherry XG, Hegde T, Sastry KVR, et al. Efficacy of stereotactic aspiration in deep-seated and eloquent-region intracranial pyogenic abscesses. Neurosurgical Focus 2008; 24(6): 13.

28. Senft C, Seifert V, Hermann E, et al. Surgical treatment of cerebral abscess with the use of a mobile ultralow-field MRI. Neurosurgical Review 2009; 32(1): 77–85.

12 Deep brain stimulation for debilitating Parkinson's disease

Jonathan A. Hyam

Expert commentary   Alexander L. Green and Tipu Z. Aziz

Case history

A 70-year-old man was referred to the functional neurosurgical service with a diagnosis of idiopathic Parkinson's disease (PD) for 16 years. His symptoms were rigidity, bradykinesia, and dyskinesias, causing disability and limitations in his activities of daily living, such as washing himself, cutting up food, writing, and safely using appliances unsupervised. He had no disturbance of awareness, sensory-perceptual function, thought, or intellectual function.

Since the time of his diagnosis his oral medications included madopar (containing L-dopa and a levodopa (L-dopa) decarboxylase inhibitor to reduce its breakdown outside the brain), selegiline (a monoamine oxidase inhibitor), pergolide (a dopaminergic agonist), and he had an apomorphine (another dopaminergic agonist) pump in situ. However, his medical therapy had resulted in dyskinesias, 6 years after the diagnosis of PD. After adjustment to sinemet and apomorphine, he experienced a medication 'off' state for 75% of the day with motor symptoms breakthrough despite medication with resulting bradykinesia and rigidity; and medication 'on' state for 25% of the day.

✪ Learning point   Pharmacological agents used in Parkinson's disease

Levodopa therapy was a breakthrough in the management of PD during the 1960s [1]. Due to the eventual motor complications of its use, a variety of other drugs have been developed for PD, which act on dopaminergic and non-dopaminergic systems. In early PD, there is no single first choice drug, and therapy with L-dopa, dopaminergic agonists, or monoamine oxidase-B inhibitors, is recommended [2]. Table 12.1 describes the range of pharmacological agents currently used in PD [3].

Table 12.1 Pharmacological agents used in PD

Type	Example	Side effects
Dopamine	L-dopa Madopar, Sinemet (L-dopa + decarboxylase inhibitor)	Motor fluctuations, dyskinesias
Dopaminergic agonist	Bromocriptine, apomorphine, pramipexole	Hallucinations, sleepiness, impulsive behaviour, e.g. gambling, hypersexuality
Anticholinergics	Benzhexol	Central/peripheral autonomic disturbance
Monoamine oxidase inhibitors	Selegiline	Sleep disturbance, light-headedness
Catechol-O-methyltransferase Inhibitors	Entacapone	Augmented dopa-induced dyskinesias,
Glutamate-antagonist; ? dopamine reuptake blocker	Amantadine	Hallucinations, depression

❝ Expert comment

There are many treatments for Parkinson's disease and DBS should be considered as one of many options, although not always the most suitable. As these are complex patients, they should be assessed by a multidisciplinary team including neurologist, surgeon, specialist nurse, neuropsychologist, and other relevant healthcare professionals

On examination, he had no arm tremor. Movements were bradykinetic. Dyskinesias, particularly on the right, and bilateral cog-wheel rigidity were present. Cranial nerve and peripheral neurological examinations were otherwise normal. Micrographia was demonstrated. Unified Parkinson's disease Rating Scale (UPDRS) scores were Part 1: 5/16; Part 2: 3/56 on, 25/56 off; Part 3: 15/104 on, 43/104 off. Formal neuropsychological evaluation using interview and battery tests did not reveal significant psychological pathology. Brain MRI was normal.

> ✪ **Learning point** Unified Parkinson's disease Rating Scale
>
> UPDRS was developed to monitor the severity and progression of PD, whereby several existing scales were incorporated into one, allowing more efficient and flexible patient assessment. It is extensively used by neurologists across the world with 87% reporting its use in trials and 70% using it in clinical practice [4]. The Movement Disorders Society judged the UPDRS as providing a comprehensive assessment of the motor aspects of PD especially, more than the non-motor aspect, although some items had low or adequate inter- and intra-rater reliability [4]. It is divided into four categories evaluating:
>
> - **I:** mentation, behaviour, and mood.
> - **II:** activities of daily living.
> - **III:** motor examination.
> - **IV:** complications of therapy.
>
> The Modified Hoehn & Yahr Staging and Schwab & England ADL Scales were added later (Table 12.2).
>
> **Table 12.2 Unified PD Rating Scale**
>
> | Part | Aspects of disease | Factors included |
> |---|---|---|
> | I | Mentation, behaviour and mood | Intellect, thought disorder, depression |
> | II | Activities of daily living* | Falls, dressing, swallowing, hygiene, utensil handling |
> | III | Motor examination | Tremor, posture, rigidity, speech, gait, bradykinesia |
> | IV | Complications of therapy | Dyskinesias, on/off fluctuations, orthostasis |
> | V | Modified Hoehn & Yahr staging | Disease severity, uni/bilateral, balance, independence |
> | VI | Schwab & England ADL Scale | Independence/dependence, showering, swallowing, bladder/bowel |
>
> *Denotes patients tested in both on and off PD states.
> Modified from Fahn et al. [5].

When discussing the aims of surgery with the patient, amelioration of the bradykinesia, dyskinesias, and rigidity were agreed to be the most important. The patient was offered and accepted bilateral subthalamic nucleus (STN) deep brain stimulation.

A stereotactic pre-operative MRI was performed to define the subcortical nuclei for electrode targeting (see Figure 12.1). At the beginning of the procedure, a stereotactic frame was applied to the patient's head under local anaesthesia and a stereotactic CT performed. CT is less susceptible to spatial artefacts and is registered with the MRI. The subthalamic nucleus was identified using the patient's imaging, and with the assistance of registration with a brain atlas to help confirm and plot the target coordinates. The patient was taken to theatre and bilateral craniostomies were fashioned under local anaesthetic. A 1.8-mm diameter radiofrequency electrode was passed to target, monitoring impedance to detect transgression of the ventricle, which can lead to electrode misplacement. The DBS electrode was then inserted in its place (Figure 12.2a). A neurologist objectively assessed the contralateral limb rigidity during test stimulation to ensure electrode position produced clinical benefit. The

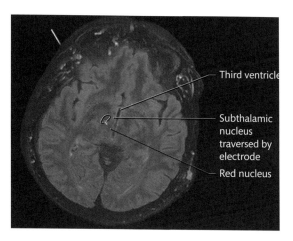

Figure 12.1 Reconstructed three-dimensional brain MRI in axial section with deep brain electrode trajectory to subthalamic nucleus (circled) planned on neuronavigation workstation.

procedure was repeated on the contralateral side. On placement of the contralateral radiofrequency electrode to target, there was an improvement in rigidity, independent of stimulation, a phenomenon known as 'stun', whereby the mechanical interruption or microlesioning of the target nucleus produces a temporary therapeutic effect. Although it confirms that the target produces clinical efficacy, it also prevents the fine-tuning of electrode placement based on further clinical examination during the procedure.

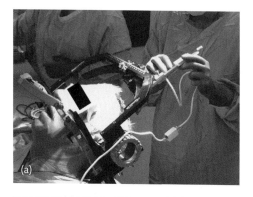

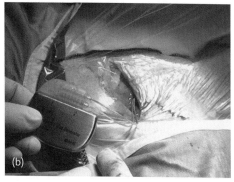

Figure 12.2 (a) Deep brain electrode implanted using stereotactic frame attached to patient. (b) Implanted pulse generator to be internalised within subclavicular pocket

A post-operative stereotactic CT head was performed with head frame and localizer still attached, which verified the electrode contacts' position in the STNs. On returning to theatre, under general anaesthesia, extension leads were connected to the electrodes and tunnelled behind the ear, into a subclavian pocket that had been fashioned. The implanted pulse generator was connected to the extension leads and placed in the pocket, which was then closed (Figure 12.2b). The patient was woken in recovery and had suffered no neurological deterioration. The stimulator was not initially activated. There was a unilateral improvement in rigidity and dyskinesia as a result of the intra-operative stun effect. Stimulation was activated 2 weeks post-operatively at 1.5V, 90 microseconds and 130Hz, allowing the acute changes of surgery including stun to settle down so that stimulation titration was performed without such a confounding factor.

Post-operative UPDRS scores at 6 months were Part 1: 1/16; Part 2: 8/56 on, 24/56 off; Part 3: 8/104 on, 34/104 off.

There was a marked improvement in Part III of the UPDRS with improvements in rigidity, dyskinesias, and bradykinesia on examination. There was no deterioration in mood or cognition detected.

Discussion

PD is a neurodegenerative disorder caused, in part, by the loss of dopaminergic neurones in the substantia nigra (pars compacta). This results in disruption of the normal oscillatory and synchronous neuronal activity between the cortex, globus pallidus interna (GPi) and STN, The three cardinal clinical manifestations of PD are bradykinesia, tremor, and rigidity. Gait and postural instability is often also seen [6]. The place of surgery in the management of PD has been cyclical. It was once the mainstay of treatment, in the form of ablative surgeries, such as pedunculotomy, and was then made largely redundant by the advent of dopaminergic drugs. However, it was found that dopaminergic drugs caused side effects including dyskinesias, which could be severely incapacitating. Once again, surgery (commonly taking the form of DBS) became an important modality in the management of PD, not only to treat the cardinal symptoms of the disease itself, but also to treat the dyskinetic side effects of medical therapy.

Patient selection

The commonest reasons for poor outcomes after DBS are: poor patient selection, poor operative electrode placement, and inadequate stimulation programming [7]. In DBS for PD, the ideal patient characteristics are a patient with idiopathic PD with an excellent response to L-dopa, particularly the medication motor 'on' state. Broadly, DBS surgery is offered to those who suffer from intractable tremor, debilitating side effects of medical therapy, such as dyskinesia, are of a younger age, and have a psychological and physical health sufficient to tolerate surgery and ongoing stimulation management as an outpatient. Patients with psychiatric diagnoses of major depression, acute psychosis, and dementia are excluded [7]. Therefore, a movement disorder neurologist and clinical psychologist/psychiatrist should form part of the DBS team, as well as the surgeon. A multidisciplinary approach is key to the management of these patients. Furthermore, identification of the most debilitating symptoms for the individual patient are critical as this determines whether non-surgical therapies have been exhausted for a given symptom profile, the location of the deep-brain stimulator placement, and allows for an estimation of the chances that DBS will be beneficial.

Location, location, location

Depending on the site targeted by DBS, a variety of symptoms can be ameliorated (see 'Learning point: Parkinson's disease symptoms and relevant deep-brain stimulation target nuclei'). It is therefore critical to tailor the targeting to the individual patient. DBS for PD is supported by the NICE Guidelines of 2006 with particular reference to STN, GPi and thalamic stimulation [2].

Subthalamic nucleus

The cardinal symptoms of PD, namely bradykinesia, rigidity, and tremor, as well as dyskinesias resulting from medication, can all be ameliorated by STN DBS to varying degrees. The STN was identified as a target in PD as a direct result of primate models [8,9]. As STN DBS diminishes these symptoms, the pharmacological therapy can be reduced together with their resulting side effects, particularly the incidence and severity of dyskinesias. Krack et al. demonstrated that STN DBS improved the motor symptoms of PD, improved activities of daily living, and reduced medication requirements [10]. The multicentre PD SURG Trial randomly assigned 366 patients with advanced PD to immediate surgery with best medical therapy or best medical therapy alone [11]. This was effectively a study of STN DBS surgery as only four patients received stimulation of a different nucleus, i.e. the GPi. The PD SURG trial found that DBS produced clear advantages compared with maximal medical therapy in clinical assessments and patient-assessed quality of life at 1 year follow-up. DBS conferred improvements in mobility and the activities of daily living domains of the PDQ-39 questionnaire, the total UPDRS, particularly part IV including time and severity of dyskinesias and 'off' periods, and a fall in daily dopaminergic drug requirement by a third. PD SURG found an adverse surgery-related event in 19% of patients. There was one procedure-related death, but no suicides [11].

Adverse effects of STN DBS attributable to the subthalamic location itself include psychiatric and cognitive disturbances, reflecting the STN's role in association and limbic circuits [12]. PD SURG found no decline in cognition as rated by the dementia rating scale (DRS-II), although its sensitivity to cognitive decline has been questioned [13]. Speech decline after surgery was detected on detailed neuropsychological testing, with a reduced verbal fluency and vocabulary [11]. Decline in cognition and mood has been inconsistently reported by other series, but appears to affect 1–2% of patients [14].

Globus pallidus interna

The GPi has been an important target in PD for the amelioration of dyskinesias. Its impact on bradykinesia and rigidity is becoming increasingly recognized. In a multicentre RCT, the cooperative studies programme (CSP) 468 Study Group demonstrated that STN and GPi DBS were more efficacious than medical therapy alone, in terms of increased time in the PD on state without dyskinesias, increased motor function, and a variety of quality of life measures [15]. After randomization between STN and GPi stimulation, they later demonstrated that both targets produced equivalent efficacy in motor function improvement measured by the UPDRS

ⓖ Expert comment

Patient selection for DBS is one of the most important aspects. A good candidate is generally one who has a good response to L-dopa, but either the side effects of the treatment are too severe (dyskinesia) or motor on–off fluctuations predominate. Tremor can also be treated successfully. Approximately 10% of patients with PD are suitable.

Part III at 24 months [16]. Although dopaminergic drug requirement was lowered to a greater degree by STN stimulation, it also led to a decline in mood and visuo-motor processing speed compared with GPi stimulation. Given that cognitive and mood disturbance was also found less after GPi compared with STN stimulation in other studies [17, 18, 19], pallidal stimulation is an important option for treating bradykinesia, rigidity, and dyskinesias in PD, and is a valid target in the case presented here.

Thalamus

Tremor amelioration is one of the oldest indications for functional neurosurgery after Irving Cooper's serendipitous observations in the 1950s [20,21]. Tremor can be treated by DBS of the motor thalamus or the STN. Thalamic DBS should be reserved for cases in which tremor is the predominant debilitating symptom and where the other cardinal symptoms of PD or drug side effects have not and are not expected to manifest [7]. Within the motor thalamus, the ventralis intermedius nucleus (VIM) is the commonest target, but the ventralis oralis nucleus (VOP), intimately related to it, is an alternative [22]. As this patient was not troubled by tremor, thalamic stimulation would not be an appropriate choice for him.

Pedunculopontine nucleus

Postural instability and gait freezing have historically not responded well to DBS nor L-dopa therapy. However, a novel target, the pedunculopontine nucleus (PPN), was identified in primate studies [23, 24, 25], as a reticular nucleus located at the junction of the mesencephalon and pons [Jenkinson et al. 2006; 26]. In humans with advanced PD, PPN stimulation results in improvements in measurements of gait, posture, and balance [27, 28, 29]. As these were not prominent symptoms in this gentleman's PD, PPN stimulation would not be an appropriate choice for him.

> ✚ **Clinical tip** Indications and patient selection for DBS in PD
>
> Patient selection is critical and only a minority of PD sufferers are appropriate for DBS. The factors recommended to confer good outcome from DBS can be divided into three broad categories relating to the PD itself and response to L-dopa, psychiatric and psychological factors, and general surgical factors.
>
> **Parkinson's disease features**
> - Idiopathic.
> - Excellent response to L-dopa.
> - Dyskinesias.
> - Intractable tremor.
>
> **Psychiatric**
> - No dementia.
> - No major depression.
> - No acute psychosis.
> - Cognition status good.
>
> **General**
> - Younger age.
> - Fitness for neurosurgery.

> ✪ **Learning point** Parkinson's disease symptoms and relevant deep-brain stimulation target nuclei
>
> Depending on the electrode target, DBS can confer benefit on a range of symptoms in PD. Establishing the symptoms most deleterious to the individual patient is therefore crucial to planning DBS in order to provide as much benefit as possible (Table 12.3). Some targets benefit a greater range of symptoms than others [2,16,27].
>
> **Table 12.3** PD symptoms and relevant deep-brain stimulation target nuclei
>
> | Symptom | Target |
> | --- | --- |
> | Tremor | Thalamus, STN |
> | Bradykinesia, rigidity | STN, GPi |
> | Dyskinesia | STN, GPi |
> | Postural instability, gait freezing | PPN |

> ✚ **Clinical tip** Accurately implanting deep brain stimulation electrodes
>
> Several measures to optimize the accuracy of deep brain electrode implantation are undertaken. Their utilization varies depending on the case and the unit.
>
> **Neuroimaging**
>
> MRI provides definition of the subcortical structures for targeting. CT provides greater spatial accuracy as it is less subject to artefacts than MRI. Fusion of the two modalities provides the advantages of both.
>
> **Intra-operative neurological assessment**
>
> Test stimulation and clinical assessment while the patient is awake provides rapid feedback on the clinical effect of stimulation and adverse effects, and allows optimization of electrode depth. The anaesthetist's role is therefore crucial. This is not suitable for patients who would not tolerate surgery while awake, such as those in whom their movement disorder is so severe.
>
> **Microelectrode recording**
>
> Localization of cell groups within the target nucleus by depth recordings from multiple fine microelectrodes provides neurophysiological targeting feedback. Disadvantages include longer operative time and a concern of increase risk of intracranial haemorrhage due to multiple electrode passes [30].

Lesional surgery

Creating a lesion, rather than chronically implanting an electrode is an important alternative for clinicians and patients to consider. Historically, deep brain ablational surgery preceded DBS, which is not suitable for all patients. Lesions of the GPi (pallidotomy) or motor thalamus (thalamotomy) can confer similar efficacy to DBS [31,32] and benefits from subthalamotomy have also been reported [17,33], and are therefore useful to consider in PD patients. DBS is an expensive therapy on account of the hardware costs of the electrode and pulse generator and also the subsequent need for follow-up and battery replacement surgeries. The advantage of a lesion is that it is a one-off therapy and does not require continued follow-up nor is there any hardware to manage. Therefore, determining factors include the patient's tolerance and compliance with intensive follow-up, and their agreement to undergo further battery change procedures to maintain stimulation, their cognitive level, expectations and level of neurological risk they deem acceptable, bilateral symptoms (bilateral thalamotomy has an unacceptably high risk of speech and swallowing disturbance [34,35], hardware and infection fears, and local economic factors. The lesion, however, is an irreversible and unmodifiable therapy. DBS electrodes have the advantage that they can be switched-off or removed if causing adverse effects and the stimulation parameters can be titrated to the patient's needs in addition to allowing adjustment over time as their tolerance or disease state changes.

A final word from the expert

There are likely to be two main future developments and these are equivalent to a 'space race' between improving technology and other biological treatments. For example, electrode design is advancing rapidly with improvements in electric field shaping and other modalities, such as optogenetics. On the other hand, there have been huge recent developments in stem cell research, viral vectors, and growth factor infusions with the aim of restoring 'normal' brain.

References

1. Cotzias GC, Papavasiliou PS, Gellene R. L-dopa in Parkinson's syndrome. New England Journal Medicine 1969; 281(5): 272.
2. National Institute for Health and Clinical Excellence (NICE). Parkinson's diseases: diagnosis and management in primary and secondary care, NICE Clinical Guideline 35. London: NICE, 2006. Available at: http://www.nice.org.uk/nicemedia/live/10984/30088/30088.pdf.
3. Kalinderi K, Fidani L, Castor Z, et al. Pharmacological treatment and the prospect of pharmacogenetics in Parkinson's disease. International Journal of Clinical Practice 2011; 65(12): 1289–94.
4. Movement Disorder Society Task Force on Rating Scales for Parkinson's Disease. The Unified Parkinson's Disease Rating Scale (UPDRS): status and recommendations. Movement Disorders 2003; 18(7): 738–50.
5. Fahn S, Elton RL, Members of the UPDRS Development Committee. Unified Parkinson's Disease Rating Scale. In: S Fahn, CD Marsden, DB Calne, et al. (eds), Recent developments in Parkinson's disease vol. 2 (pp. 153–64). Florham Park, NJ: Macmillan Health Care Information 1987.
6. Williams D, Tijssen M, van Bruggen G, et al. Dopamine-dependent changes in the functional connectivity between basal ganglia and cerebral cortex in humans. Brain 2002; 125: 1558–69.
7. Volkmann J. Selecting appropriate Parkinson's patients for deep brain stimulation. In:P Bain, T Aziz, X Liu, et al. (eds), Deep brain stimulation (pp. 75–83). Oxford: Oxford University Press, 2009.
8. Aziz TZ, Peggs D, Sambrook MA, et al. Lesion of the subthalamic nucleus for the alleviation of 1-methyl-4-phenyl-1,2,3,6-tetrahydropyridine (MPTP)-induced parkinsonism in the primate. Movement Disorders 1991; 6: 288–92.
9. Bergman H, Wichmann T, Delong MR. Reversal of experimental parkinsonism by lesion of the subthalamic nucleus. Science 1990; 249: 1436–8.
10. Krack P, Batir A, Van Blercom N, et al. Five year follow-up of bilateral stimulation of the subthalamic nucleus in advanced Parkinson's disease. New England Journal of Medicine 2003; 349: 1925–34.
11. Williams A, Gill S, Varma T, et al., on behalf of the Parkinson's disease Surgical Collaborative Group. Deep brain stimulation plus best medical therapy versus medical

therapy alone for advanced Parkinson's disease (PD SURG trial): a randomized, open-label trial. Lancet Neurology 2010; 9 (6): 581–91.

12. Hamani C, Saint-Cyr SA, Fraser J, et al. The subthalamic nucleus in the context of movement disorders. Brain 2004; 127: 4–20.

13. Rodriguez-Oroz MC. Deep brain stimulation for advanced Parkinson's disease. Lancet Neurology 2010; 9(6): 558–9.

14. Woods SP, Fields JA, Troster AI. Neuropsychological sequelae of subthalamic nucleus deep brain stimulation in Parkinson's disease: a critical review. Neuropsychology Reviews 2002; 12: 111–26.

15. Weaver FM, Follett K, Stern M, et al. Bilateral deep brain stimulation vs best medical therapy for patients with advanced Parkinson disease: a randomized controlled trial. Journal of the American Medical Association 2009; 301(1): 63–73.

16. Follett KA, Weaver FM, Stern M, et al. Pallidal versus subthalamic deep-brain stimulation for Parkinson's disease. New England Journal of Medicine 2010; 362(22): 2077–91.

17. Walter BL, Vitek JL. Surgical treatment for Parkinson's disease. Lancet Neurology 2004; 3: 719–28.

18. Volkmann J, Alert N, Voges J, et al. Safety and efficacy of pallidal or subthalamic nucleus stimulation in advance PD. Neurology 2001; 56: 548–51.

19. Rodriguez-Oroz MC, Obeso JA, Lang AE, et al. Bilateral deep brain stimulation in Parkinson's disease: a multicentre study with 4 years follow-up. Brain 2005; 128: 2240–9.

20. Cooper IS. Effect of anterior choroidal artery ligation on involuntary movements and rigidity. Transactions of the American Neurological Association 1953; 3(78th meeting): 6–7.

21. Das K, Benzil DL, Rovit RL, et al. Irving S. Cooper (1922–1985): a pioneer in functional neurosurgery. Journal of Neurosurgery 1998; 89(5): 865–73.

22. Hyam J, Owen SLF, Kringelbach ML, et al. Contrasting connectivity of the ventralis intermedius and ventralis oralis posterior nuclei of the motor thalamus demonstrated by probabilistic tractography. Neurosurgery 2012; 70(1): 162–9.

23. Jenkinson N, Nandi D, Miall RC, et al. Pedunculopontine nucleus stimulation improves akinesia in a Parkinsonian monkey. NeuroReport 2004; 15: 2621–4.

24. Jenkinson N, Nandi D, Oram R, et al. Pedunculopontine nucleus electric stimulation alleviates akinesia independently of dopa-minergic mechanisms. NeuroReport 2006; 17: 639–41.

25. Nandi D, Aziz TZ, Giladi N, et al. Reversal of akinesia in experimental parkinsonism by GABA antagonist microinjections in the pedunculopontine nucleus. Brain 2002; 125(11): 2418–30.

26. Zrinzo L, Zrinzo LV, Tisch S, et al. Stereotactic localization of the human pedunculopontine nucleus: atlas-based coordinates and validation of a magnetic resonance imaging protocol for direct localization. Brain 2008; 131(6): 1588–98.

27. Plaha P, Gill SS. Bilateral deep brain stimulation of the pedunculopontine nucleus for Parkinson's disease. NeuroReport 2005; 16: 1883–7.

28. Moro E, Hamani C, Poon YY, et al. Unilateral pedunculopontine stimulation improves falls in Parkinson's disease. Brain 2010; 133(1): 215–24.

29. Thevathasan W, Coyne TJ, Hyam JA, et al. Pedunculopontine nucleus stimulation improves gait freezing in Parkinson's disease. Neurosurgery 2011; 69: 1248–54.

30. Zrinzo L, Foltynie T, Limousine P, et al. Reducing hemorrhagic complications in functional neurosurgery: a large case series and systematic literature review. Journal of Neurosurgery 2012; 116(1): 84–94.

31. Bittar RG, Hyam J, Nandi D, et al. Thalamotomy versus thalamic stimulation for multiple sclerosis tremor. Journal of Clinical Neuroscience 2005; 12(6): 638–42.

32. Gross RE. What happened to posteroventral pallidotomy for Parkinson's disease and dystonia? Neurotherapeutics 2008; 5: 281–93.

33. Alvarez L, Macias R, Lopez G, et al. Bilateral dorsal subthalamotomy in Parkinson's disease (PD): initial response and evolution after 2 years. Movement Disorders 2002; 17(Suppl. 5): S95.
34. Alusi SH, Aziz TZ, Glickman S, et al. Stereotactic lesional surgery for the treatment of tremor in multiple sclerosis: a prospective case-controlled study. Brain 2001; 124(8): 1576–89.
35. Samra K, Waltz JM, Riklan M, et al. Relief of intention tremor by thalamic surgery. Journal of Neurology Neurosurgery and Psychiatry 1970; 33(1): 7–15.

Endoscopic resection of a growth hormone-secreting pituitary macroadenoma

Alessandro Paluzzi

⊕ Expert commentary Paul Gardner

Case history

A 61-year-old male presented with a 2-year history of fatigue, erectile dysfunction, and increasing hand and shoe sizes (size 9 to size 11). He also complained of visual problems affecting his driving. His wife had reported that he had started snoring at night, and had noticed that his nose and jaw had grown to change his facial features significantly compared with photographs of him several years before.

His previous medical history was unremarkable except for hypertension.

✪ Learning point The signs and symptoms of acromegaly

The acral changes (from *Gr* akron = extremity) are the most common clinical signs that lead to the diagnosis. Hands and feet are broadened, and the fingers and toes are thickened and stubby. The nose is widened, and the cheekbones and forehead become prominent, sometimes with frontal bossing. Prognathism, maxillary widening, dental diastasis, and macroglossia are also common.

In addition to the typical dysmorphic facial and body features, acromegaly is associated with a number of systemic complications, including hypertension, caradiomyopathy, diabetes mellitus, sleep apnoea syndrome, and colon cancer. These account for the associated mortality risk in acromegalic patients compared with the normal population [1]. Treatment of each specific co-morbidity greatly improves the general prognosis of the patients [2]. Furthermore, the systemic comorbidities, together with the presence of macroglossia and jaw malocclusion, need to be taken into account pre-operatively before removal of a pituitary adenoma, since they increase the anaesthetic risk of these patients.

On examination, the features of acromegaly were noted. His blood pressure was 170/102 on lisinopril/hydrocholorthyazide and random blood glucose was 8.3mmol/L (normal range 3.9–5.5mmol/L). Visual field assessment demonstrated gross bitemporal hemianopia, and this was confirmed on Humphrey visual field automated testing (Figure 13.2e).

Endocrine tests showed a random growth hormone (GH) level of 58ng/mL (normal range 0–5 ng/mL) and IGF-1 level of 667ng/mL (reference range: 71–290ng/mL). Other endocrine tests revealed hypothyroidism with decreased free T4 at 0.48ng/dL (normal range 0.8–1.8ng/dL) and normal TSH at 0.520μIU/mL

(normal range 0.300–5000µIU/mL). He also displayed hypogonadotropic hypo-
gonadism with decreased LH at 0.3mIU/mL (normal range 1–5.6mIU/mL) and
FSH at 1.5mIU/mL (normal range 1.5–14.3mIU/mL) and undetectable testosterone <1ng/dL (normal range 250–1100ng/dL). His AM cortisol was also low at
1µg/dL (normal AM range 7–25µg/dL) with an ACTH of 15pg/mL (normal range
9–46pg/mL).

T1-weighted MRI with contrast revealed a large sellar lesion with suprasellar
extension consistent with pituitary macroadenoma measuring 3.3 × 2.6 × 3.7cm
(Figure 13.1). The tumour extended laterally beyond the lateral wall of the cavernous
internal carotid artery, suggesting a high probability of cavernous sinus invasion
(Knosp grade III) (Figure 13.1 a, c, e).

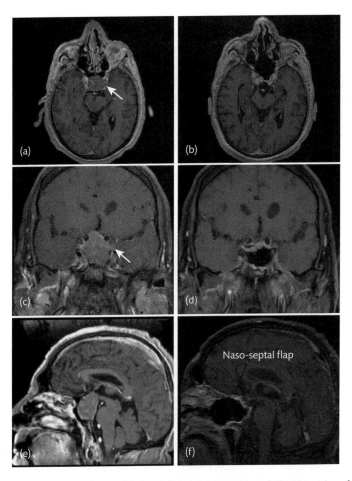

Figure 13.1 Pre- and post-operative (12 months) gadolinium-enhanced T1 MR imaging of
the macroadenoma. (a, b) Axial views. The arrow points to the portion of the adenoma invading
the left cavernous sinus. (c, d) Coronal views. On the pre-operative scan (c) the most lateral border
of the adenoma on the left side extends beyond the lateral edge of the carotid artery indicating,
according to the Knosp classification, high probability of cavernous sinus invasion. (e, f) sagittal
views. In the post-operative scan (f) the enhancing tissue at the level of the planum sphenoidale
corresponds to the muco-perichondrial naso-septal flap used to repair the intra-operative
dural opening.

> **★ Learning point** Knosp classification
>
> In 1991, Engelbert Knosp proposed a radiological classification to predict the likelihood of cavernous sinus invasion from a pituitary adenoma. He studied the pre-operative MRI scans of 25 pituitary adenomas that were confirmed surgically to have invaded the cavernous sinus space. Five 'Knosp grades' were defined by the relationship of the adenoma's lateral edge with the internal carotid artery, as shown on the most representative coronal post-contrast T1 slice. Grade 0 represents the normal condition, and Grade 4 corresponds to the total encasement of the intracavernous carotid artery. According to this classification, surgically proven invasion of the cavernous sinus space was present in all Grade 4 and 3 cases and in all but one of the Grade 2 cases; no invasion was present in Grade 0 and Grade 1 cases.

In view of the recent history of visual deterioration and the diagnosis of acromegaly from a GH-secreting adenoma the patient was advised to undergo surgical intervention. He consented to an expanded endonasal approach (EEA) for resection of the pituitary macradenoma.

During the operation, marked expansion of the sella was noticed. After initial bony exposure of the sella and both cavernous sinuses (Figure 13.2a), the tumour was debulked using a '2-sucker technique' (Figure 13.2b). The adenoma was found to have invaded the medial wall of the left cavernous sinus and to extend into the medial compartment of the cavernous sinus. Complete resection of this component of the tumour was achieved with the help of a 45-degree angled endoscope. The inferior hypophyseal artery was identified and coagulated (Figure 13.2c). To avoid herniation of arachnoid through the enlarged diafragma sellae during the initial steps of the tumour debulking, the suprasellar portion of the tumour was addressed only at the end, using again a 45-degree angled endoscope (Figure 13.2d). Both superior hypophyseal arteries were visualized and preserved. Gross total resection of the tumour was achieved. The repair of the dural defect was carried out using a pedicled muco-perichondrial naso-septal flap (Figure 13.1f).

The patient made a satisfactory post-operative recovery. His vision subjectively improved immediately post-operatively and formal visual field assessment 2 weeks and 6 months later demonstrated an objective substantial decrease in the visual field defects bilaterally (Figure 13.2f). Post-operative MRI scans at 3, 6, and 12 months (Figure 13.1b, d, f) demonstrated gross total resection without any evidence of residual or recurrent tumour.

His GH on the first post-operative day was down to 0.74ng/mL (normal range 0–5 ng/mL), while the IGF-1 was still abnormal at 412ng/mL (reference range: 71–290ng/mL). Two weeks later, both levels were normal, with a random GH of 0.40ng/mL and IGF-1 of 113ng/mL and the MRI scan at 1 month showed no evidence of residual adenoma. Both endocrinological and radiographic results were taken with caution at this stage, since it is well known that during the first 3 months post-operatively they can be misleading. During subsequent follow-up, the clinical features of acromegaly gradually improved and biochemical cure was maintained at 7 months and at his last follow-up 1 year post-operatively.

The patient was also medically treated with oral hydrocortisone 10mg bd, transdermal testosterone 5g/day, and levothyroxine 100µg/day for panhypopituitarism that was present preoperatively.

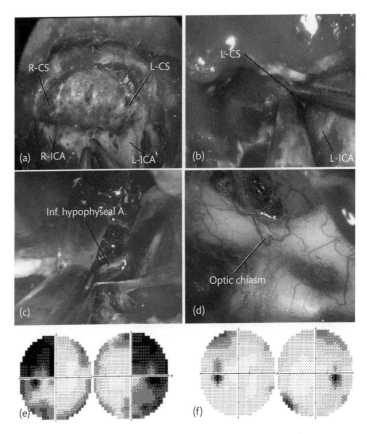

Figure 13.2 (a) Intra-operative endoscopic picture of the initial bony exposure from cavernous sinus to cavernous sinus. (b) Intra-operative picture with a 45-degree angled endoscope of the left medial cavernous sinus opened; two angled suction tubes are used to remove the tumour from this compartment. The left cavernous internal carotid artery is exposed. (c) During dissection of the medial cavernous sinus, the left inferior hypophyseal artery is identified. Failure to recognize it can lead to its avulsion from the internal carotid artery and arterial bleeding difficult to control. (d) Intra-operative picture with a 45-degree angled endoscope after the suprasellar component of the adenoma has been removed. It is possible to appreciate the decompressed optic chiasm. (e) Pre-operative Humphrey's visual field test displaying a bi-temporal hemianopsia. (f) Post-operative examination 6 months after the operation showing a dramatic improvement.

R-CS = right cavernous sinus; L-CS = left cavernous sinus; R-ICA = right internal carotid artery; L-ICA = left internal carotid artery; Inf. Hypophyseal A. = inferior hypophyseal artery.

Discussion

Pituitary tumours represent the third most common primary brain tumour after gliomas and meningiomas [3]. Autopsy studies confirmed a frequency in the population of 14.4% [4]. The prevalence of acromegaly is in the order of 40–125 cases per million and its annual incidence is 3 or 4 cases per million [5,6] although recent studies suggest that it might as high as 1034 cases per million [7,8].

Apart from the classic dysmorphic features of acromegaly or gigantism (if the over-secretion takes place before the growth plates have closed), patients develop systemic complications over time including hypertension, cardiomyopathy, diabetes,

⊗ **Learning point** Incidence of pituitary adenomas

Pituitary adenomas represent the third most common primary brain tumour after gliomas and meningiomas, with a frequency in the population of 14.4% from autopsy studies.

sleep apnoea, arthritis, carpal tunnel syndrome, and colon cancer. These account for the associated 2–2.5 times increased mortality risk in acromegalic patients compared to the normal population [1].

Mass effect from macroadenomas can lead to visual field defects, hypopituitarism, headache, and oculomotor nerve deficit. Due to the insidious development of these signs and symptoms, it is estimated that the interval between their onset and the diagnosis of acromegaly is about 7–8 years [9], although a more recent study reports that this delay has now reduced to 2–3 years [10]. The delay in the diagnosis might explain why the majority of GH-secreting pituitary adenomas are macroadenomas (>1cm in diameter).

MRI represents the gold-standard imaging for the diagnosis of a pituitary adenoma. The typical appearance is of a well-circumscribed lesion isointense to grey matter on non-contrasted sequence. On T1-weighted sequence, the normal posterior lobe of the pituitary gland looks brighter, possibly due to the presence of myelin. The heterogenous appearance in macroadenomas often reflects the presence of haemorrhage, necrosis, or proteinaceous material within cystic degeneration. After contrast injection, pituitary adenomas classically enhance to a lesser extent than the surrounding normal gland. The ability to discriminate between normal gland and adenoma, however, is limited by a reduced size of tumour, often being challenging in the case of small microadenomas.

> **✓ Evidence base** Natural history of pituitary adenomas [11]
>
> The only evidence about the natural history of untreated pituitary adenomas comes from studies on pituitary incidentalomas (PIs) or non-functioning-pituitary adenomas (NFPAs) managed conservatively. A recent systematic review and meta-analysis pooled together patients from eleven such studies, all of them being non-comparative cohort studies. The median follow-up was 3.9 years (range 1–15). The differentiation between PIs and NFPAs was not feasible and the quality of these studies was judged to be suboptimal and with several methodological limitations. The conclusions were that the incidence of tumour growth in PIs/NFPAs is higher in macroadenomas and solid lesions in comparison with microadenomas and cystic lesions. There was a trend that did not reach statistical significance for greater incidence of pituitary apoplexy and new endocrine dysfunction worsening in macroadenomas compared with microadenomas.

The treatment of GH secreting pituitary adenomas aims to:

- **Achieve biochemical cure:** the normalization of GH and/or IGF-1 levels has been shown to reduce the mortality risk to the one of the normal population [12]. The most recent criteria for biochemical cure are a normal IGF-1 and GH < 0.4ng/mL or a random GH < 1.0ng/mL. 11 Most of the papers in the literature, however, still reports the old criteria set in previous guidelines of normal IGF-1 and GH < 1ng/mL after OGTT or random GH < 2.5ng/mL at least 3 months post-operatively [13]
- **Control the signs and symptoms of acromegaly:** improve physical appearance, voice, mouth occlusion, etc.
- **Reduce mass effect from the tumour:** improve visual fields and pituitary function

> **❝ Expert comment** Mortality in acromegaly
>
> Patients with acromegaly due to a GH-secreting pituitary adenoma have a risk of mortality that is 2–2.5 times that of the normal population [1].

> **❝ Expert comment**
>
> The clinical suspicion of acromegaly needs to be confirmed biochemically. An increased serum GH level that is not suppressed by oral glucose tolerance testing (OGTT) to less than 1mg/L (3mIU/L) and increased IGF-1 above the age-adjusted normal range are diagnostic. For a woman aged between 40 and 60, the normal range is 237–246ng/mL, for a man it is 211–251ng/mL. More recent guidelines suggest that the cut-off of GH nadir during OGTT should be decreased to 0.4mg/L (1mIU/L), in view of the fact that modern assays have become extremely sensitive [10].

> **✪ Learning point** Remission criteria for acromegaly
>
> The 2011 guidelines by the American Association of Clinical Endocrinologists (AACE) recommend that in order to achieve surgical cure, the following criteria need to be met at least 3 months post-operatively:
>
> - IGF-I value within normal range for age and gender.
> - GH value less than 0.4ng/mL after glucose load or a random GH value less than 1.0ng/mL.

The AACE guidelines recommend surgery as the primary mode of therapy in all GH-secreting microadenomas and all macroadenomas with mass effect. Surgical debulking to improve the response of subsequent medical therapy is also advocated in patients with macroadenomas without mass effect and with low likelihood of surgical cure (e.g. cavernous sinus invasion) [10]

The trans-sphenoidal (sublabial and transeptal microscopic or endonasal endoscopic) route is widely accepted as the standard approach for the majority of pituitary adenomas, while the role of craniotomy, even for large suprasellar tumours, is gradually being replaced by the EEA.

In the UK, the NICE recommends the use of endoscopic trans-sphenoidal removal of pituitary adenomas, since it results in comparable surgical outcomes to conventional surgery, may shorten operation time, and the complication rate is less than that of conventional surgery [14]. These guidelines were issued based on the evidence available in 2003. Since then, further larger studies, all retrospective reviews, have confirmed the efficacy and safety of the procedure with comparable or better results than microscopic surgery in terms of outcome [15–22].

𝄞 Expert comment

Compared with traditional microscopic trans-sphenoidal approaches, the endoscopic approach offers technical advantages in particular situations:

- **Extension to or invasion of the cavernous sinus (CS):** by removing the bone covering at least the medial part of both cavernous sinuses, it becomes possible to retract them laterally to reach the areas normally difficult to visualize with the microscope. This is facilitated by the wide angle view and proximity of the endoscope, and can be augmented by the used of angled endoscopes (usually 45 degrees). In the case of secreting tumours with CS invasion it is possible to excise the medial cavernous wall and aim for complete resection of the adenoma, provided this does not extend to the lateral CS wall, where the oculomotor nerves are located. The use of intra-operative neurophysiological monitoring electromyelography (EMG) plays an important role in avoiding injury to these nerves.
- **Suprasellar extension:** for adenomas with suprasellar extension that do not descend into the sella (fibrous, dumb-bell shaped, previous radiation or pharmacological therapy), the endoscopic trans-tuberculum approach offers improved access to the suprasellar cistern and its contents. This is particularly important for visualizing the superior hypophyseal arteries, hence preserving the blood supply to the stalk and the optic chiasm.
- **Pars intermedia/posterior lobe lesions:** in less common situations where a functioning microadenoma is located in the pars intermedia or in the posterior lobe, an 'infrasellar' approach with a 45-degree endoscope allows access to these lesions from a caudo-rostral direction without the need to damage or split an intact anterior lobe

✚ Clinical tip Follow-up tests

The ideal time to assess whether the resection has been complete and the patient is in biochemical remission is about 3 months post-operatively. Before then the radiological, as well as endocrinological investigations can be misleading [26]

𝄞 Expert comment

In patients who have failed surgical resection, or without radiological evidence of residual tumour, but persistently elevated biochemical markers, the use of somatostatin analogues (SSAs) and/or GH antagonists can be recommended as adjuvant therapy. In selected cases, these drugs have also a role as primary medical therapy, namely in those patients in whom surgery is contraindicated or is unlikely to achieve satisfactory results [10]

To assess whether biochemical cure has been achieved it is advisable to wait 3–6 months before conducting the above mentioned biochemical tests [23,24]. For reasons that are unclear, it takes months for the IGF-1 levels to normalize even after complete resection of the adenoma [25]. A similar rule applies to post-operative MRI. Early MRI is often difficult to interpret due to the presence of blood products, absorbable gelatin materials or fat, all of which take several weeks to disappear. For this reason the first post-operative scan should be performed about 3 months after surgery [26].

> ✪ **Learning point** Somatostatin analogues and growth hormone (GH) receptor antagonists [10]
>
> Octreotide and lanreotide are the two most common SSAs used in acromegaly, they have similar efficacy profiles and newer formulations for im or deep sc injections enable them to be administered once a month. SSAs are effective in normalizing IGF-I and GH levels in approximately 55% of patients. The clinical and biochemical responses to SSAs are inversely related to tumour size and degree of GH hypersecretion. SSAs reduce pituitary tumour size modestly in approximately 25–70% of patients, therefore, they should not be relied on for decompression of local structures in the presence of mass effects. Their side effects include gastrointestinal upset, malabsorption, constipation, gallbladder disease, hair loss, and bradycardia. They can cross the placenta and, although a sc injection of octreotide can cause an acute decrease in uterine artery blood flow, longer use of octreotide does not appear to cause adverse effects on the course of pregnancy, on delivery, or on foetal development. There have been a number of cases in which octreotide was used in pregnant patients and most of these pregnancies were uneventful. In a few cases of pregnant patients given SSA therapy, the resultant infants were small for gestational age, although the causality was not clear.
>
> Pegvisomant is a GH receptor antagonist that seems to be effective regardless of baseline tumour size or degree of GH hypersecretion. It normalizes IGF-I values in more than 90% of the patients, including patients who are partially or completely resistant to other medical therapies, and it is effective at improving glucose homeostasis in patients with associated diabetes mellitus. Side effects of pegvisomant, include flu-like illness, allergic reactions, and increase in liver enzymes. Tumour enlargement has been infrequently associated with use of pegvisomant, therefore, serial monitoring with pituitary MRI scans is suggested. Specific recommendations for the use of pergvisomant during pregnancy cannot be made since the experience is limited to a single case in which pegvisomant administration was well tolerated, the patient's condition was well controlled, and the infant was normal in size and health.

Compared with conventional adjuvant radiotherapy for residual disease, stereotactic radiosurgery has the theoretical advantage of potentially stabilizing the disease and reducing tumour size, while sparing the optic apparatus and the pituitary function, provided the adenoma is more than 5mm away from them [27]. Another advantage of stereotactic radiosurgery over conventional radiotherapy seems to be the shorter mean time to achieve biochemical remission (2 years) [28] The biochemical remission rates reported in the literature vary between 17 and 50%, although the follow-up is limited to a period between 2 and 5 years [29–34]. In terms of tumour control, up to 75% of the patients treated with radiosurgery achieve a decrease in tumour size, a result similar to conventional radiotherapy [30–33].

A final word from the expert

There is not enough evidence to favour surgery versus conservative management in asymptomatic patients with non-functioning adenomas, since their life-time risk of developing visual field defects, hypopituitarism, or pituitary apoplexy is not known. However, these studies seem to suggest that patients with macroadenomas are at a higher risk than patients with microadenoamas to develop such events.

References

1. Terada T, Kovacs K, Stefaneanu L, et al. Incidence, pathology, and recurrence of pituitary adenomas: study of 647 unselected surgical cases. Endocrine Pathology 1995; 6: 301–10.
2. Ezzat S, Asa SL, Couldwell WT, et al. The prevalence of pituitary adenomas: a systematic review. Cancer 2004; 101: 613–19.
3. Holdaway IM, Rajasoorya C. Epidemiology of acromegaly. Pituitary 1999; 2: 29–41.
4. Alexander L, Appleton D, Hall R, et al. Epidemiology of acromegaly in the Newcastle region. Clinical Endocrinology (Oxford) 1980; 12: 71–79.
5. Daly AF, Rixhon M, Adam C., et al. High prevalence of pituitary adenomas: a cross-sectional study in the province of Liege, Belgium. Journal of Clinical Endocrinology and Metabolism 2006; 91: 4769–75.
6. Schneider HJ, Sievers C, Saller B., et al. High prevalence of biochemical acromegaly in primary care patients with elevated IGF-1 levels. Clinical Endocrinology 2008; 69: 432–435.
7. Swearingen B, Barker FG II, Katznelson L, et al. Long-term mortality after transsphenoidal surgery and adjunctive therapy for acromegaly. Journal of Clinical Endocrinology and Metabolism 1998; 83: 3419–26.
8. Rajasoorya C, Holdaway IM, Wrightson P, et al. Determinants of clinical outcome and survival in acromegaly. Clinical Endocrinology (Oxford) 1994; 41: 95–102.
9. Nachtigall L, Delgado A, Swearingen B, et al. Changing patterns in diagnosis and therapy of acromegaly over two decades. Journal of Clinical Endocrinology and Metabolism 2008; 93: 2035–41.
10. Katznelson L, Atkinson JL, Cook DM, et al. American Association of Clinical Endocrinologists Medical Guidelines for Clinical Practice for the Diagnosis and Treatment of Acromegaly—2011 update: executive summary. Endocrine Practice 2011; 17 (4): 636–46.
11. Karavitaki N, Collison K, Halliday J, et al. What is the natural history of nonoperated nonfunctioning pituitary adenomas? Clinical Endocrinology (Oxford) 2007; 67 (6): 938–43.
12. Holdaway IM, Bolland MJ, Gamble GD. A meta-analysis of the effect of lowering serum levels of GH and IGF-I on mortality in acromegaly. European Journal of Endocrinology 2008; 159: 89–95.
13. Cook DM, Ezzat S, Katznelson L, et al. AACE medical guidelines for clinical practice for the diagnosis and treatment of acromegaly. Endocrine Practice 2004; 10: 213–25. [Published corrections appear in Endocrine Practice 2005; 11: 144; and 2008; 14: 802–3.]
14. National Institute of Health and Clinical Excellence. Endoscopic transsphenoidal pituitary adenoma resection, NICE interventional procedures guidance IPG32. Available at: http://guidance.nice.org.uk/IPG32 (accessed on 24 January 2012).
15. Messerer M, De Battista JC, Raverot G, et al. Evidence of improved surgical outcome following endoscopy for nonfunctioning pituitary adenoma removal. Neurosurgical Focus 2011; 30 (4): E11.
16. Dorward NL. Endocrine outcomes in endoscopic pituitary surgery: a literature review. Acta Neurochirugia (Wien) 2010; 152 (8): 1275–9.
17. Gondim JA, Schops M, de Almeida JP, et al. Endoscopic endonasal transsphenoidal surgery: surgical results of 228 pituitary adenomas treated in a pituitary center. Pituitary 2010; 13 (1): 68–77.
18. D'Haens J, Van Rompaey K, Stadnik T, et al. Fully endoscopic transsphenoidal surgery for functioning pituitary adenomas: a retrospective comparison with traditional transsphenoidal microsurgery in the same institution. Surgical Neurology 2009; 72 (4): 336–40.
19. Tabaee A, Anand VK, Barrón Y, et al. Endoscopic pituitary surgery: a systematic review and meta-analysis. Journal of Neurosurgery 2009; 111 (3): 545–54.
20. Dehdashti AR, Ganna A, Karabatsou K, et al. Pure endoscopic endonasal approach for pituitary adenomas: early surgical results in 200 patients and comparison with previous microsurgical series. Neurosurgery 2008; 62 (5): 1006–15.

21. Frank G, Pasquini E, Farneti G, et al. The endoscopic versus the traditional approach in pituitary surgery. Neuroendocrinology 2006; 83 (3-4): 240–8.

22. Kabil MS, Eby JB, Shahinian HK. Fully endoscopic endonasal vs. transseptal transsphenoidal pituitary surgery. Minimally Invasive Neurosurgery 2005; 48 (6): 348–54

23. Carmichael JD, Bonert VS, Mirocha JM, et al. The utility of oral glucose tolerance testing for diagnosis and assessment of treatment outcomes in 166 patients with acromegaly. Journal of Clinical Endocrinology and Metabolism 2009; 94: 523–7.

24. Melmed S, Colao A, Barkan A, et al. Guidelines for acromegaly management: an update. Journal of Clinical Endocrinology and Metabolism 2009; 94: 1509–17.

25. Espinosa-de-Los-Monteros AL, Sosa E, Cheng S, et al. Biochemical evaluation of disease activity after pituitary surgery in acromegaly: a critical analysis of patients who spontaneously change disease status. Clinical Endocrinology (Oxford) 2006; 64: 245–9.

26. Dina TS, Feaster SH, Laws ER Jr, et al. MR of the pituitary gland postsurgery: serial MR studies following transsphenoidal resection. American Journal of Neurological Research: American Journal of Neuroradiology 1993; 14: 763–9.

27. Minniti G, Gilbert DC, Brada M. Modern techniques for pituitary radiotherapy. Reviews in Endocrine and Metabolic Disorders 2009; 10: 135–44.

28. Pollock BE, Jacob JT, Brown PD, et al. Radiosurgery of growth hormone-producing pituitary adenomas: factors associated with biochemical remission. Journal of Neurosurgery 2007; 106: 833–8.

29. Castinetti F, Taieb D, Kuhn JM, et al. Outcome of gamma knife radiosurgery in 82 patients with acromegaly: correlation with initial hypersecretion. Reviews in Endocrine and Metabolic Disorders 2005; 90: 4483–8.

30. Attanasio R, Epaminonda P, Motti E, et al. Gamma-knife radiosurgery in acromegaly: a 4-year follow-up study. Reviews in Endocrine and Metabolic Disorders 2003; 88: 3105–12.

31. Jezková J, Marek J, Hána V, et al. Gamma knife radiosurgery for acromegaly—long-term experience. Clinical Endocrinology (Oxford) 2006; 64: 588–95.

32. Pollock BE, Jacob JT, Brown PD, et al. Radiosurgery of growth hormone-producing pituitary adenomas: factors associated with biochemical remission. Journal of Neurosurgery 2007; 106: 833–8.

33. Vik-Mo EO, Oksnes M, Pedersen PH, et al. Gamma knife stereotactic radiosurgery for acromegaly. European Journal of Endocrinology 2007; 157: 255–63.

34. Zhang N, Pan L, Wang EM, et al. Radiosurgery for growth hormone-producing pituitary adenomas. Journal of Neurosurgery 2000; 93 (Suppl. 3): 6–9.

14 Trigeminal neuralgia

Isaac Phang

ⓘ **Expert commentary** Nigel Suttner

Case history

A 59-year-old man presented to clinic with a 9-month history of recurrent excruciating left jaw and cheek pain, described as lancinating in nature. At worst, five or six episodes were clustered together per day with spontaneous resolution. Pain episodes were triggered by eating and shaving, and severe enough to limit his lifestyle and impact on his psychological well-being. The diagnosis was of trigeminal neuralgia (TN) of the V2 and V3 distributions.

Clinical neurological examination was unremarkable.

He was initially commenced on carbamezapine, but this was soon discontinued due to a rise in his liver transaminase. He was then started on gabapentin 900mg tds with phenytoin 50mg tds added for better control, although he did have some side effects of drowsiness and dizziness. He continued, however to have episodes of breakthrough pain and, after surgical assessment and discussion, opted for percutaneous balloon compression (PBC) of the left trigeminal ganglion. The procedure was performed under a short general anaesthetic. The foramen ovale was navigated using intraoperative X-ray screening with Niopam 300 radio-opaque dye and standard anatomical landmarks. A jaw twitch was noted just prior to penetration of the foramen ovale, and CSF and a small amount of venous blood were obtained once the needle was in place. Inflation of the Fogarty 4 balloon was performed for 90 seconds (Figure 14.1). He obtained complete pain relief within 24 hours of surgery and was discharged home.

He was reviewed in clinic 2 months after the procedure. Relief from the initial pain persisted and he had been weaned off all analgesia. He had transient masticatory weakness post-balloon compression, but this resolved completely.

Two weeks after this assessment, however, he had a recurrence of his trigeminal neuralgia. Ultrafast gradient echo 3D MRI brain at this juncture did not show any compression of the left trigeminal nerve from a space-occupying lesion/neurovascular conflict, nor demyelinating disease. There was, however, atrophy of the left trigeminal nerve (Figure 14.2). A resolving left temporal contusion was noted adjacent to Meckel's cave, as a result of the percutaneous balloon compression.

He now opted for microvascular decompression, as he did not want to go back onto medication. Suboccipital (retrosigmoid) craniectomy, exploration of the left trigeminal nerve from the root entry zone to Meckel's cave, was carried out. This revealed compression from a loop of anterior inferior cerebellar artery (AICA), but also significantly from a loop of superior cerebellar artery (SCA) and a vein related to part of the root entry zone (Figure 14.3). The loop of AICA also compressed the VII/VIII complex more distally. The vein was cauterized and divided. Merocel® sponges were placed between the loop of SCA and the nerve, as well as between the

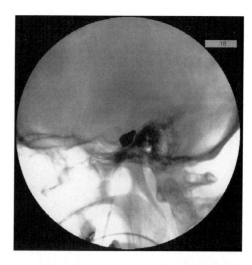

Figure 14.1 Intra-operative fluoroscopy (lateral basal skull X-ray) showing intra-operatively inflated pear-shaped Fogarty catheter for balloon compression in the management of trigeminal neuralgia.

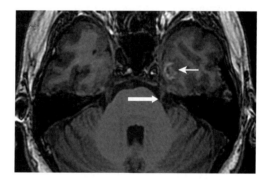

Figure 14.2 T1-weighted axial MRI showing atrophy of left trigeminal nerve (big arrow). A resolving small contusion is noted in the adjacent temporal lobe due to inadvertent injury during prior percutaneous balloon compression (small arrow).

loop of AICA and the nerve. Recovery was uneventful and he was discharged home on post-operative day 4.

Post-operative review at 2 months revealed continued pain relief off analgesia. There was an area of subjective decrease in sensation over his left V2 region.

Discussion

The incidence of TN is approximately 4 in 100,000 [1]. The age of onset is typically in the sixth to eighth decade, and women are more affected than men with a ratio of 3:2. The right side of the face is affected more often than the left. TN occurs bilaterally in 5% of patients. Family history may be positive in 5%.

The diagnosis of TN is made on clinical history alone. There are no diagnostic tests. It can be divided into typical/classical TN (TN1) or atypical TN (TN2) [2]. Janetta [3] breaks down further into typical, atypical, and mixed TN. Mild sensory changes occur clinically in the trigeminal distribution in up to 30% of patients with TN, invariably in the area of facial pain [3]. This is despite the diagnostic criteria of the International Headache Society.

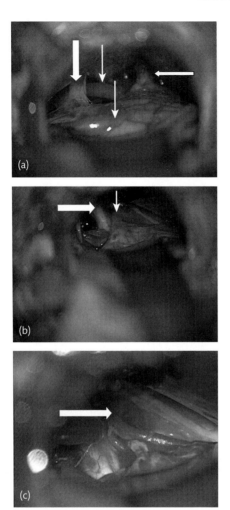

Figure 14.3 (a) Microvascular decompression of left trigeminal nerve. Intra-operative photograph showing a loop of AICA (small vertical arrows) coursing around the left VII/VIII complex (big vertical arrow). The superior petrosal vein is seen superiorly (horizontal arrow). (b) Microvascular decompression of left trigeminal nerve. Intra-operative photograph showing the trigeminal complex exposed (large arrow), with a vein (small arrow) coursing over the dorsal root entry zone. (c) Microvascular decompression of left trigeminal nerve. Intra-operative photograph showing the vein divided and a loop of SCA (large arrow) abutting the trigeminal nerve.

⊕ **Learning point** Definition of trigeminal neuralgia

The International Classification of Headache Disorders III (ICHD-3) for trigeminal neuralgia.

I. Classical trigeminal neuralgia: diagnostic criteria

A. At least three attacks of unilateral facial pain fulfilling criteria B and C
B. Occurring in one or more divisions of the trigeminal nerve, with no radiation beyond the trigeminal distribution
C. Pain has at least three of the following four characteristics:
   1. recurring in paroxysmal attacks lasting from a fraction of a second to 2 minutes
   2. severe intensity
   3. electric shock-like, shooting, stabbing or sharp in quality
   4. precipitated by innocuous stimuli to the affected side of the face[1]

(continued)

D. No clinically evident neurological deficit
E. Not better accounted for by another ICHD-3 diagnosis.

II. Classical trigeminal neuralgia with concomitant persistent facial pain: diagnostic criteria

A. Recurrent attacks of unilateral facial pain fulfilling criteria for classical trigeminal neuralgia
B. Persistent facial pain of moderate intensity in the affected area
C. No better accounted for by another ICHD-3 diagnosis.

Corroborating features are:

- Pain usually starts in the second or third division, affecting the cheek or the chin. In <5% of patients the first division is affected.
- Pain never crosses to the opposite side.
- Between paroxysms, the patient is usually asymptomatic, but a dull background pain may persist in some long-standing cases.
- Following a painful paroxysm, there is usually a refractory period during which pain cannot be triggered.
- The pain often evokes spasm of the muscle of the face on the affected side (**tic douloureux**).
- Classical trigeminal neuralgia is usually responsive, at least initially, to pharmacotherapy.

Burchiel [2] classifies trigeminal neuralgia into type 1 (TN1) where the pain is sharp, shooting, episodic pain and type 2 (TN2), where the pain is aching or throbbing more than 50% of the time, and the pain is constant. Although the natural history of trigeminal neuralgia has not been fully elucidated, it is postulated that the character of classical trigeminal neuralgia may over time change into that of type 2 pain [3].

Pathogenesis

The ignition hypothesis [4] proposes electrophysiological mechanisms, which explain the triggering, amplification, and stop mechanism of paroxysmal pain in trigeminal neuralgia. Injured neurons become hyperexcitable and generate impulses autonomously, creating ectopic pacemaker sites. Spontaneous firing may induce a burst of firing—an after-discharge in the injured neuron, with recruitment of surrounding neurons. Thus, this provides the 'ignition', explaining the sudden nature of the pain. The amplification is attributed to resonance of intrinsic oscillations in membrane potential of the dorsal root ganglion cells. Normally, only a few of the dorsal root ganglion cells demonstrate this characteristic, but injured cells may acquire this property. Moreover, the oscillations resonate, causing impulses to fire in a sustained manner, thus providing the sustained amplification of pain. This is encouraged by ephaptic transmission and crossed after discharge between damaged neurons. This spread of activity from large myelinated afferents to unmyelinated C nociceptors explains why innocuous stimuli elicit paroxysmal pain. The refractory period is explained by hyperpolarization due to an influx of Ca^{2+}-activated K^+ channels.

The vascular conflict theory proposed by Janetta suggests that compression of the Obersteiner–Reidleich transition zone of central to peripheral myelination of the trigeminal nerve causes demyelination of the trigeminal nerve, and hence TN, and explains the success of microvascular decompression in the treatment of TN. Histological studies of compressed trigeminal nerves in patients with TN1 show demyelination at areas of maximal compression, with adjacent areas of less severe damage [4]. Histological studies of PBC specimens in New Zealand rabbits have shown preferential destruction of large myelinated fibres serving touch, while sparing the unmyelinated fibres that mediate nociceptive pain transmission [5]. The pain relief following PBC suggests that the large myelinated fibres are central to the pathogenesis of paroxysmal pain.

> **❻ Expert comment** Theories of pathogenesis of TN
>
> The precise cause and mechanisms of pain in trigeminal neuralgia are not fully understood. Most commonly pulsatile compression from neurovascular conflict peripherally at the root entry zone (REZ) of the nerve has been cited as the cause of idiopathic TN [6,7], which leads to demyelination. Tumours compressing the trigeminal nerve in the posterior fossa and demyelination of the nerve at the REZ in multiple sclerosis support a peripheral mechanism. This is confirmed histopathologically [4] and explains the ephaptic transmission between axons leading to amplification of sensory input. The Ignition hypothesis [8] attempts to explain the underlying mechanisms involved.
>
> However, not all of the features of TN can be explained on a peripheral basis. A central origin cannot be ignored. Pain and temperature fibres extend downwards into the nucleus caudalis of the spinal nucleus of V. Lesions here produce facial analgesia supporting a central area for pain transmission [9].

> **✪ Learning point** Imaging in trigeminal neuraligia
>
> It is known that MR imaging has good sensitivity in predicting neurovascular compression [10, 11, 12]. There are two main schools of thought regarding pre-operative vascular imaging in TN. The first suggests that the lack of neurovascular compression seen on MR vascular imaging has poor specificity and low negative predictive value [11]. Therefore, the decision to proceed to microvascular decompression should take into account both clinical and radiological findings [11] as certain vessels are beyond the resolution of contemporary imaging [13,14]. The second school of thought suggests that there is good correlation between imaging and intraoperative findings of neurovascular compression not only with high sensitivity but specificity as well [15,16] with modern MRI sequences.

> **❻ Expert comment** Imaging in trigeminal neuralgia
>
> There are two reasons to image patients with TN. First, a secondary cause, such as multiple sclerosis or tumours should be excluded. Secondly, anatomical variation prior to microvascular decompression should be considered.
>
> Standard MRI protocols include cisternal MRI axial and coronal T1-weighted pre- and post-gadolinium and T2-weighted sequences. In order to best visualize the vascular conflict, heavily T2W sequences, which provide a high contrasting picture between the CSF and structures passing through the cisterns are required [9], or balanced steady state free precession (bSSFP) images. They have similar appearances, but are named according to the manufacturer of the MRI scanner, e.g. Philips, Siemens, GE. These include balanced fast field echo (BFFE), true fast imaging with steady-state precession (FISP), and fast imaging employing steady state acquisition (FIESTA).
>
> 3D time of flight (TOF) angiography can further delineate arterial compression of the nerve, and in combination with bSSFP may increase the sensitivity and specificity [17].

Surgical treatment of trigeminal neuralgia

First-line medical therapy is carbamezapine or oxcarbazepine. Second-line treatment is based on Class III/IV evidence and includes add-on therapy with lamotrigine or a switch to lamotrigine, baclofen, or pimozide [18]. Although medical treatment works initially in about 75% of patients, it may fail over time. Surgery for TN is reserved for patients who have failed medical therapy or cannot tolerate its side effects.

Table 14.1 A comparison between the various destructive procedures for trigeminal neuralgia

	PTR	PGR	PBC	SRS
Results	99% initial pain relief 21% recurrence at 15 years [19]	90% initial pain relief 23% recurrence at 11 years	30% recurrence at 10 years	96% initial pain relief 25% recurrence at 3 years [20]
Side effects	15% troublesome numbness 3% corneal analgesia			
Comments	Trade-off between longer-term pain relief and dysaesthesia. Requires patient co-operation	Cisternal fibrosis due to repeated procedures may not allow glycerol into Meckel's cave [22]	Bradycardia occurs more frequently. Ipsilateral masticatory weakness more frequent. Lower incidence of anaesthesia dolorosa [21]	Median time to pain relief is 4 weeks

Surgery for TN can be divided into decompressive, destructive, and palliative procedures. The choice of procedure depends on the comorbidity and age of the patient, adversity to risk, pre-existing symptoms from TN and underlying cause of TN (Table 14.1). If the patient is fit enough for microvascular decompression, then this is the surgical treatment of choice, as it has the best prognosis for long-term pain relief. Destructive procedures, while usually providing immediate pain relief, is associated with residual sensory disturbances, which in the case of anaesthesia dolorosa, can be more severe than the initial TN itself.

Destructive procedures for trigeminal neuralgia
These are procedures that damage the trigeminal ganglion in Meckel's cave. They include PBC, percutaneous thermal radiofrequency rhizotomy and percutaneous glycerol rhizotomy. Stereotactic radiosurgery (SRS) targets the root entry zone of the trigeminal nerve. With the exception of SRS, they generally provide immediate pain relief and have a higher incidence of facial numbness. However, as they ameliorate only the symptoms of TN and not the cause, recurrence of TN symptoms is fairly high. Moreover, as they rely on the destruction of trigeminal ganglion, some sensory fibres will be damaged, producing numbness and dysaesthesia in the trigeminal distribution. This may range initially from a mild dysaesthesia to anaesthesia dolorosa.

Direct comparisons between large patient cohorts have been made, showing that the initial results and recurrence rates are similar in the percutaneous rhizotomy procedures [19, 20, 21, 22]. The choice of a percutaneous procedure depends not only on the suitability of the patient, e.g. anaesthesia considerations, presence of cisternal fibrosis, or pre-existing deficits, but also on the surgeon's experience.

Decompressive procedures for trigeminal neuralgia
Microvascular decompression (MVD) as pioneered by Janetta in 1967 [23] remains the mainstay for decompression of the trigeminal nerve. There is a vast body of surgical experience, and with advances in neuroanaesthesia, patients with comorbidities and advanced age have been treated successfully. It treats the underlying

> **⊗ Learning point**
> Anaesthesia dolorosa
>
> It refers to persistent and painful anaesthesia or hyperaesthesia in the distribution of the trigeminal nerve. It is frequently described as a constant burning, crawling, or itching sensation in the denervated area, worse than the original TN. It is a rare complication of surgical treatment for TN and is often refractory to medical or surgical therapy.

pathophysiology of TN, has good immediate pain relief, and the incidence of facial numbness is less than that of destructive procedures. However, working in the cerebellopontine angle exposes the patient to the potential risks of facial weakness, diplopia, hearing disturbances, CSF leak, and cerebellar damage, in addition to the risks of a craniotomy. The incidence of pain relief off medication in the largest series thus far is 70% at 10 years. The commonest cause of compression was the SCA at 75% with the AICA at 10% [16,24].

The approach is well-described in standard neurosurgical texts and is carried out via a suboccipital/retromastoid craniotomy, exposing the junction of the transverse and sigmoid sinuses. With gentle retraction of the cerebellum, the VII/VIII complex, superior petrosal sinus and finally the trigeminal complex are identified. Decompression is achieved by insertion of a Merocel® sponge between the offending artery/vein and the trigeminal nerve. Waxing of the mastoid air cells and a watertight fascial closure minimizes the risk of CSF leak.

⊕ **Clinical tip** Microvascular decompression

- Once the arachnoid space is entered, patience is required for CSF drainage to aid cerebellar relaxation.
- Superomedial retraction of the cerebellum with gentle advancement of the retractor first exposes the VII/VIII complex, then the superior petrosal vein and, finally, the trigeminal complex. A superiorly placed retractor may tear bridging tentorial veins, whereas a laterally placed retractor puts undue traction on the VII/VIII complex. The goal of cerebellar retraction is to elevate it slightly towards the surgeon and not to merely compress it medially.
- Inspection of the entire length of the trigeminal nerve is necessary to look for potential pathology.
- Surface veins should be decompressed, rather than cauterized and divided due to recollateralization and, hence, recurrence of pain.

A final word from the expert

90% of recurrent TN occurs in the original distribution. Repeat percutaneous destructive procedures can be attempted if there is preservation of facial sensation. In the case of a failed microvascular decompression, Janetta recommends repeat exploration [25], with care taken to inspect for vessels that may have been displaced during surgical positioning or sponge slippage. However, Burchiel does not favour re-exploration unless there is a high degree of suspicion of residual compression, either by high resolution MR imaging or a previous inadequate decompression [16]. Other pathology may be encountered such as granuloma secondary to sponge placement, new vessel compression and recanalization of veins.

References

1. Katusic S, Beard CM, Bergstralh E, et al. Incidence and clinical features of trigeminal neuralgia, Rochester, Minnesota, 1945–1984. Annals of Neurology 1990; 27(1): 89–95.
2. Burchiel KJ. A new classification for facial pain. Neurosurgery 2003; 53(5): 1164–7.
3. Janetta PJ. Typical and atypical symptoms. In: PJ Janetta (ed.), Trigeminal neuralgia (pp. 41–5). Oxford: Oxford University Press, 2011.
4. Devor M, Govrin-Lippmann R & Rappaport ZH. Mechanism of trigeminal neuralgia: an ultrastructural analysis of trigeminal root specimens obtained during microvascular decompression surgery. Journal of Neurosurgery 2002; 96(3): 532–43.

5. Brown JA, Hoeflinger B, Long PB, et al. Axon and ganglion cell injury in rabbits after percutaneous trigeminal balloon compression. Neurosurgery 1996; 39: 993–1003.

6. Dandy WE. Concerning the cause of trigeminal neuralgia. American Journal of Surgery 1934; 24: 447–55.

7. Jannetta PJ. Vascular compression is the cause of trigeminal neuralgia. APS Journal 1993; 2(4) 217–27.

8. Devor M, Amir R, Rappaport ZH. Pathophysiology of trigeminal neuralgia: the ignition hypothesis. Clinical Journal of Pain 2002; 18(1): 40–13.

9. Borges A, Casselman J. Imaging the trigeminal nerve. European Journal of Radiology 2010; 74(2): 323–40.

10. Anderson VC, Berryhill PC, Sandquist MA, et al. High-resolution three-dimensional magnetic resonance angiography and three-dimensional spoiled gradient-recalled imaging in the evaluation of neurovascular compression in patients with trigeminal neuralgia: a double-blind pilot study. Neurosurgery 2006; 58(4): 666–73.

11. Vergani F, Panaretos P, Penalosa A, et al. Preoperative MRI/MRA for microvascular decompression in trigeminal neuralgia: consecutive series of 67 patients. Acta Neurochirugia (Wien) 2011; 153(12): 2377–81.

12. Yoshino N, Akimoto H, Yamada I, et al. Trigeminal neuralgia: evaluation of neuralgic manifestation and site of neurovascular compression with 3D CISS MR imaging and MR angiography. Radiology 2003; 228: 539–45.

13. Miller J, Acar F, Hamilton B, et al. Preoperative visualization of neurovascular anatomy in trigeminal neuralgia. Journal of Neurosurgery 2008; 108(3): 477–82.

14. Sekula RF, Jr, Janetta PJ. The evaluation of the pre-operative patient. In: P. Janetta (eds for more than one names) Trigeminal neuralgia (pp. 87–100). Oxford University Press, 2011.

15. Leal PR, Hermier M, Souza MA, et al. Visualization of vascular compression of the trigeminal nerve with high-resolution 3T MRI: a prospective study comparing preoperative imaging analysis to surgical findings in 40 consecutive patients who underwent microvascular decompression for trigeminal neuralgia. Neurosurgery 2011; 69(1): 15–26.

16. Elias WJ, Burchiel KJ. Microvascular decompression. Clinical Journal of Pain 2002; 18: 35–41.

17. Anderson VC, Berryhill PC, Sanquist DP, et al. High resolution three dimensional magnetic resonance angiography and three dimensional spoiled gradient-recalled imaging in the evaluation of neurovascular compression in patients with trigeminal neuralgia: a double-blind pilot study. Neurosurgery 2006; 58(4): 666–73.

18. Obermann M. Treatment options in trigeminal neuralgia. Therapeutic Advances in Neurological Disorders 2012; 3(2): 107–15.

19. Taha JM, Tew JM, Jr, Buncher CR. A prospective 15-year follow up of 154 consecutive patients with trigeminal neuralgia treated by percutaneous stereotactic radiofrequency thermal rhizotomy. Journal of Neurosurgery 1995; 83(6): 989–93.

20. Linskey ME, Ratanatharathorn V, Penagaricano J. A prospective cohort study of microvascular decompression and gamma knife surgery in patients with trigeminal neuralgia. Journal of Neurosurgery 2008; 109: 160–72.

21. Skirving DJ, Dan NG. A 20-year review of percutaneous balloon compression of the trigeminal ganglion. Journal of Neurosurgery 2001; 94(6): 913–17.

22. Kouzounias K, Lind G, Schectmann G, et al. Comparison of percutaneous balloon compression and glycerol rhizotomy for the treatment of trigeminal neuralgia. Journal of Neurosurgery 2010; 113(3); 486–92.

23. Janetta PJ. Structural Mechanisms of trigeminal neuralgia. Arterial compression of the trigeminal nerve at the pons in patients with trigeminal neuralgia. J Neurosurg 1967; 26(1 pt2): 159–162.

24. Barker FG, Jannetta PJ, Bissonette DJ, et al. The long-term outcome of microvascular decompression for trigeminal neuralgia. New England Journal of Medicine 1996; 334: 1077–84.

25. Janetta PJ, Bissonette DJ. Management of the failed patient with trigeminal neuralgia. Clinical Neurosurgery 1985; 32: 334–47.

15 Cerebral metastasis

Melissa C. Werndle

❝ **Expert commentary** Henry Marsh

Case history

A 59-year-old woman presented to her local A&E department with a 2-week history of gradual onset worsening headache, with a few days of associated blurred vision. Her past medical history was significant for breast cancer, diagnosed in 2007, treated with bilateral mastectomies, adjuvant chemotherapy, and hormone therapy. On examination, she was alert and orientated with no focal neurological deficit. Fundoscopy revealed bilateral papilloedema.

MRI pre- and post-contrast revealed a 2.5-cm heterogeneously enhancing, defined lesion at the grey white junction in the left frontal lobe. There was significant surrounding vasogenic oedema (Figure 15.1). CT chest/abdomen/pelvis did not reveal any other secondary spread.

Given her symptoms and the imaging appearances, the patient was commenced on dexamethasone, and treatment options were discussed.

The patient's headaches improved with dexamethasone, but she continued to complain of blurred vision. On day 2 after admission, she underwent a left frontal craniotomy and gross total removal of the lesion.

> ❝ **Expert comment** Operative considerations
>
> Most solitary metastases can be resected using an image-guided 'mini-craniotomy' and linear incision. From the scan, it is easy to mistakenly think that a metastasis is on the surface of the brain and yet find, on opening the dura, that the tumour is not visible, so using guidance in most cases is sensible. If the tumour is beneath the surface and must be approached via a cortical incision, it is important to realize that retractors and instruments can push the lesion away and the computer navigation becomes unreliable. Brain swelling on opening the dura may also disorientate the surgeon with respect to image guidance. If the lesion is not easy to find it may be better to take the patient to the CT scanner and obtain a scan having left a suitable marker in place, rather than to poke blindly around in the deep white matter.
>
> As metastases are often superficial, care must be taken with major draining veins if the lesion is adjacent to the venous sinuses, to avoid post-operative venous infarct or venous haemorrhage.

Histology revealed pleomorphic polygonal cells, forming trabeculae, acini, and cribiform patters with necrosis. The tumour was infiltrating cortex, white matter, and leptomeninges. The appearances were of a metastatic adenocarcinoma consistent with a breast origin.

The patient had an uneventful post-operative recovery and was referred to the oncologists for adjuvant therapy.

> ✪ **Learning point**
> Differentiating abscess from tumour on MRI
>
> Although usually a shorter history, it can be very challenging to differentiate abscess from tumour, both clinically and on CT. MR is helpful: tumours show unrestricted diffusion, whereas abscesses show restricted diffusion. Restricted diffusion is indicated by hyperintensity on diffusion weighted imaging (DWI), and low ADC (Apparent Diffusion Coeffecient).

> ✪ **Learning point**
> Dexamethasone—how it works
>
> Dexamethasone revolutionized the outcome of surgery for brain tumours following Galicich's seminal paper on alleviating oedema in brain tumours in 1960s [1]. The clinical improvement in patients with symptoms and signs of oedema from tumours is often rapid and obvious. The exact mechanism of action remains an unknown; however, the principles are a decrease in the blood–tumour barrier permeability, decreased tumoural perfusion, decreased tumoural diffusivity resulting in reduced intracranial pressure, and improved cerebral perfusion pressure.

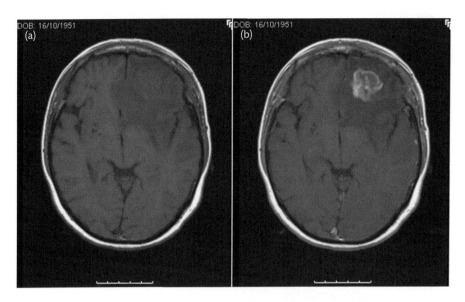

Figure 15.1 T1-weighted MR (a) pre- and (b) post-gadolinium images, showing left frontal isointense intrinsic lesion with surrounding oedema, which enhances heterogeneously.

Discussion

The incidence of cerebral metastases, which is the most common type of adult brain tumour, is up to 40% in patients diagnosed with a primary systemic cancer [2]. The common primary sites are lung, breast, melanoma, renal, and colorectal [3]. Most systemic treatments for primary malignancies do not cross the blood–brain barrier; therefore, we are seeing an increase in brain metastases in patients who previously would not have survived their primary disease.

Classical imaging characteristics of a cerebral metastasis are of a contrast enhancing well-defined lesion at the gray–white junction with significant surrounding oedema. Hyperdensity on CT indicates a haemorrhagic metastasis, commonly melanoma. Lesions may be single or multiple. CT underestimates the number of lesions compared with MRI (by a measure of 2–3-fold), especially lesions under 5mm in diameter, and therefore MRI is the preferred mode of imaging [4]. MRI features of the lesion are iso- to mild hypointensity on T1, hyperintensity on T2, and enhancement post-gadolinium.

The current treatment options available for brain metastases are radiotherapy, stereotactic radiosurgery, and surgery (open surgical resection). The treatment combination is determined by a number of factors, which include:

- Underlying malignancy.
- Performance status.
- Location of cerebral metastasis.
- Number of cerebral metastases.
- Systemic staging and prognosis.
- Age.

Although these principles apply universally, management may vary from country to country and even from centre to centre, in terms of how aggressively the patient

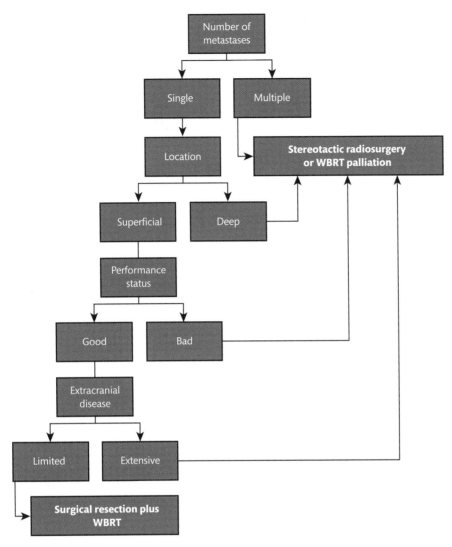

Figure 15.2 Treatment algorithm.

is treated. A challenge is to balance prolongation of life with maximizing quality of life. At times, these principles are at odds and each case must be considered individually. In general, in patients with a good performance status (Karnofsky over 70, or performance status 0, 1, 2) and controlled extracranial disease, surgical resection followed by whole brain radiotherapy confers the maximum survival [5,6] (see Figure 15.2) This is superior to whole-brain radiotherapy alone.

❝ Expert comment Aim of surgery

The aim should be to remove the metastasis completely. There is normally a good plane, and a combination of debulking and dissection of the tumour–white matter plane using a curved instrument, such as a Penfield number 2 makes this usually an easy operation.

✔ Evidence base

There are varying levels of evidence for different treatment modalities. There is a succinct series of systematic reviews published in *Journal of Neurooncology* [7-10]. It is important to note this review applied to good performance status patients with a single brain metastasis.

- Radiotherapy: whole brain radiotherapy is used adjunctively following surgery/stereotactic radiosurgery to decrease the rate of recurrence and increase length of time to recurrence. As a single modality treatment for palliation, whole brain radiotherapy (WBRT) improves symptoms and survival by 3 months compared with supportive care only.
- Surgery: when compared to WBRT alone, surgery (followed by WBRT) improves survival by 4–6 months.
- Stereotactic radiosurgery: stereotactic radiosurgery (SRS) plus radiotherapy is equally effective when compared to surgery plus radiotherapy (retrospective studies only) for small lesions (<3cm) with no midline shift over 1cm.

In patients with a single 'unresectable' metastasis, a stereotactic radiosurgery boost following WBRT improves survival compared to WBRT alone [11]. Consider SRS for unresectable or multiple metastases.

- Chemotherapy: limited benefit in brain metastases.

ⓕ Expert comment Selection of patients for treatment

Solitary metastases on the surface of the brain in patients without a significant neurological deficit after steroid treatment and with a prognosis of more than a few months are suitable for image-guided resection. If the lesion is small and there is extensive white matter oedema, it is probably wise to give steroids for several days before surgery to reduce the risk of severe intra- or post-operative brain swelling. Solitary deep lesions within the brain, if less than 3cm in size, should usually be treated with stereotactic radiotherapy. It is a question of judgement as to when stereotactic radiotherapy should be used instead of surgery.

The natural history of brain metastases, if left untreated, is a median survival in the order of weeks to months. If this heterogenous group is subdivided, those with an unfavourable combination of the aforementioned factors (underlying malignancy small cell lung cancer, poor performance status, 'inoperable' location, multiple lesions, extensive extracranial disease, and older age) have a prognosis of under 3 months. A 'favourable' combination improves median survival to 18 months [12].

A final word from the expert

With a constant improvement in treatment available for underlying primaries, where patients are now surviving longer, there is an onus on developing targeted therapies for cerebral metastases.

Anti-angiogenic therapy

Angiogenesis is an integral part of brain tumour formation, including cerebral metastases. The process is led by over-expression of the signal protein VEGF. Experimentally, obstruction of the angiogenic VEGF pathway inhibits the formation of cerebral metastases in lung, breast, and colorectal models [13], with promising results. Several anti-angiogenic agents are being studied in a number of Phase I and II human trials.

Cancer-specific targeted therapies

There are a range of agents being studied in cerebral metastases from breast, melanoma, and lung cancer. The most promising include inhibitors of (1) BRAF (v-RAF murine sarcoma viral oncogene homolog B1) for melanoma, and (2) epithelial growth factor receptor for non-small cell lung cancer [13].

References

1. Galicich JH, French LA, Melby JC. Use of dexamethasone in treatment of cerebral edema associated with brain tumors. Lancet 1961; 81: 46–53.
2. Gavrilovic IT, Posner JB. Brain metastases: epidemiology and pathophysiology. Journal of Neurooncology 2005; 75(1): 5–14.
3. Schouten LJ, Rutten J, Huveneers HA, et al. Incidence of brain metastases in a cohort of patients with carcinoma of the breast, colon, kidney, and lung and melanoma. Cancer 2002; 94(10): 2698–705.
4. Seute T, Leffers P, ten Velde GP, et al. Detection of brain metastases from small cell lung cancer: consequences of changing imaging techniques (CT versus MRI). Cancer 2008; 112(8): 1827–34.
5. Vecht CJ, Haaxma-Reiche H, Noordijk EM, et al. Treatment of single brain metastasis: radiotherapy alone or combined with neurosurgery? Annals of Neurology 1993; 33(6): 583–90.
6. Patchell RA, Tibbs PA, Walsh JW, et al. A randomized trial of surgery in the treatment of single metastases to the brain. New England Journal of Medicine 1990; 322(8): 494–500.
7. Gaspar LE, Mehta MP, Patchell RA, et al. The role of whole brain radiation therapy in the management of newly diagnosed brain metastases: a systematic review and evidence-based clinical practice guideline. Journal of Neurooncology 2010; 96(1): 17–32.
8. Kalkanis SN, Kondziolka D, Gaspar LE, et al. The role of surgical resection in the management of newly diagnosed brain metastases: a systematic review and evidence-based clinical practice guideline. Journal of Neurooncology 2010; 96(1): 33–43.
9. Linskey ME, Andrews DW, Asher AL, et al. The role of stereotactic radiosurgery in the management of patients with newly diagnosed brain metastases: a systematic review and evidence-based clinical practice guideline. Journal of Neurooncology 2010; 96(1): 45–68.
10. Mehta MP, Paleologos NA, Mikkelsen T, et al. The role of chemotherapy in the management of newly diagnosed brain metastases: a systematic review and evidence-based clinical practice guideline. Journal of Neurooncology 2010; 96(1): 71–83.
11. Andrews DW, Scott CB, Sperduto PW, et al. Whole brain radiation therapy with or without stereotactic radiosurgery boost for patients with one to three brain metastases: phase III results of the RTOG 9508 randomised trial. Lancet 2004; 363(9422): 1665–72.
12. Jakola AS, Gulati S, Nerland US, et al. Surgical resection of brain metastases: the prognostic value of the graded prognostic assessment score. Journal of Neurooncology 2011; 105(3): 573–81.
13. Preusser M, Capper D, Ilhan-Mutlu A, et al. Brain metastases: pathobiology and emerging targeted therapies. Acta Neuropathologica 2012; 123(2): 205–22.

16 The surgical management of the rheumatoid spine

Robin Bhatia

Expert commentary Adrian Casey

Case history

A 52-year-old woman was referred to the spinal outpatients' clinic with a 5-year history of neck pain, loss of hand dexterity, and gait deterioration. The previous medical history was remarkable for rheumatoid arthritis (RA) affecting the hand and knee joints symmetrically, and pulmonary nodules diagnosed on chest radiography. She had previous multiple small joint replacements in her hands and a hip replacement.

The loss of hand dexterity manifested itself as increasing difficulty fastening buttons and using cutlery to eat. In the year prior to presentation, the patient's walking distance had progressively deteriorated, and she required a zimmer frame to mobilize. She taking methotrexate (5mg/week) and NSAIDs. The visual analogue score of neck pain at presentation was 7/10 (where 0/10 corresponded to no pain, and 10/10 was the worst pain imaginable), and her sleep was disturbed nightly.

Examination revealed bilateral hand deformities consistent with rheumatoid disease, with a gross grip strength of 3/5 (MRC grading). Proximal upper limb power was limited by neck pain and shoulder girdle rigidity. Power was globally 4/5 in the lower limbs with marked hypertonia, and exaggerated knee and ankle reflexes. Plantar reflexes were bilaterally up-going, with 3 beats of clonus at the right ankle. Her pre-operative Ranawat class was IIIa, based on the clinical findings. The Myelopathy Disability Index (MDI) was 85%, and Neck Disability Index (NDI) was 75%.

⊗ Learning point Functional measures in rheumatoid cervical spine disease

The Ranawat Class classifies neurological function in rheumatoid spine disease into four broad categories, as shown in Table 16.1. This measure is simple to use and has been widely accepted. In the original publication of 1979, Ranawat et al. applied the classification scheme to 33 patients

Table 16.1 Classification of neurological function in rheumatoid disease according to Ranawat et al. [1]

Ranawat Class	Description
I	No neurological deficit
II	Subjective weakness/dysaesthesia +/–hyperreflexia
IIIa	Objective weakness with long tract signs and ambulatory
IIIb	Quadraparetic and non-ambulatory

Data from: Ranawat CS, O'Leary P, Pellicci P, Tsairis P, Marchisello P, Dorr L: Cervical spine fusion in rheumatoid arthritis. J Bone Joint Surg Am 1979;61:1003–1010

(continued)

with rheumatoid cervical spine disease, including atlanto-axial subluxation, superior odontoid peg migration and subaxial subluxation. Two patients improved from Class III to II after spinal fusion, five patients improved within Class III, i.e. they became ambulatory, but the remaining patients showed no change in class or deterioration post-operatively [1].

The Myelopathy Disability Index (MDI), as developed by Casey et al. in 1996, described a functional scale of myelopathic disability based on an abridged form of the Stanford Health Assessment Questionnaire (HAQ). Responses to ten questions relating to rising, eating, walking, self-hygiene, gripping, and getting into and out of a car, were scored in terms of level of difficulty, with the overall score out of 30 converted to a percentage. MDI showed excellent correlation ($r = 0.98$) to the original Stanford HAQ, and was an accurate predictor of functional outcome in 194 rheumatoid spine patients operated on in comparison to the Ranawat and Steinbrocker grades [2].

The Neck Disability Index (NDI) was developed by Howard Vernon in 1989, as a modification of the Oswestry Low Back Pain Disability Index. The NDI primarily tests for pain-related functional deficits in categories such as personal care, lifting, driving, reading, sleeping, work, and recreation. The overall score is out of 50 converted to a percentage. The NDI showed moderate to high correlations ($r = 0.6$ and $r = 0.7$) to the visual analogue score and McGill Pain Questionnaire respectively, in small groups of conservatively-managed whiplash-injured patients [3].

Plain lateral radiographs in flexion and extension revealed atlanto-axial subluxation with atlanto-dental interval (ADI) of 5mm and posterior atlanto-dental interval (PADI) of 15.5mm. CT of the craniocervical junction and upper thoracic spine revealed basilar impression with a Redlund-Johnell measurement of 25mm, and odontoid bony erosion with generalized osteopaenia (Figure 16.1). MRI imaging confirmed basilar impression, but without overt brainstem compression, and cervical canal stenosis at C4 and, to a lesser extent, at C5 due to anterior disc-osteophyte bars and posterior buckling of ligamentum flavum. There was intramedullary signal change of the spinal cord at the C4 and C5 levels on the T2-weighted imaging (Figure 16.2).

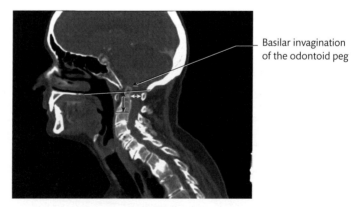

Basilar invagination of the odontoid peg

Figure 16.1 Sagittal CT image through the lower skull and cervicothoracic spine. The markedly degenerate and osteopenic rheumatoid spine shows basilar invagination, cervical canal stenosis, and subaxial cervical disease. The Redlund-Johnell measurement (purple arrow: 25mm) and the posterior atlanto-dental interval (white arrow: 15mm) are demonstrated.

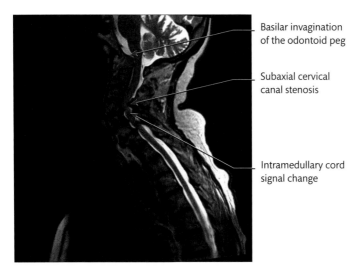

Basilar invagination
of the odontoid peg

Subaxial cervical
canal stenosis

Intramedullary cord
signal change

Figure 16.2 Sagittal T2-weighted MRI demonstrating spinal cord compression in the subaxial region particularly C4 /C5, with intramedullary cord signal change. The abnormally high position and proximity of the odontoid tip to the cervicomedullary junction is noted.

> ⊗ **Learning point** Measuring basilar migration
>
> The terms basilar invagination and basilar impression are more or less used interchangeably with 'upward migration', 'vertical translocation', and 'cranial settling'. Multiple eponymous measurements were developed to describe the degree of basilar impression/invagination on radiographic imaging. One reason for this was the unreliability of eroded bony landmarks as a consequence of the disease process.
>
> In 1939, Chamberlain stated that if the odontoid peg protruded more than 3mm above a line between the hard palate and the opisthion, then this was diagnostic of invagination [4]. McGregor, in 1948, defined a line between posterior hard palate and the most inferior point of the occipital curve (over 4.5mm odontoid projection was positive for basilar invagination) [5]. Wackenheim in 1974 defined invagination if there was odontoid protusion posterior to a line drawn along the superior surface of the clivus [6]. Ranawat described a line from the midpoint of the odontoid peg to a transverse line through the atlas (positive if <15mm in males or <13mm in females) [1]. Redlund-Johnell and Peterson drew a line from the midpoint of the caudal surface of C2 body to McGregor's line, defining significant basilar invagination if the distance was <34mm in males and <29mm in females, as shown in Figure 16.2 [7]. Clark's stations refer to the division of the sagittally-imaged odontoid peg into three equal parts; if the ring of the atlas was level with the middle or caudal third, then basilar invagination was diagnosed [8].
>
> The modern era of early MRI has made many of these measurements obsolete, since clinicians can now view ligamentous integrity and the direct impact of basilar migration on the craniocervical junction. Riew et al. examined cervical radiographs in 131 rheumatoid patients and found that the only three measurements with over 90% sensitivity were the Redlund-Johnell, Clark's stations, and the Ranawat measurement, with a combined sensitivity of 94% and negative predictive value of 91% [9].

Given the severity of her presenting symptomology, and clinical progression, the decision was made to proceed to posterior occipito-cervicothoracic fixation and C4/C5 laminectomy. Methotrexate was stopped 2 weeks prior to surgery. After induction, the patient was positioned prone in Mayfield head pins, and

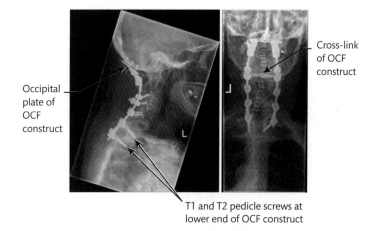

Occipital plate of OCF construct

Cross-link of OCF construct

T1 and T2 pedicle screws at lower end of OCF construct

Figure 16.3 Lateral and AP radiographs immediately post-occipito-cervicothoracic fixation with rigid occipital plate/rod construct.

intra-operative X-ray imaging revealed satisfactory atlanto-axial and subaxial cervical alignment, with a neutral head position in order to maintain horizontal vision. Intravenous third generation cephalosporin (1.5g cefuroxime) and steroid (8mg dexamethasone) were administered on induction. Somatosensory- and motor-evoked potential spinal cord monitoring was used throughout the operation. A midline incision was made extending between the external occipital protuberance (EOP) and T4 posterior spinous process. After bilateral subperiosteal paraspinal muscle strips (extending laterally enough to reveal the facet joints), bilateral C3, C4, and C5 poly-axial lateral mass screws, and bilateral T1 and T2 pedicle screws were inserted under intra-operative image guidance. An occipital plate was applied by drilling two holes into the midline keel of the occiput beneath the EOP, and affixed using bicortically purchasing screws. C4 and C5 laminectomies were then carried out. The occipital plate was attached to bilateral lordotic titanium rods, positioned and torque-affixed into the heads of the cervical and thoracic screws. A cross-link was also affixed to the rods between C3 and C4. Morcelized own-bone fragments from the laminectomies and demineralized synthetic bone graft were applied lateral to the rods, and the wound was closed in layers of vicryl with clips to skin.

Immediate post-operative assessment revealed that the patient's neurological deficit was unchanged, and the patient was once again mobilizing on day 2 with her zimmer frame. Plain X-rays revealed satisfactory placement of intrumentation and occipitocervical alignment (Figure 16.3). The patient was discharged from hospital after 12 days. Follow-up at 6 months revealed the persistence of long tract signs and MRC 4/5 global lower limb power (Ranawat IIIa, still mobilizing with a zimmer frame). However, NDI had significantly improved to 45% (with particular improvements in sleeping, eating, and reading), and MDI had improved to 50%. Her post-operative visual analogue score of neck pain was 4/10, with appropriate reductions in her analgesia. Repeat X-ray imaging did not reveal evidence of bony fusion at this stage. She recommended methotrexate 4 weeks postoperatively, and remained without exacerbation of her rheumatoid disease in this period.

Discussion

RA affects approximately 1% of the population and, of those affected, approximately 50% will have cervical spine involvement [14]. Conlon et al. reported that 295/333 (88%) rheumatoid patients complained of cervical symptoms [15], but only 2/609 (0.3%) in a study by da Silva et al. required cervical spine fusion between 1955 and 1995 [16]. Therefore, there appears to be a significant difference at present in the numbers of rheumatoid spine patients managed by rheumatologists and those managed by spinal surgeons.

There is a female predominance of RA, with F:M ratio of approximately 3:1. RA is an autoimmune disease, the target of which is primarily joint synovium leading ultimately to articular cartilage and bone destruction with the development of synovial cysts and ligamentous laxity; atlanto-axial instability follows transverse ligament laxity, and basilar invagination is secondary to alar ligament and occipital condyle destruction. Cardiovascular, respiratory, skin, renal, vascular, and ocular systems may be affected by extra-articular rheumatoid disease. In general, the longer the disease, the more extensive and severe the articular and systemic involvement, although in recent years disease-modifying anti-rheumatoid drugs (DMARDs) have positively influenced disease progression [17].

The spinal neurosurgeon needs to address the following fundamental questions when managing the rheumatoid cervical spine.

What are the pathologies commonly encountered?

Broadly and clearly, these commonly co-exist and comprise atlanto-axial (horizontal) subluxation, vertical translocation giving rise to basilar invagination, pannus-related craniocervical stenosis/ligamento-osseous erosion, and subaxial instability/stenosis, as shown in Figure 16.4.

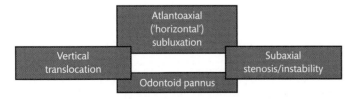

Figure 16.4 Basic concepts in rheumatoid cervical spine pathology. There is a relationship and interplay between different pathologies.

At what point in the disease process (from asymptomatic to clinically severe brainstem and spinal cord compression) should we surgically intervene?

The natural history of cervical rheumatoid disease is not entirely known, and the decision to operate balances the risks of intervention with the likelihood of preventing/improving neurological and functional decline. Moreover, using neurological examination parameters to guide operative decision-making reliably is difficult due to the peripheral joint and nervous involvement of RA.

The development of surgical techniques to manage the rheumatoid cervical spine was mirrored by the development of instrumentation. Although this case highlights the use of occipitocervical fixation for severe disease, spinal surgeons may also chose to carry out 'segment-saving surgery', or C1–C2 fixation.

✪ Learning point C1–C2 fixation

Atlanto-axial subluxation presents earlier in the disease process of rheumatoid cervical spine disease, with a prevalence range of 10–25% at a mean of 3.9 years after the diagnosis of RA [18]. There is now common acceptance for early surgical intervention to help neck pain and occipital neuralgia, prevent (occasionally catastrophic) spinal cord damage due to instability, and possibly to slow down disease progression, i.e. the development of vertical translocation at the craniocervical junction. However, there is no clear consensus on the relationship between the ADI and/or PADI, and the absolute requirement for surgical intervention.

Historically, the Gallie fusion described in 1939, and later modified by Brookes and Jenkins, employed sublaminar wires passed under the C1 arch and around the C2 spinous process [19], or under the C2 lamina with bone blocks between C1 and C2 [20]. There were risks of accidental durotomy and spinal cord damage on sublaminar wire passage, however, and commonly patients were subsequently managed in a halo brace.

The 1980s saw the rise of interlaminar clamps, such as the Halifax clamp described by Tucker [21], with improved stability in rotation and extension. However, there was a high incidence of posterior element fracture, MRI artefact, and pseudoarthrosis with these devices.

In 1987, Magerl described C1–C2 fixation using posterior trans-articular screws [22]. This result enhanced rigidity, particularly in rotation, since the screws are passed through the articulating surfaces between C1 and C2. Added rigidity in flexion and extension can be obtained by Gallie-type C1–C2 wiring, although one major advantage of the Magerl C1–C2 fixation was the opportunity afforded to posteriorly decompress the craniocervical junction without affecting the construct. However, despite high reported fusion rates with this procedure (90–98% [22], the variable anatomy of the vertebral

(continued)

artery can sometimes preclude safe screw placement; indeed, pre-operative vascular imaging, such as CT angiography, is required therefore.

An alternative to the two screw fixation described by Magerl was reported by Goel in 1994 (and later modified by Harms in 2001) using four screws to fix the lateral masses of C1 to the pedicles of C2 [23,24]. The screws are secured by rods bilaterally. The development of poly-axial screws greatly aided this operative procedure. The Goel–Harms procedure is particularly advantageous when the atlanto-axial subluxation will not reduce, precluding the passage of trans-articular screws, when there is aberrant vertebral anatomy, or when the posterior elements are fractured or required to be decompressed. If C2 pedicle screws are not feasible due to bony anatomy, then C2 pars or translaminar screws can be placed. The C2 nerve root is an important landmark, and there is a debate about whether to section or retract the nerve root during the insertion of the C1 lateral mass screw; 'long shank' screws avoid screw thread irritation of the nerve in this regard.

Does early C1–C2 fixation alter the pathological process in the rheumatoid spine? This question at present remains definitively unanswered, but there is a school of thought that early C1–C2 fixation can arrest the progression to vertical or basilar translocation, as well as reduce pannus formation [25]. However, it may also exacerbate the development of subaxial cervical disease [18].

What are the systemic issues related to the underlying diagnosis of RA, and how do these impact on peri-operative morbidity and mortality?

The peri-operative management of the patient with RA requires a multidisciplinary approach, and sufficient time pre-operatively to optimize the patient's general medical status.

Cardiovascular system abnormalities include pericarditis (30–80%), arrhythmia, mitral valvular disease (30–80%), coronary vasculitis, and cardiomyopathy [26]. Hakala reported a poor prognosis in rheumatoid patients admitted with interstitial lung fibrosis [27]. Generalized osteopenia may compromise bony fusion and is compounded by chronic steroid use.

Rheumatoid patients also have more fragile skin making them susceptible to pressure sores, and poor wound healing. Rheumatoid patients undergoing cervical surgery often require post-operative management on the High Dependency Unit, given their poor pre-operative status and limited physiological reserve.

Expert comment

The risk benefit profile for the RA patient is best for those with pain alone or minimal neurology. Careful attention to tissue handling, patient warming, prophylactic antibiotics, and pre-operative optimization of medication (stop steroids and DMARDs) and nutrition will potentially reduce complications. Rheumatoid pulmonary interstitial fibrosis and a higher apparent incidence of bronchiectasis are challenges for the anaesthetist, particularly in the prone position. Tracheostomy is rarely needed, even in those patients who need trans-oral decompression of the odontoid process. Mouth opening may be limited in the presence of temporomandibular (synovial joint) rheumatoid disease. Awake fibre-optic intubation is often required in the presence of the combined airway issues and an unstable cervical spine.

What has been the impact of disease-modifying drugs on the natural history of rheumatoid spinal disease, and what are the risks associated with continued use during the peri-operative period?

Biologic disease-modifying antirheumatic drugs (bDMARDs) extend the treatment choices for RA patients with suboptimal response or intolerance to a conventional

DMARD, such as methotrexate. Adalimumab, etanercept, and infliximab are examples of tumour necrosis factor (TNF) inhibitors, and are effective treatments compared with placebo in the control of symptoms, improving physical function, and slowing radiographic changes in joints [28]. Other DMARDs include interleukin-1 receptor antagonists (e.g. anakinra) and anti-CD20 monoclonal antibodies (e.g. rituximab). These drugs hold promise, but are relatively new and the long-term benefits, particularly with regards to alteration of the natural history of rheumatoid disease in the spine is unknown. Moreover, they are not free of side effects; there may be an increased risk of bacterial infection associated with TNF inhibitor therapy [29].

⭐ **Learning point** Disease-modifying drugs in the perioperative period

Although the side-effects of NSAIDs and glucocorticoids in the peri-operative period are well-described in the literature, less is known about the effects of biologic response-modifying medications, such as methotrexate, tumour necrosis factor-inhibitors (e.g. infliximab), interleukin-1 receptor antagonists (e.g. anakinra), and anti-CD20 monoclonal antibodies (e.g. rituximab).

Sany et al. conducted a randomized unblinded prospective trial on sixty-four rheumatoid patients receiving methotrexate therapy, half of whom stopped taking methotrexate pre-operatively. There were no infections in either group, with comparable numbers of delayed wound healing [30]. Carpenter et al., on the other hand, reported increased local infection rates in patients continuing methotrexate compared with those stopping, in a prospective study of thirty-two patients undergoing hip arthroplasty [31]. A larger prospective randomized study by Grennan et al (n = 388), failed to show any significant increase in infection rate or wound complications in those on methotrexate compared with those stopping in the peri-operative period (in fact, the rates of local sepsis were lower in those continuing methotrexate), with no differences in rates of rheumatoid flare-ups [32].

No formal trials have addressed the peri-operative complications associated with continuing other disease-modifying drugs. Based on the extrapolation of limited studies in rheumatoid patients on infliximab undergoing abdominal surgery, and animal studies, Rosandich et al. and Pieringer et al. tentatively proposed discontinuation of these medications 2 weeks pre-operatively and restarting after a similar period of time, although further clinical data is required [33,34].

What is the optimal way of decompressing and fusing the rheumatoid cervical spine, and when should we consider (two-stage) anterior and posterior decompression? What type of instrumentation should one use and what is the capability of the underlying bony substrate in this disease to support fusion?

The application of occipitocervical fixation (OCF) constructs is challenging because of the unique 3D anatomy of the craniocervical region. The major considerations include the varying thickness of the occipital bone and the unusual load requirements on the construct, which is in essence supporting the head [35]. Historically, occipitocervical fusion using on-lay morcelized or fibular strut grafting with halo placement [36] was superceded by the internal rod and sublaminar wire technique, popularized in the last two decades of the twentieth century [37,38]. Roy-Camille introduced the concept of rigid occipitocervical fusion with skull base screws, plates, and lateral mass screws in 1989 [39], and in 1991 Grob et al. reported a technique of rigid occipitocervical (OC) fixation using an occipital Y-plate and lateral mass screws (including trans-articular atlanto-axial screws) for a variety of pathologies in fourteen patients, all of whom achieved solid bony fusion and satisfactory clinical outcomes [40]. Furthermore, biomechanical cadaveric studies were supportive of rigid OC fixation over semi-rigid rod and wire systems [41,42], although in clinical practice fusion rates were similar and neither technique requires post-operative halo fixation.

⊘ Evidence base A systematic review of OCF

In 2010, Winegar et al. published an extensive literature review of occipitocervical fixation with regards to techniques and outcomes. Their search generated 799 adult patients who underwent OC fixation between 1969 and 2011. The mean age +/– SD of patients undergoing OCF was 54 +/– 17 years (range 18–87 years). The indications for OCF were classified into five groups: inflammatory diseases (of which RA was the most common), congenital abnormalities, tumour, trauma, and other, non-specific indications. There were six types of instrumentation employed:

- Posterior wires/rods.
- Screws/rods.
- Hooks/rods.
- Screws/plates.
- Wires/plates.
- Wire/on-lay grafts.

The highest rates of fusion were for systems employing wires/rods and screws/rods, although the latter technique was more effective in RA. Most occipitocervical fusions occurred over a period of 4 months, excepting tumours in which only 45% fused over that period of time. Fusion was associated with neurological improvement and improved patient satisfaction overall.

Although only 16% of articles in the review documented adverse complications, the overall rate was 52%, divided into instrumentation misplacement, vascular injury, thecal sac injury, anaesthetic complications, and unspecified. There was a 22% rate of intrumentation failure, posterior wiring notably was associated with 10% failure rate compared with 6.2% with screws [43].

One of the largest series of non-rigid OC fixations for RA specifically was published by Zygmunt et al., who reported 163 rheumatoid patients over a mean follow-up period of 54 months [44]. The most common presenting symptom in patients with RA and cervical subluxation was neck pain, often with associated occipital neuralgia, but a wide spectrum of symptoms and signs secondary to brainstem, cranial nerve, and cord or cervical root compression were also reported. The Brattstrom–Granholm method of occipital burr hole-to-C2 fixation using wires, C2 spinous process pin, and PMMA cement was employed. The indication for surgery was atlanto-axial subluxation (defined as ADI > 3mm). Seventy-four per cent of patients reported significant improvements in pain and neurological deficit. Complications in this large series included wire breakages in 21/163, eight of whom required revisional surgery, five wound infections, five cerebellar injuries related to occipital burr hole wire passage, nine patients had progressive postoperative myelopathy, two cases had progressive vertical subluxation of the odontoid peg. Thirty-seven of 163 patients developed progressive subaxial subluxation at the levels below fixation (typically C4/C5). Therefore, wire-based constructs do have the additional risks of wire breakage, bone abrasion, and accidental durotomy/neurological injury when being passed [35].

➕ Clinical tip The optimal construct for occipital cervical fixation

According to Nockels et al., the optimal implant for OCF would allow for:

- Rigid fixation of the occiput to the subaxial cervical spine without the requirement for halo bracing.
- The ability to perform atlanto-axial screw fixation and posterior decompression.
- The ability of the construct to conform to the individual anatomy.
- Ease of use.
- Means to correct deformity.
- Overall low profile.
- The ability to tolerate biomechanical forces unique to the region over a long-term basis.

Nockels believed that rigid fixation systems best met these goals [35].

A controversial point is whether to operate on patients with severe cervical rheumatoid disease. The decision must weigh up the benefits and risks to the patient. Moskovich et al. reported that 40% of patients improved in Ranawat class, and a significant number had prolonged improvements in neck pain score in a group of 150 rheumatoid patients undergoing OCF using the Ransford loop and sublaminar wires. However, there was a 10% mortality rate and 11% re-operation rate due to disease progression and post-operative complications [38]. Rheumatoid patients with severe disease (Ranawat Class IIIb) at baseline have the worst post-operative prognosis. Casey et al. reported mortality rates up to 30%, with little improvement in disability in this subgroup, suggesting that OC fixation as a procedure to help patients is carried out 'too little and too late' [10]. On the other hand, it may be reasonable to observe closely rheumatoid patients who are asymptomatic with fixed basilar invagination and no spinal cord compression. In those with MRI T2-weighted signal change in the cord or syrinx surgery can be considered to prevent future neurological decline or sudden death. It is important that the surgery is carried out in specialist units with a high turnover of RA patients and by spinal surgeons who are experienced in the management of the rheumatoid spine.

A final word from the expert

The rheumatoid patient presents many challenges in diagnosis, pre-operative optimization, and selection of levels to instrument. The fixation and bony healing is in a challenging environment with immunosuppressive agents and often osteoporosis from the historical use of steroids. The results of surgery for pain relief and preservation of neurological function are good, provided that it is not left too late. If the patient is no longer ambulant, surgery may be too much, too late, with high complication rates. Surgical fixation for atlanto-axial fixation for those patients who can still walk has a lot to offer patients in terms of neurological protection and pain relief, and is a rewarding area.

References

1. Ranawat CS, O'Leary P, Pellicci P, et al. Cervical spine fusion in rheumatoid arthritis. Journal of Bone Joint Surgery American 1979; 61: 1003–10.
2. Casey AT, Bland JM, Crockard HA. Development of a functional scoring system for rheumatoid arthritis patients with cervical myelopathy. Annals of Rheumatic Diseases 1996; 55: 901–6.

3. Vernon H, Mior S. The Neck Disability Index: a study of reliability and validity. Journal of Manipulative Physiological Therapeutics 1991; 14: 409–15.

4. Chamberlain WE. basilar impression (platybasia): a bizarre developmental anomaly of the occipital bone and upper cervical spine with striking and misleading neurologic manifestations. Yale Journal of Biology and Medicine 1939; 11: 487–96.

5. McGreger M. The significance of certain measurements of the skull in the diagnosis of basilar impression. British Journal of Radiology 1948; 21: 171–81.

6. Wackenheim A. Roentgen diagnosis of the craniovertebral region. New York: Springer, 1974.

7. Redlund-Johnell I, Pettersson H. Radiographic measurements of the cranio-vertebral region. Designed for evaluation of abnormalities in rheumatoid arthritis. Acta Radiologica. Diagnosis (Stockholm) 1984; 25: 23–8.

8. Clark CR, Goetz DD, Menezes AH. Arthrodesis of the cervical spine in rheumatoid arthritis. Journal of Bone Joint Surgery American 1989; 71: 381–92.

9. Riew KD, Hilibrand AS, Palumbo MA, et al. Diagnosing basilar invagination in the rheumatoid patient. The reliability of radiographic criteria. Journal of Bone Joint Surgery American 2001; 83-A: 194–200.

10. Casey AT, Crockard HA, Bland JM, et al. Surgery on the rheumatoid cervical spine for the non-ambulant myelopathic patient-too much, too late? Lancet 1996; 347: 1004–7.

11. Bhatia R, Haliasos N, Vergara P, et al. The surgical management of the rheumatoid spine: Has the evolution of surgical intervention changed outcomes? Journal of the Craniovertebral Junction and Spine 2014; 5 (1): 38–43.

12. Bhatia R, DeSouza, R, Bull J, et al. Rigid occipitocervical fixation: indications, outcomes, and complications in the modern era Journal of Neurosurgery of the Spine 2013; 18 (4): 333–9.

13. Vergara P, Singh J, Casey A, et al. C1–C2 posterior fixation: are 4 screws better than 2? Neurosurgery 2012; 71: ON S86–95.

14. Krauss WE, Bledsoe JM, Clarke MJ, et al. Rheumatoid arthritis of the craniovertebral junction. Neurosurgery 2010; 66: 83–95.

15. Conlon PW, Isdale IC, Rose BS. Rheumatoid arthritis of the cervical spine. An analysis of 333 cases. Annals of Rheumatic Diseases 1966; 25: 120–6.

16. da Silva E, Doran MF, Crowson CS, et al. Declining use of orthopedic surgery in patients with rheumatoid arthritis? Results of a long-term, population-based assessment. Arthritis & Rheumatology 2003; 49: 216–20.

17. Hamilton JD, Gordon MM, McInnes IB, et al. Improved medical and surgical management of cervical spine disease in patients with rheumatoid arthritis over 10 years. Annals of Rheumatic Diseases 2000; 59: 434–8.

18. Werle S, Ezzati A, El Saghir H, et al. Is inclusion of the occiput necessary in fusion for C1–2 instability in rheumatoid arthritis? Journal of Neurosurgery of the Spine 2013; 18: 50–6.

19. Gallie WE. Skeletal traction in the treatment of fractures and dislocations of the cervical spine. Annals of Surgery 1937; 106: 770–6.

20. Brooks AL, Jenkins EB. Atlanto-axial arthrodesis by the wedge compression method. Journal of Bone Joint Surgery American 1978; 60: 279–84.

21. Tucker HH. Technical report: method of fixation of subluxed or dislocated cervical spine below C1–C2. Canadian Journal of Neurological Sciences 1975; 2: 381–2.

22. Magerl F, Sceman PS. Stable posterior fusion at the atlas and axis by trans-articular screw fixation. In: P Kehr, A Weidner,(eds for more than one name), Cervical spine (pp. 322–7). New York: Springer-Verlag, 1987.

23. Goel A, Laheri V. Plate and screw fixation for atlanto-axial subluxation. Acta Neurochirugia (Wien) 1994; 129: 47–53.

24. Harms J, Melcher RP. Posterior C1–C2 fusion with poly-axial screw and rod fixation. Spine (Phila Pa 1976) 2001; 26: 2467–71.

25. Landi A, Marotta N, Morselli C, et al. Pannus regression after posterior decompression and occipito-cervical fixation in occipito-atlanto-axial instability due to rheumatoid arthritis: case report and literature review. Clinical Neurology and Neurosurgery 2013; 115: 111–16.

26. Voskuyl AE. The heart and cardiovascular manifestations in rheumatoid arthritis. Rheumatology (Oxford) 2006; 45 (Suppl. 4): iv4–7.

27. Hakala M. Poor prognosis in patients with rheumatoid arthritis hospitalized for interstitial lung fibrosis. Chest 1988; 93: 114–18.

28. Chen YF, Jobanputra P, Barton P, et al. A systematic review of the effectiveness of adalimumab, etanercept and infliximab for the treatment of rheumatoid arthritis in adults and an economic evaluation of their cost-effectiveness. Health Technology Assessment 2006; 10: iii–iv, xi-xiii, 1–229.

29. Nam JL, Winthrop KL, van Vollenhoven RF, et al. Current evidence for the management of rheumatoid arthritis with biological disease-modifying antirheumatic drugs: a systematic literature review informing the EULAR recommendations for the management of RA. Annals of Rheumatic Diseases 2010; 69: 976–86.

30. Sany J, Anaya JM, Canovas F, et al. Influence of methotrexate on the frequency of postoperative infectious complications in patients with rheumatoid arthritis. Journal of Rheumatology 1993; 20: 1129–32.

31. Carpenter MT, West SG, Vogelgesang SA, et al. Postoperative joint infections in rheumatoid arthritis patients on methotrexate therapy. Orthopedics 1996; 19: 207–10.

32. Grennan DM, Gray J, Loudon J, et al. Methotrexate and early postoperative complications in patients with rheumatoid arthritis undergoing elective orthopaedic surgery. Annals of Rheumatic Diseases 2001; 60: 214–17.

33. Rosandich PA, Kelley JT, 3rd, Conn DL. Perioperative management of patients with rheumatoid arthritis in the era of biologic response modifiers. Current Opinion Rheumatology 2004; 16: 192–8.

34. Pieringer H, Stuby U, Biesenbach G. Patients with rheumatoid arthritis undergoing surgery: how should we deal with antirheumatic treatment? Seminars in Arthritis Rheumatics 2007; 36: 278–86.

35. Nockels RP, Shaffrey CI, Kanter AS, et al. Occipitocervical fusion with rigid internal fixation: long-term follow-up data in 69 patients. Journal of Neurosurgery of the Spine 2007; 7: 117–23.

36. Newman P, Sweetnam R. Occipito-cervical fusion. An operative technique and its indications. Journal of Bone Joint Surgery (British volume) 1969; 51: 423–31.

37. Moskovich R, Crockard HA, Shott S, et al. Occipitocervical stabilization for myelopathy in patients with rheumatoid arthritis. Implications of not bone-grafting. Journal of Bone Joint Surgery American 2000; 82: 349–65.

38. Chen HJ, Cheng MH, Lau YC. One-stage posterior decompression and fusion using a Luque rod for occipito-cervical instability and neural compression. Spinal Cord 2001; 39: 101–8.

39. Roy-Camille R, Saillant G, Mazel C. Internal fixation of the unstable spine by a posterior osteosynthesis with plate and screws. Cervical Spine Research Society 1989: 390–404.

40. Grob D, Dvorak J, Panjabi M, et al. Posterior occipitocervical fusion. A preliminary report of a new technique. Spine (Phila Pa 1976) 1991; 16: S17–24.

41. Sutterlin CE, 3rd, Bianchi JR, Kunz DN, et al. Biomechanical evaluation of occipitocervical fixation devices. Journal of Spinal Disorders 2001; 14: 185–92.

42. Oda I, Abumi K, Sell LC, et al. Biomechanical evaluation of five different occipito-atlanto-axial fixation techniques. Spine (Phila Pa 1976) 1999; 24: 2377–82.

43. Winegar CD, Lawrence JP, Friel BC, et al. A systematic review of occipital cervical fusion: techniques and outcomes. Journal of Neurosurgery of the Spine 2010; 13: 5–16.

44. Zygmunt SC, Christensson D, Saveland H, et al. Occipito-cervical fixation in rheumatoid arthritis-an analysis of surgical risk factors in 163 patients. Acta Neurochirugia (Wien) 1995; 135: 25–31.

17 Cervical spondylotic myelopathy

Ellie Broughton

 Expert commentary Nick Haden

Case history

A 60-year-old, right-handed male presented to his GP with a 1-year history of gradual decline in his gait and dexterity. In the last 6 months he had also been experiencing right-sided arm pain radiating into his hand. He was unable to perform fine motor tasks, such as doing up buttons, and had started feeling unsteady on his feet.

His past medical history included hypertension only. He was otherwise well and a retired accountant. Examination findings included right arm numbness in C5 distribution, and loss of co-ordination in his hands and feet. He was hyperreflexic throughout with up-going plantars. Power in his legs was reduced to 4+ in hip flexion bilaterally.

MRI of his cervical spine revealed marked degeneration at C5/6 with cord impingement and foraminal stenosis on the right. There was also less severe degenerative changes at C6/7. His overall spinal alignment was straight (see Figure 17.1).

Given this history and the findings on MRI, a diagnosis of CSM was made. The patient went on to have a two-level anterior cervical discectomy with fusion at the level C5/6 and C6/7.

Post-operatively the patient had resolution of his right-sided arm pain and some improvement in his right arm numbness. Immediate post-operative imaging revealed

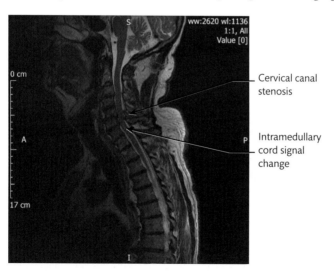

Figure 17.1 T2-weighted MRI cervical spine of the patient showing canal stenosis at C5/6 and C6/7, with intramedullary cord signal change.

Cervical canal stenosis

Intramedullary cord signal change

⭐ **Learning point** Clinical presentation of cervical spondylotic myelopathy

The course of cervical spondylotic myelopathy (CSM) is one of slow and/or stepwise decline [1]. Symptoms include motor and sensory disturbance, diminished balance and dexterity, spasticity, paralysis and sphincter disturbance [2,3]. Additionally, there can be radicular symptoms from nerve root compression.

⭐ **Learning point** Cord signal change

Increased signal on T2 and decreased signal on T1-weighted MRI is correlated with patients who are older, have a longer duration of disease, worse neurology, and worse long-term recovery [3,4]. It is suggested that these changes therefore indicate irreversible cord damage [3]. Focal T2 hyperintensity had better outcomes than multisegment hyperintensity and T1 hypointensity [5,6]. Post-operative expansion of intramedullary high signal on T2 has also been observed and has a worse prognosis for recovery [3].

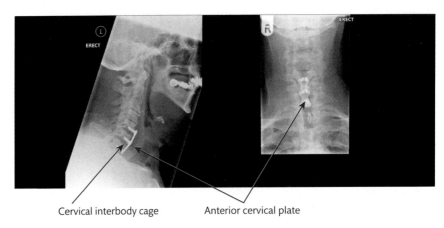

Cervical interbody cage   Anterior cervical plate

Figure 17.2 Post-operative imaging of 2 level ACDF.

satisfactory placement of instrumentation (Figure 17.2). At 6-month follow-up his walking improved. Follow-up imaging revealed no evidence of further kyphosis or instability in the spine, and fusion was obtained.

Discussion

CSM is a progressive degenerative process, resulting in motion abnormalities, loss of disc height, ligamentous redundancy, arthrosis of uncovertebral and facet joints, and formation of osteophytes [3]. This can result in circumferential spinal canal narrowing and nerve root compression [3]. Although this case focuses on the most common cause of myelopathy, degenerative spondylosis, compression can also result from other aetiologies, such as traumatic injuries, tumours, and ossification of the posterior longitudinal ligament [2].

Surgical intervention follows in the case of failed conservative management, or in patients with intractable pain and/or progressive neurology [7]. The prognosis is variable and, if stenosis has been present for many years, then demyelination and necrosis of gray and white matter can lead to irreversible deficits [1,7]. Matz et al. showed that mild CSM can be treated conservatively for up to 3 years with equivalent results to surgery, but it is a progressive disease and severe CSM always requires surgical management [8].

Surgical management of CSM is a challenging concept to neurosurgeons as there are many different factors to consider with each patient to determine the correct operative approach.

The options for treatment including the approach (anterior, posterior, or combined), the number of levels that should be treated and what should be done with the disc space (graft, arthroplasty, or nothing). These choices will be influenced by pathological and patient factors, in addition to the surgeon's overall experience and skill set. It is also important to consider what is achievable, as the aim is to address the pathology while also limiting morbidity and optimizing long-term outcome [9].

Expert comment Principles of treating cervical spondylotic myelopathy

- Neurological decompression and alleviation of symptoms.
- Maintaining stability of the spine.
- Correcting or preserving deformity.

In addition to these key principles, some surgeons advocate maintaining motion.

The pathological factors that were relevant in this case were, first, that the disease was mostly anterior, the alignment was straight overall, and there were both radiculopathic and myelopathic symptoms. The patient factors to consider were his young age, no co-morbidities or neck deformity that might limit the approach and good overall bone quality.

Approach
The first aspect of treatment to consider is the approach.

> **⊕ Learning point** Techniques used in surgical treatment of cervical spondylotic myelopathy
>
> Surgery can be anterior, posterior, or combined. There is no significant difference in outcome with any approach and they all are successful in the treatment of CSM [8,10–13]. The approaches include;
>
> • **Anterior cervical discectomy and fusion** (ACDF).
> • **Anterior cervical corpectomy and fusion** (ACCF).
> • **Anterior cervical discectomy and arthroplasty**.
> • **Laminectomy and fusion:** laminectomy has been associated with late deterioration with kyphosis and, therefore, is only recommended in combination with fusion [10,14].
> • **Laminoplasty:** single or double-door.

The majority of spondylotic disease cases, as in this one, is located anterior and is easier to treat with an anterior approach, where the pathology can be directly visualized and removed without manipulating the spinal cord. This fulfils the first principle of neurological decompression and is the most common approach for CSM [7]. Anterior approaches show good neurological outcome, excellent stability, and carry a low morbidity [5]. When disease is at the extremes of the cervical spine, an anterior approach can become more challenging [7]. Dysphagia, odynophagia, and dysphonia are the most common complications in anterior surgery, but are almost always only in the early post-operative period [11].

ACDF and ACCF are both suitable anterior approaches for decompression and with use of a plate have equivalent fusion rates, although corpectomy has higher rates of graft complication [2,10,15]. ACDF removes soft disc and bony osteophytes and is usually effective in decompressing the spinal canal [3]. Multiple levels can be treated in this way, but if there is disease behind the vertebral body, then ACCF may allow a more complete decompression [10]. This can be particularly important in kyphotic spines, where the cord is draped over osteophyte-disc bars which may not be fully removed with ACDF (see Figure 17.3)[7]. However, some authors report that not only can multilevel ACDF decompress, as well as ACCF, but that there is the additional benefit of improved restoration of lordosis due to increased distraction points and smaller inter-body grafts [16]. This is why multilevel discectomy was chosen in this case, although there is no denying that it can be more difficult and time-consuming than a corpectomy and, therefore, must be the surgeon's choice.

> **⊕ Clinical tip** Factors in surgical decision making
>
> **Pathological factors**
> • Location of pathology.
> • Overall and segmental alignment.
> • Multilevel vs. single-level.
> • Myelopathy vs. radiculopathy.
>
> **Patient factors**
> • Age, co-morbidities.
> • Previous surgery.
> • Pre-existing neck deformity.
> • Bone quality (osteoporosis/ Ankylosing spondylitis (AS)).

> **❝ Expert comment** The anterior approach
>
> An anterior approach is excellent for decompressing the cord, thereby relieving myelopathic symptoms. This patient also had radicular symptoms and, therefore, wide foraminotomies with removal of uncinate spurs should be performed to alleviate this. Some consider it easier and safer (with direct visualization) to decompress the foramina with a posterior approach. However, in this patient, with a straight spine and anterior pathology, I would still advocate an anterior approach.

> **⊕ Clinical tip** Corpectomy
>
> When performing corpectomy the space can be filled with an auto- or allograft material. Allograft is normally bone harvested from the patient's hip. In some centres titanium cages are preferred due to the potential risks of iliac bone harvesting, such as infection, haematoma, and the rare lateral femorocutaneous nerve neuralgia [5]. Some surgeons maintain that autograft bone is superior, in particular tricortical iliac crest bone [16].

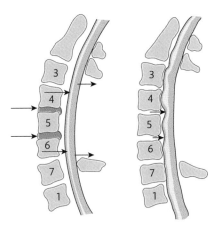

Figure 17.3 Normal lordosis of spine on left image with dorsal migration of cord following laminectomy. The right-hand picture shows a straighter spine with prevention of migration of cord and, therefore, persistent compression after laminectomy.

> **❝ Expert comment**
>
> Post-operative kyphosis is one of the most feared complications of cervical spine surgery; therefore, it is important to have an understanding of a patient's spinal alignment and how surgery can affect it.
>
> Sagittal balance can be assessed on MRI or CT and lateral flexion/extension X-rays will evaluate the degree of instability [17]. In straight or kyphotic spines, an anterior approach is advocated to allow proper distraction and extension, correcting alignment and improving lordosis [2,7,17]. Conversely, posterior approaches in straight or kyphotic spines can worsen the kyphosis, cause instability and restrict neurological improvement [2,7,17,18]. The latter occurs because the spinal cord is tented over anterior pathology and lordosis is required for dorsal migration of the cord away from anterior compression, which cannot occur in a kyphotic spine.

In this case, the spinal alignment was straight overall, with some loss of the natural lordosis of the cervical spine and the pathology was anterior; therefore, an anterior approach is ideal. If there is no anterior pathology then laminectomy with good instrumentation or laminoplasty can be performed in a kyphotic spine, with debate as to whether this increases risk of kyphosis and instability [2,17].

> **✔ Evidence base** How approach affects kyphosis
>
> In forty-eight CSM patients, where twenty-four were fixed anteriorly (corpectomy and cage) and twenty-four posteriorly (laminectomy and lateral mass screws), an initial improvement in lordosis of 8.8 degrees was seen in the anterior group and a decline of 6.5 degrees in the posterior group. Over time, the lordotic correction declined in the anterior group, possibly due to subsidence of the cage before fusion has occurred [18]. Another study of forty-three patients with >10 degrees of kyphosis pre-operatively showed a significant decrease in kyphosis in twenty-eight patients fused anteriorly, compared with fifteen patients with en-bloc C3–7 posterior laminoplasty. However, at long-term follow-up (mean 3.3 years), there was no significant difference in neurological function [19]. Thus, posterior fixation leads to a more constant, but kyphotic alignment than anterior fixation, which may not affect clinical outcome in early follow-up.

The use of curved rods and screws with smaller heads, which can fit closer together, may help with posterior cervical surgery and sagittal balance [18]. However, ultimately anterior spondylotic osteophytes may prevent adequate distraction, decompression, and realignment; in such cases, a combined approach can be considered [9,18,20]. Combined approaches are useful if there is a fixed kyphosis (where there is ankylosis of segments and kyphosis cannot be corrected posturally or with traction), and in cases where there is high risk of multicolumn instability [21].

✪ **Learning point** Fixed kyphosis

One review of sixteen patients demonstrated that combined approaches can correct an average deformity of +38 degrees (kyphosis) to –10 degrees (lordosis), rendering 75% lordotic and 25% straight post-operatively [21].

Combined approaches can be performed in one- or two-stage operations. They offer higher fusion rates for multilevel disease and lower complication rates, particularly in relation to anterior plate/fusion failure and graft dislodgement seen with anterior approach alone [9]. The latter is probably due to the fact that the additional posterior fusion takes the load off the anterior system [20].

Posterior procedures allow dorsal migration of the cord, decreased axial tension and improved vascular perfusion leading to neurological improvement in 70–95% of patients [12,22]. The advantages over anterior surgery include adequate long-segment decompression, wider decompression than anterior approaches (due to limit of vertebral arteries), and no complications of dysphagia or vocal cord palsy [23,24]. This makes them more attractive when performing multisegment surgery. However, the potentials of hardware failure, loss of alignment (kyphosis) or instability are recognized and feared complications in multilevel procedures [12,22].

There are different ways to approach laminectomy, and fusion and lateral mass fixation has been advocated as the procedure of choice, due to its biomechanical properties, simplicity, and low complication rate [23,25].

✔ **Evidence base** Laminectomy

Sekhon et al. looked at fifty patients with CSM, treated with wide posterior decompression (laminectomy) and lateral mass instrumentation with alignment maintained in 96% and fusion in >90% [23]. Kyphotic spines were excluded. The authors also suggest that posterior fusion can result in regression of spondylotic disease, and that there is a low rate of adjacent segment disease (2% at 25.6 months follow-up), due to posterior tension banding allowing micromotion anteriorly and shielding the intervertebral discs from stress of fusion [23].

Bapat et al. reviewed 129 CSM patients, comparing anterior, posterior, and combined approaches [11]. Overall, good outcome was achieved in 86% of patients, allowing a return to work or original levels of activity [11]. A further study of seventy CSM patients decompressed anteriorly showed that 94.2% had some improvement in functional status post-operatively, whilst 5.8% were unchanged and none worsened [5].

Laminoplasty is a good alternative to laminectomy for multilevel disease, with the aim to preserve lordosis and reduce post-op kyphosis [22,24,26]. Motion and stability are maintained and the clinical results at least match, and in some cases are better than that of laminectomy and anterior fusions [13,22,24,26]. It is, however, contraindicated in patients with a fixed kyphosis and anterior pathology due to the anterior tenting discussed previously [26]. Other criticisms are that it causes axial pain and limits the range of motion, although these have not been proven [22].

✔ **Evidence base** Combined approaches

One study of forty patients with anterior and posterior CSM, treated with a combined approach (corpectomy or discectomy anteriorly then fusion +/– laminectomy posteriorly) showed relief of neurological symptoms in all patients at 1-year follow-up with 97.5% radiological fusion [20]. Another study of thirty-five patients with single-stage combined approach showed no cases of pseudoarthrosis or graft/instrumentation related complications [9].

Petraglia reviewed forty patients with CSM who underwent laminoplasty. None developed kyphosis at 31 months follow-up and 90% improved in myelopathic symptoms [24]. Kaminsky et al. reviewed twenty patients with laminoplasty for CSM against twenty-two patients with laminectomies and found a greater improvement in myelopathy and pain in the laminoplasty group [22]. Laminoplasty was also associated with fewer complications compared with laminectomy, largely related to post-operative kyphosis and instability [22].

Number of levels treated

A challenging aspect in some cases can be the decision regarding how many levels to fuse. In this case, although the most severe and symptomatic disease was at C5/6, the neighbouring C6/7 level had also degenerated. Multiple levels can often be affected in CSM, as is the nature of the condition, and deciding on whether to treat only the worst affected/symptomatic levels or to treat other affected levels within the same operation can be difficult. The risk with the former is that adjacent segment disease (ASD) can occur post-operatively, resulting in progressive, symptomatic disease at already degenerate levels. To avoid this, all affected levels (C5/6 and C6/7) could be treated in one operation, increasing the length and complexity of the operation, but potentially preventing ASD. This was the chosen management plan in this patient.

Older patients with a higher degree of ASD evident on pre-operative imaging have higher rates and earlier onset of symptomatic ASD post-operatively, supporting the case for a naturally progressing condition [27,28]. Rates of symptomatic ASD have been reported from 2 to 17%, strongly influenced by the follow-up time, as the average delay can be around 6.5 years [11,15,27]. One long-term follow-up study showed a yearly incidence around 2.9% and, therefore, a 10-year prevalence of 19% [28]. The levels most commonly affected are C4/5, C5/6, and C6/7, and paradoxically multilevel fusion has shown to be lower risk than single level, which may be related to multisegment fusions covering the higher risk levels [27,28]. However, there is concern that long-rigid constructs produced with combined approaches can cause instability [9]. Use of disc prosthesis to maintain motion at operated segments has been recommended as a potential method of reducing ASD, and this will be discussed further [29].

If multiple levels are more attractive to treat, due to minimizing ASD, then one must weigh this up against the risks of multilevel surgery and how this might affect the chosen approach.

> **⑥ Expert comment** Considering multilevel surgery
>
> An anterior approach is successful at treating one or two diseased levels, but more than two levels becomes more controversial, due to the higher risk of complications (dysphagia, dysphonia), and a higher incidence of non-union and graft-related problems [2,19]. Multilevel disease is more classically approached posteriorly, as this is considered to be quicker and carry less morbidity than its anterior counterpart [17]. However, one study of seventy anterior approaches, including single-, double-, and triple-level surgery, showed that the number of levels had no impact on functional recovery [5]. If an anterior approach is used for multiple levels then a corpectomy and fusion may by preferred to multiple ACDFs as discussed earlier.

Deciding on the number of levels to treat will also be strongly influenced by patient factors. In this case, the patient was young and fit, and could tolerate a longer and more complex multilevel operation. There would also be easy access to most levels, as he had good range of movement in the neck and no fixed deformity. His age means there are potentially many more years of wear and tear for his neck to withstand, and the two-level surgery may help prevent ASD progressing over time, causing him symptoms from the lower already-diseased level.

The disc space

Fusion can be achieved with either graft or an empty disc space with an anterior plate. The benefit of fusion is to eliminate painful motion at the spondylotic segment treated and improve stability and sagittal alignment [2]. However, as previously discussed, the fear with cervical fusion is that reduction of normal cervical spine movement results in increased stress at adjacent levels [30,31].

Arthroplasty is an alternative to fusion that, by restoring disc height and segmental motion at the operated level, preserves normal motion at neighbouring levels [30,32]. However, it is not clear currently whether emphasis should be placed on maintenance of motion, as this in itself has the potential to exacerbate myelopathic symptoms and disease progression [26].

> **⑥ Expert comment** Arthroplasty
>
> It should also be remembered that, while ACDF is a relatively standardized procedure, arthroplasty is still new, and there are a variety of types and techniques being used, which undoubtedly influence the outcome. There is no good evidence of efficacy in kyphotic spines and long-term follow-up data are limited. Ultimately, the surgeons own preference and experience must be used.

⚡ **Evidence base** Arthroplasty

Du et al. followed twenty-five arthroplasty patients over an average of 15.3 months, 48% of whom had straight spines [30]. Post-operatively, there was significant functional improvement, significant increase in global lordosis, and no complications with the arthroplasty such as subsidence [30].

Quan et al. did one of the longest follow-up studies (over 8 years) looking at twenty-seven disc arthroplasties for spondylosis induced radiculopathy [31]. No patient required further surgery on the same or adjacent levels and physiological mobility was maintained in 78% (22% became fused) [31]. Nineteen percent showed evidence of adjacent segment degeneration, but 75% of these were from the fused group and all had pre-operative signs of degeneration at adjacent levels [31].

Coric et al. showed that radiographic ASD was only 9% in arthroplasty patients compared with 25% in ACDF patients [32].

Clinical improvement in arthroplasty is at least equivalent to that achieved with discectomy and fusion [31, 32, 33]. Additionally, complications from plating, pseudarthosis, and the need for external orthosis are avoided [30].

⭐ **Learning point** Complications of arthroplasty

- **Heterotopic ossification:** can restrict movement and has been shown to increase with time, especially if more than 1 level is treated [31].
- **Kyphosis:** has been recognized to develop over time and therefore many of the studies exclude kyphotic spines [30,31]. However, some studies show improved lordosis, and it is suggested that good technique with optimum preparation of end plates is crucial in preventing anterior displacement of the arthroplasty and subsequent kyphosis [30,34].
- **Other spinal deformities:** ensuring central placement of the arthroplasty should prevent coronal plane deformities and unequal loading of facets resulting in arthrosis [33].

Arthroplasty implants can deteriorate over time and become misplaced [29].

A final word from the expert

There are quite clearly many issues when deciding on how to approach the spine, and these must be weighed up again one another, so that there is minimal risk, but maximal neurological benefit for the patient. Deciding on the direction of approach, number of levels and graft materials to use is a complex and challenging area in the treatment of cervical spondylotic myelopathy.

Immediate outcome from CSM surgery are in general very good. The best predictor of lower functional score post-operatively is low score pre-operatively [5,22]. This is unsurprising and supports early treatment to maintain neurology for as long as possible. Changes in cord signal at presentation also carry prognostic information and can be helpful in predicting outcome.

References

1. Matz. The natural history of cervical spondylotic myelopathy. Journal of Neurosurgery of the Spine 2009; 11: 104–11.
2. Edwards CC, Riew KD, Anderson PA, et al. Cervical myelopathy: current diagnostic and treatment strategies. Spine Journal 2003; 3: 68–81.
3. Yagi M, Ninomiya K, Kihara M, et al. Long-term surgical outcome and risk factors in patients with cervical myelopathy and a change in signal intensity of intramedullary

spinal cord on magnetic resonance imaging. Journal of Neurosurgery of the Spine 2010; 12: 59–65.

4. Zhang P, Shen Y, Zhang YZ, et al. Significance of increased intensity on MRI in prognosis after surgical intervention for cervical spondylotic myelopathy. Journal of Clinical Neuroscience 2011; 18: 1080–3.

5. Chibbaro S, Benvenuti L, Carnesecchi S, et al. Anterior cervical corpectomy for cervical spondylotic myelopathy: experience and surgical results in a series of 70 consecutive patients. Journal of Clinical Neuroscience 2006; 13: 233–8.

6. Fernandez de rota JJ, Meschian S, Fernández de Rota A, et al. Cervical spondylotic myelopathy due to chronic compression: the role of signal intensity changes in magnetic resonance images. Journal of Neurosurgery of the Spine 2007; 6: 17–22.

7. Medow JE, Trost G, Sandin J. Surgical management of cervical myelopathy: indications and techniques for surgical corpectomy. Spine Journal 2006; 6: 233S–41S.

8. Matz PG, Holly LT, Mummaneni PV, et al. Anterior cervical surgery for the treatment of cervical degenerative myelopathy. Journal of Neurosurgery of the Spine 2009; 11: 170–3.

9. Kim PF, Alexander JT. Indications for circumferential surgery for cervical spondylotic myelopathy. Spine Journal 2006; 6: 299S–307S.

10. Mummaneni PV, Kaiser MG, Matz PG, et al. Cervical surgical techniques for the treatment of cervical spondylotic myelopathy. Journal of Neurosurgery of the Spine 2009; 11: 130–41.

11. Bapat MR, Chaudhary K, Sharma A., et al. Surgical approach to cervical spondylotic myelopathy on the basis of radiological patterns of compression: prospective analysis of 129 cases. European Spine Journal 2008; 17 (12): 1651–3.

12. Anderson. Laminectomy and fusion for the treatment of cervical degenerative myelopathy. Journal of Neurosurgery of the Spine 2009; 11: 150–6.

13. Matz PG, Anderson PA, Groff MW, et al. Cervical laminoplasty for the treatment of cervical degenerative myelopathy. Journal of Neurosurgery of the Spine 2009; 11: 157–69.

14. Ryken TC, Heary RF, Matz PG, et al. Cervical laminectomy for the treatment of cervical degenerative myelopathy. Journal of Neurosurgery of the Spine 2009; 11: 142–9.

15. Andaluz N, Zuccarello M, Kuntz C. Long-term follow-up of cervical radiographic sagittal spinal alignment after 1- and 2-level cervical corpectomy for the treatment of spondylosis of the subaxial cervical spine causing radiculomyelopathy or myelopathy: a retrospective study. Journal of Neurosurgery of the Spine 2012; 16 (1): 2–7.

16. Hillard VH, Apfelbaum RI. Surgical management of cervical myelopathy: indications and techniques for multilevel cervical discectomy. Spine Journal 2006;6(6 Suppl.): 242S–51S.

17. Wiggins GC, Shaffrey CI. Dorsal surgery for myelopathy and myeloradiculopathy. Neurosurgery 2007; 60: S71–S81.

18. Cabraja M, Abbushi A, Koeppen D, et al. Comparison between anterior and posterior decompression with instrumentation for cervical spondylotic myelopathy: sagittal alignment and clinical outcome. Neurosurgical Focu S 2010; 28 (3): E15.

19. Uchida K, Nakajima H, Sato R, et al. Cervical spondylotic myelopathy associated with kyphosis or sagittal sigmoid alignment: outcome after anterior or posterior decompression. Journal of Neurosurgery of the Spine 2009; 11: 521–8.

20. Konya D, Ozgen S, Gercek A, et al. Outcomes for combined anterior and posterior surgical approaches for patients with multisegmental cervical spondylotic myelopathy. Journal of Clinical Neuroscience 2009; 16 (3): 404–9.

21. O'Shaughnessy BA, Liu JC, Hsieh PC, et al. Surgical Treatment of Fixed Cervical Kyphosis With Myelopathy. Spine (Phil Pa 1976) 2008; 33 (7): 771–8.

22. Kaminsky SB, Clark CR, Traynelis VC. Operative treatment of cervical spondylotic myelopathy and radiculopathy. A comparison of laminectomy and laminoplasty at five year average follow-up. Iowa Orthopedic Journal 2004; 24: 95–105.

23. Sekhon LH. Posterior cervical decompression and fusion for circumferential spondylotic cervical stenosis: review of 50 consecutive cases. Clinical Neuroscience 2006; 13 (1): 23–30.

24. Petraglia AL, Srinivasan V, Coriddi M, et al. Cervical laminoplasty as a management option for patients with cervical spondylotic myelopathy: a series of 40 patients. Neurosurgery 2010; 67 (2): 272–7.
25. Komotar RJ, Mocco J, Kaiser MG. Surgical management of cervical myelopathy: indications and techniques for laminectomy and fusion. Spine Journal 2006; 6: 252S–67S.
26. Hale JJ, Gruson KI, Spivak JM. Laminoplasty: a review of its role in compressive cervical myelopathy. Spine Journal 2006; 6: 289S–98S.
27. Ishihara H, Kanamori M, Kawaguchi Y, et al. Adjacent segment disease after anterior cervical interbody fusion. Spine Journal 2004; 4: 624–8.
28. Hilibrand AS, Carlson GD, Palumbo MA, et al. Radiculopathy and myelopathy at segments adjacent to the site of a previous anterior cervical arthrodesis. Journal of Bone and Joint Surgery 1999; 81-A(4): 519–28.
29. Seo M, &Choi D. Adjacent segment disease after fusion for cervical spondylosis; myth or reality? British journal of neurosurgery 2008; 22 (2): 195–199.
30. Du J, Li M, Liu H, et al. Early follow-up outcomes after treatment of degenerative disc disease with the discover cervical disc prosthesis. Spine Journal 2011; 11 (4): 281–9.
31. Quan GM, Vital JM, Hansen S, et al. Eight-year clinical and radiological follow-up of the Bryan cervical disc arthroplasty. Spine (Phila Pa 1976) 2011; 36 (8): 639–46.
32. Coric D, Nunley PD, Guyer RD, et al. Prospective, randomized, multicenter study of cervical arthroplasty: 269 patients from the Kineflex|C artificial disc investigational device exemption study with a minimum 2-year follow-up: clinical article. Journal of Neurosurgery of the Spine 2011; 15 (4): 348–58.
33. Cardoso MJ, Rosner MK. Multilevel cervical arthroplasty with artificial disc replacement. Neurosurgery FocuS 2010; 28 (5): E19.
34. Woo Kim, Jae Hyuk Shin, Jose Joefrey Arbatin, et al. Effects of a cervical disc prosthesis on maintaining sagittal alignment of the functional spinal unit and overall sagittal balance of the cervical spine. European Spine Journal 2008; 17 (1): 20–9.

18 Brainstem cavernous malformation

Harith Akram

Ⓒ Expert commentary Mary Murphy

Case history

A 53-year-old Caucasian woman presented with sudden onset occipital headache with double vision, right-sided facial numbness and loss of balance, which developed over a few minutes. She was found to have a right-sided gaze palsy and a right internuclear opthalmoplegia (one-and-a-half syndrome), right-sided upper motor neuron (UMN) facial weakness and associated right-sided limb ataxia. A plain CT scan of the head showed a large right-sided pontine haemorrhage (see Figure 18.1). A brain MRI showed a 30 × 25 × 25mm right-sided pontine multicystic space-occupying lesion with surrounding haemorrhage. The ventricular system was of normal size with no signs of hydrocephalus (see Figure 18.2a–c).

The patient made a slow, but meaningful neurological recovery over a period of months. She experienced four further episodes of spontaneous bleeding over a course of 3 years. Each episode typically resulted in neurological deterioration followed by slow improvement. The patient had no previous family history of cerebral cavernous malformations.

✪ Learning point Brainstem gaze centres and the medial longitudinal fasiculus

A simplified model of gaze would involve three regions—the frontal gaze centres with control of saccadic eye movements, the occipital gaze centres for pursuit and accommodation, and the brainstem gaze centres. These form a complicated internuclear connection network between the oculomotor, trochlear, and abducent nuclei, the vestibular brainstem nuclei and the mesencephalic nucleus of trigeminal nerve which provides feedback concerning head movement. The horizontal gaze centre is located in the abducent nucleus and possibly the parapontine reticular formation. The medial longitudinal fasiculus (MLF) connects the ipsilateral abducent nucleus with the contralateral oculomotor nucleus. Damage to the MLF results in internuclear opthalmoplegia (INO). Damage to the abducent nucleus, in addition, would result in 'one-and-a-half' syndrome, where there is complete paralysis of horizontal pursuit movement in the ipsilateral eye (the eye is fixed), and ipsilateral horizontal conjugate gaze palsy with preserved convergence.

Note that the nucleus of the facial nerve is in the proximity of the abducent nucleus.

The case was discussed at the local neurovascular Multidisciplinary team (MDT) meeting. Surgical excision of the lesion was proposed to the patient, but the patient was inclined to explore a non-operative management option. Therefore, the case was referred to the radiosurgery MDT meeting and the patient was deemed an appropriate candidate for treatment with radiosurgery. An application to the Primary Care Trust (PCT) was made to fund the treatment.

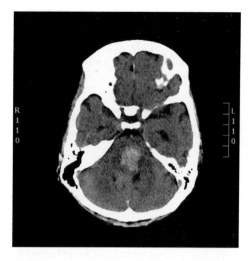

Figure 18.1 A plain CT scan of head showing hyperdensity in the pons in keeping with an acute haemorrhage.

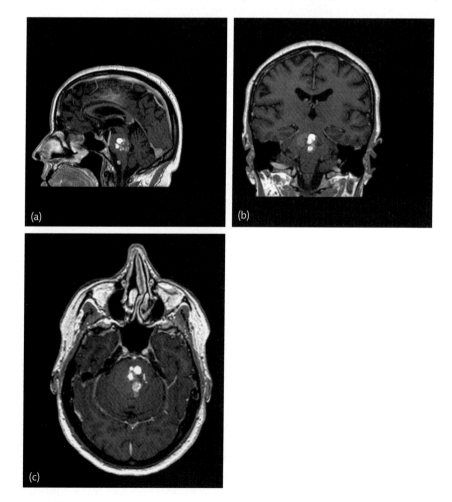

Figure 18.2 (a,b,c) Sagittal, coronal, and axial MRI scans showing a multicystic lesion (cavernoma) in the pons.

Discussion

Cavernous malformations or cavernomas are angiographically occult vascular malformations that affect the brain and spinal cord. Walter Dandy described the first surgical excision of a brainstem cavernous malformation in 1928 in a 31-year-old man, who presented with 'stiffness in his right leg in spells'; Dandy stated that the patient 'was living and well' at follow up [1].

The true incidence of cavernous malformation became clear only following the development of MRI, as the vast majority of lesions are not detectable on angiography. Cavernomas of the CNS affect 0.4–0.9% of the population and account for 8–15% of all vascular malformations with 9–35% of cavernomas affecting the brainstem [2]. Post-mortem studies suggest that nearly 4% of the population have cavernous malformations [3], but with the ready availability of MRI in modern practice, the detection of incidental lesions (incidentalomas) has become more common, leading to an increasing number of referrals to neurosurgeons.

Cavernous malformations were thought to be purely congenital lesions; however, this has proven not to be the case as long-term follow-up especially of the familial variety showed that some lesions can develop de novo. Follow-up has also shown that those lesions are not static and can increase in size with time [3].

Cavernomas are histologically composed of sinusoidal layers of immature vascular endothelium, with evidence of chronic haemorrhage with haemosiderin-laden macrophages in the periphery of the lesion. There is no brain parenchyma within the lesion and no shunting. Gliotic changes are seen around the lesion. Occasionally, cystic formation signifying previous bleeding can be seen and some lesions have calcium deposits within them [4].

Presentation depends on the location of the lesion. Supratentorial lesions present with seizures in 50% of cases, focal neurological deficit in 30% of patients, and headache in 25% of patients. Patients can also present acutely with intracerebral haemorrhage and symptoms due to mass effect.

Infratentorial lesions very rarely present with seizures (3%) and usually present with focal neurological deficit due to haemorrhage, which can lead to mass effect and occasionally obstructive hydrocephalus. Brainstem and spinal cord cavernomas have a variety of presentations. Due to the fact that the brainstem and the spinal cord are composed of densely packed nuclei and tracts cavernomas present early with neurological deficit depending on the location and size of the lesion. There is a spectrum of deficit from gaze palsy, long tract signs to coma, and death from brainstem damage.

Bleeding risk is difficult to ascertain, especially as these lesions exhibit micro-haemorrhages, explaining the presence of haemosiderin around the lesions even when there are no documented episodes of haemorrhage. The estimated risk of clinically significant haemorrhage in non-brainstem cavernomas is 0.1–1% per lesion per year. The risk of rebleeding is 4.5% if a single haemorrhage has occurred, but is much higher if there have been two or more clinically significant bleeds. Brainstem cavernomas have a higher rate of haemorrhage, this is largely due to the fact that even minor haemorrhages are symptomatic due to the tightly packed nuclei and tracts in the brainstem. The estimated risk of bleeding is 5% per year with a documented risk of rebleeding as high as 30% per year, the interval between haemorrhages is unpredictable [2].

A familial form of CCM has been described and linked to genetic mutations affecting the long arm of chromosome 7 (7q) [CCM1], the short arm of chromosome 7 (7p)

❝ Expert comment

Developmental venous anomalies (DVAs) can be useful radiological landmarks, but are not useful operatively, when one is generally trying to avoid them.

❂ Learning point

When cavernomas bleed, the haematoma tends to be 'intralesional', which leads to expansion of the lesion and resultant mass effect in contrast to arteriovenous malformations (AVMs), which cause bleeding into the brain tissue and or the subarachnoid space. For this reason cavernomas do not generally present with subarachnoid haemorrhage (SAH).

❝ Expert comment

Cavernomas can change dramatically in their radiological appearance over time due to repeated haemorrhages. This may have the effect of making them seem to 'grow' in a particular direction. Having said that, this phenomenon can result in an improvement in the suitability for operative resection.

[CCM2], and the long arm of chromosome 3 (3q) [CCM3] [5]. This entity is common amongst Hispanic Americans and can often present with multiple lesions. It is now believed that more than 55% of patients with cerebral cavernomas have familial tendencies [6]. Radiological follow-up of those patients shows that the lesions can change in size with time and new lesions can appear de novo [3].

❂ Learning point Imaging

The development of MRI played a major role in defining and understanding cavernous malformations, which were often termed angiographically occult or cryptic vascular malformations. Occasionally, a focal capillary blush can be seen on angiography. A developmental venous anomaly is a common finding adjacent to a cavernous malformation. CT imaging is often negative, except when there is an associated haematoma or calcification. The lesions have a characteristic 'popcorn' appearance on MRI and a signal loss is almost always seen surrounding the lesion on T2* (gradient echo) sequences representing haemosiderin deposition from chronic bleeding. The lesions can sometimes be multicystic due to previous bleeding episodes [7].

❂ Learning point Cavernomas and developmental venous anomalies

Developmental venous anomalies (DVA) are thought to be caused by a foetal vascular accident resulting in an anomalous vein draining the surrounding brain tissue. The lesions have a 'caput medusa' appearance on imaging. They are benign and do not result in bleeding. DVAs must be preserved during surgery as they drain normal brain tissue and damaging them can lead to a venous infarct. DVAs are often associated with cavernous malformations especially in the posterior fossa. Porter et al. found a 100% association with brainstem cavernomas intra-operatively. Therefore, they hypothesized that DVAs may play a role in the formation of brainstem cavernomas and their postoperative recurrence because of this intimate association [2].

Brainstem cavernomas pose a challenging pathological entity. The commonest location is the pons in 60% followed by the midbrain, then the medulla oblongata. Due to the fact that the brainstem contains tightly-packed cranial nerve nuclei and long tract fibres, the slightest damage could lead to a catastrophic deficit. Therefore, brainstem cavernomas tend to present earlier and with much smaller haematomas than cavernomas in other locations in the CNS. They can present due to progressive neurological deficit from mass effect or direct damage to neural structures. Patients can also present acutely due to haemorrhage and/or obstructive hydrocephalus, which can lead to coma and death. Posterior fossa cavernomas do not present with seizures. Natural history studies have shown the risk of rebleeding from brainstem cavernomas to be significantly higher than cavernomas elsewhere in the CNS and can be as high as 30% per year. Cavernomas that present with haemorrhage are more likely to bleed again when compared with incidental cavernomas [2,8,9].

Management of cavernomas varies considerably with the location and size of the lesion, the symptoms associated with it, and patient specific factors, i.e. age and other comorbidities. Asymptomatic (incidental) lesions can be treated conservatively with clinical and radiological follow-up. Patients who present with epilepsy may benefit from surgical excision of the lesion with the surrounding haemosiderin ring, although surgery is not guaranteed to stop the seizures.

Patients who present with mass effect or obstructive hydrocephalus from acute haemorrhage may require emergency evacuation of the haematoma, excision of the cavernoma and CSF diversion if required. In general, deep-seated lesions or lesions in eloquent locations are best treated conservatively if safe surgical excision is not possible.

The management of brainstem cavernomas and spinal cord cavernomas differs from the management of cavernomas elsewhere in the CNS due to the much higher risk of rebleeding, and the fact that very little mass effect or haemorrhage can lead to catastrophic consequences. Some authors recommend surgical excision through skull base approaches to lesions that abut the pial surface or only have a thin layer of tissue covering in symptomatic patients with two or more previous episodes of haemorrhage or one episode of haemorrhage that did not lead to a full recovery. Asymptomatic patients or patients with one previous episode of haemorrhage who go on to make a full recovery, could be treated conservatively along with patients with deep-seated brainstem lesions [2,10–13].

Another relatively modern treatment modality is stereotactic radiosurgery, i.e. Gamma knife or Cyberknife to lesions in eloquent locations when surgery is contraindicated, or is expected to result in significant morbidity or mortality. Hasegawa et al. published long-term follow-up results of eighty-two patients with high risk cavernomas treated with gamma knife in the University of Pittsburgh, Pennsylvania, between 1987 and 2000. They showed a significant reduction of the annual risk of bleeding, which was most pronounced after 2 years of treatment with minimal side effects from the treatment itself [14].

To date, there is no Class 1 evidence that stereotactic radiosurgery works, due to the difficulty in performing such a study. Advocates of surgery remain sceptical about this form of treatment [2,10].

> ✚ **Clinical tip** Surgical approaches to brainstem cavernomas—the two-point method
>
> Surgical approaches to brainstem cavernomas require a highly-skilled surgical team with meticulous pre-operative planning, including specialised imaging modalities such as tractography, which may play an increasing role in the future planning of surgical approaches. It is absolutely crucial to plan the entry point to the brainstem pre-operatively and not to rely heavily on neuronavigation systems as even a minimal amount of brain shift can be misleading. This is generally not a problem when dealing with large lesions that reach the surface.
>
> A good planning strategy is to draw a line from the centre of the lesion to the most superficial point and out through the skull. This line can be used as a guide to decide on the best surgical corridor to use in order to avoid retraction and minimize injury to neural tissue. The approaches commonly utilized are the retrosigmoid, the suboccipital, the far lateral, and the subtemporal approaches [11–13,15,16].

> ✚ **Clinical tip**
>
> When operating, ensure you have the best equipment available. Do not compromise on the patient's position, the quality of dissectors, retractors, bipolar coagulation forceps, suction, or microscope. For a brainstem cavernoma operation, everything needs to be working at its best, especially the surgeon!

A final word from the expert

Never operate on brainstem cavernomas if avoidable; many neurovascular surgeons wait for more than one symptomatic bleed. Timing is crucial—the patient must have some salvageable neurology that one would expect to be irreversibly lost if surgery was not undertaken.

References

1. Brown DL, Archer SB, Greenhalgh DG, et al. Inhalation injury severity scoring system: a quantitative method. Journal of Burn Care & Rehabilitation 1996; 17: 552–7.
2. Porter RW, Detwiler PW, Spetzler RF, et al. Cavernous malformations of the brainstem: experience with 100 patients. Journal of Neurosurgery 1999; 90: 50–8.
3. Zabramski JM, Wascher TM, Spetzler RF, et al. The natural history of familial cavernous malformations: results of an ongoing study. Journal of Neurosurgery 1994; 80: 422–32.
4. Gault J, Sarin H, Awadallah NA, et al. Pathobiology of human cerebrovascular malformations: basic mechanisms and clinical relevance. Neurosurgery 2004; 55: 1–16; discussion 16–17.
5. Mindea SA, Yang BP, Shenkar R, et al. Cerebral cavernous malformations: clinical insights from genetic studies. Neurosurgery Focus 2006; 21: e1.
6. Gunel M, Awad IA, Finberg K, et al. A founder mutation as a cause of cerebral cavernous malformation in Hispanic Americans. New England Journal of Medicine 1996; 334: 946–51.
7. Rigamonti D, Drayer BP, Johnson PC, et al. The MRI appearance of cavernous malformations (angiomas). Journal of Neurosurgery 1987; 67: 518–24.
8. Fritschi JA, Reulen HJ, Spetzler RF, et al. Cavernous malformations of the brain stem. A review of 139 cases. Acta Neurochirugia (Wien) 1994; 130: 35–46.
9. Zimmerman RS, Spetzler RF, Lee KS, et al. Cavernous malformations of the brain stem. Journal of Neurosurgery 1991; 75: 32–9.
10. Abla AA, Lekovic GP, Garrett M, et al. Cavernous malformations of the brainstem presenting in childhood: surgical experience in 40 patients. Neurosurgery 2010; 67: 1589–98; discussion 1598–9.
11. Abla AA, Turner JD, Mitha AP, et al. Surgical approaches to brainstem cavernous malformations. Neurosurgery Focus 2010; 29: E8.
12. Garrett M, Spetzler RF. Surgical treatment of brainstem cavernous malformations. Surgical Neurology 2009; 72 (Suppl. 2): S3-9; discussion S9–10.
13. Wang CC, Liu A, Zhang JT, et al. Surgical management of brain-stem cavernous malformations: report of 137 cases. Surgical Neurology 2003; 59: 444–54; discussion 454.
14. Hasegawa T, McInerney J, Kondziolka D, et al. Long-term results after stereotactic radiosurgery for patients with cavernous malformations. Neurosurgery 2002; 50: 1190–7; discussion 1197–8.
15. Brown AP, Thompson BG, Spetzler RF. The two-point method: evaluating brain stem lesions. Barrow Neurological Institute Quarterly 1996; 12: 20–4.
16. Degn J, Brennum J. Surgical treatment of trigeminal neuralgia. Results from the use of glycerol injection, microvascular decompression, and rhizotomia. Acta Neurochirugia (Wien) 2010; 152: 2125–32.

19 Peripheral nerve injury

Sophie J. Camp

⊕ Expert Commentary Rolfe Birch

Case history

Whilst serving abroad, a 23-year-old, right-handed, male soldier sustained life-threatening injuries from an improvised explosive device (IED) blast. These included a closed head injury (petechial haemorrhage in the basal ganglia), a right mandibular fracture, a comminuted left olecranon fracture, soft tissue damage to the left forearm, bilateral hand injuries (soft tissue damage to all fingers of the right hand, right ring proximal phalanx fracture, soft tissue damage to all fingers of the left hand), abdominal wound to the left iliac fossa, perineal injury, an open pelvic fracture, a right anterior acetabular fracture, and severe lower limb injuries, requiring bilateral below knee amputations.

The patient had no previous past medical history and was not taking any regular medication. He had no family history of note and lived with his parents. He smoked 20 cigarettes per day, and regularly drank large amounts of alcohol.

The patient underwent multiple surgical procedures of relevance to the upper limbs: open reduction and internal fixation (ORIF) to the left olecranon with debridement of the distal left humerus, debridement of the left upper limb with local fasciocutaneous flap to cover the instrumentation at the left elbow, left ulnar nerve graft at the elbow (7cm defect in the nerve) using the right common peroneal nerve taken from the amputated limb, right-hand debridement with closure of wounds on the index, middle, ring, and little fingers, and closed reduction of a proximal phalanx fracture of the right ring finger with K wire and rotation flap, split skin graft to the left forearm, and removal of plate from proximal left ulna due to infection.

The patient had a prolonged stay in the Intensive Therapy Unit. He reported that at no stage did he feel pain in his upper limb. There was a history of quadriplegia initially. However, the patient noted sensation and strong movement of the lower limbs within 7 days. With regard to the upper limbs, he was unable to move or feel both of these for 6–7 weeks. Recovery of sensation started in the right upper limb at 7 weeks from injury and followed thereafter in the left upper limb. This proceeded from distal to proximal in both upper limbs. Movement had commenced in the right hand by 9 weeks, and in the left 11–12 weeks.

> **⊕ Clinical tip** Symptoms to note
>
> When taking the history it is imperative to note the nature and distribution of pain, abnormal sensation, alteration or loss of sensibility, weakness, motor paralysis, and impairment of function. There may be no pain or it may be delayed in onset. It may be episodic or continuous. The presence of severe crushing or burning pain, typically in the forearm, and hand or leg and foot, and shooting pain in the distribution of the nerve(s) indicates neuropathic pain. Associated abnormal sensations suggest continued action of the noxious agent [1].

The patient was first reviewed in the War Nerve Injuries Clinic 40 weeks post-injury, and then subsequently at monthly intervals. Appearance of the proximal right upper limb was unremarkable. Clawing of the right metacarpophalangeal (MCP) joints was noted, with deformity of the right ring finger (proximal phalanx fracture), and bilateral scarring of the fingers (soft tissue injuries). The left forearm sustained massive, circumferential, soft tissue destruction, with extensive muscle loss (split skin graft noted). However, pulses were preserved throughout the left upper limb. The left elbow was ankylosed. No Horner's sign was detected or clinical evidence of phrenic nerve injury.

Neurological examination of the right upper limb revealed intact sensation to light touch and pin prick. Temperature sense and joint position sense were preserved in the right upper limb. Sensation to light touch and pin prick were present in the left upper limb, except in the left forearm containing the split skin graft and in the distribution of the left ulnar nerve, where it was abnormal to light touch and absent to pin prick. Temperature sense was impaired in the left upper limb. Joint position sense (at the thumb) was preserved. These findings did not change during the subsequent clinic reviews (over an 8-week period).

With regard to the motor examination, tone was normal in the upper limbs. Power gradings at first clinic review and at a later time point are detailed in Table 19.1.

Table 19.1 Medical Research Council (MRC) power grading of selected muscles in the upper limbs at two time points

Muscle: innervation	Right		Left	
	T0	T1	T0	T1
Trapezius: CN XI	4	5	5	5
Serratus anterior: C5,6,7	5	5	5	5
Supraspinatus: C5,(6)	4	4	3	4
Infraspinatus: C5,(6)	4	4	4	4
Latissimus dorsi: C7	5	5	4	4
Deltoid (all heads): C(5),6	2	3	1	1
Clavicular head of pectoralis major: C6,(7)	5	5	5	5
Sternal head of pectoralis major: C7,(8)	4	4	0	0
Triceps (all heads): C6,7,8	3	4	0	0
Biceps: C6	5	5	Present, but difficult to examine due to ankylosis	
Brachioradialis: C6	5	5		
Extensor carpi radialis longus and brevis (ECRL & B): C6,(7)	4	4	Active, but complete loss of continuity of extensor muscles	
Abductor pollicis longus (APL): C8	5	5	0	0
Extensor pollicis longus (EPL): C8	5	5	0	0
Flexi carpi radialis (FCR): C(6),7	5	5	0	0
Flexi carpi ulnaris (FCU): C(7),8	4	4	0	0
Flexor digitorum superficialis (FDS): C(7),8 index	4	5	3	4
middle	4	5	3	3
ring	0	1	2	2
little	0	2	0	0
Flexor digitorum profundus (FDP): C8,T1 index	4	4	3	3
middle	3	3	2	2
ring	0	0	1	1
little	0	0	0	0
Flexor pollicis longus (FPL): C8 index	3	4	3	4
Flexor pollicis brevis (FPB): T1	3	4	3	3
Interossei: T1	0	0	0	0

T0: time zero (first clinic review); T1: 8 weeks later; CNXI: cranial nerve XI (spinal accessory nerve)

Reflexes were present in the upper limbs. Tinel's sign was negative over the supra-clavicular and infraclavicular brachial plexus bilaterally. A positive Tinel's sign was noted at the proximal repair line of the left ulnar nerve and, again, present 15cm distal to the medial epicondyle. Initially, the proximal Tinel's sign was stronger. Eight weeks later, the distal Tinel's sign had progressed distally and was stronger. Sudomotor function was normal in the right upper limb, but absent on the left.

Examination of the shoulders on first clinic review revealed fixed deformity bilaterally. The passive inferior scapulohumeral angle (a measure of elevation at the glenohumeral joint) was 70 degrees on the right, 40 degrees on the left. Eight weeks later, following intensive physiotherapy, this had improved to 130 degrees on the right and 110 degrees on the left. The active values at the later review were 130 and 90 degrees on the right and left, respectively.

✚ Clinical tip Detailed examination

When undertaking the clinical examination it should be possible to ascertain the level and depth of the lesion. A sound grasp of the level of the branches of the trunk nerve and of the contribution to that nerve coming from the individual spinal nerves is a prerequisite [1]. To this end, the latest (4th) edition of *Aids to the Examination of the Peripheral Nervous System* by Michael O'Brien (2010) is invaluable [2]. The DVD companion 'Examination of the Limb Muscles' by Birch [1] *Surgical Disorders of the Peripheral Nerves* is also useful.

✪ Learning point Types of brachial plexus injury

Brachial plexus injuries can be divided into preganglionic and postganglionic lesions. Preganglionic injuries have been further classified by Bonney [3]:

- **Type A:** roots torn central to transition zone; true avulsion.
- **Type B:** roots torn distal to transition zone.
  - ○ Dura torn within spinal canal; dorsal root ganglion (DRG) displaced into neck.
  - ○ Dura torn at mouth of foramen; DRG more or less displaced.
  - ○ Dura not torn; DRG not displaced.
  - ○ Dura not torn; DRG not displaced; either ventral or dorsal root intact.

Post-ganglionic lesions, as for all peripheral nerves, can be subdivided using Seddon's classification [4]:

- **Neurapraxia:** due to blunt trauma; myelin injury or ischemia; complete recovery without degeneration.
- **Axonotmesis:** axonal loss; complete peripheral degeneration occurs, but recovery follows due to preservation of axon sheaths and the internal architecture.
- **Neurotmesis:** epineurium disrupted; loss of anatomical and functional continuity.

❝ Expert comment Tinel's sign [5]

Tinel's sign, elicited by percussion along the course of a nerve from distal to proximal, is signified by pins and needles, or abnormal sensations, which may be painful, in the distribution of the nerve. It is an important aid to diagnosis. In the conscious patient, it may be strongly positive on the day of injury, indicating the torn or ruptured axons. Absence of a Tinel's sign over a spinal nerve that is not working suggests either conduction block or avulsion. Over time, Tinel's sign continues to provide much information, including:

- In axonotmesis, or after a repair that is going to be successful, the centrifugally moving Tinel's sign is persistently stronger than that at the suture line.
- After a repair that is going to fail, the Tinel's sign at the suture line remains stronger that that at the growing point.
- Failure of distal progression of the Tinel's sign in a closed lesion indicates rupture or other injury not susceptible of recovery by natural process.
- A positive Tinel's sign means the lesion is degenerative, not a conduction block, for at least a significant number of axons within the nerve [1].

MRI of the cervical spine and brachial plexus bilaterally (Figures 19.1 and 19.2) showed oedema along the C5 and C6 nerve roots bilaterally, worse on the left than the right, extending into the supraclavicular fossae. However, there was no pseudo-meningocele to indicate nerve root avulsion.

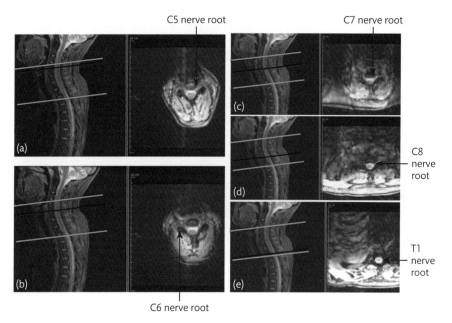

Figure 19.1 T2-weighted STIR MRI axial images showing the spinal nerves as they emerge from the cervical cord (a:C5; b:C6; c:C7; d:C8; e:T1).

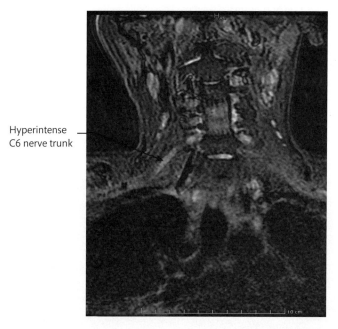

Figure 19.2 Coronal T2-weighted STIR MRI of the brachial plexus, illustrating the oedema along the upper brachial plexus nerve roots.

> ❂ **Learning point** Imaging of the brachial plexus
>
> - MRI of the brachial plexus has been used to discriminate pre- and post-ganglionic lesions. Features of preganglionic injury include: spinal cord oedema, lateral displacement of the spinal cord, a syrinx, absence of root in the canal or intervertebral foramina, traumatic meningocele, haemorrhage/scarring in the spinal canal, and denervation of erector spinae muscles (shown by wasting and fatty infiltration over a timescale of ≥15 days). Spinal cord oedema is thought to signify root avulsion central to the transition zone. Post-ganglionic injuries can also be identified, appearing as swelling of the nerve trunks on T1-weighted imaging and increased signal intensity on T2-weighted imaging [6,7].
> - CT myelography allows demonstration of the intradural nerve roots [8]. Root avulsion can be identified by the absence of continuity of the root with the cord. Traumatic meningoceles are also visible. However, the C8 and T1 roots can be difficult to visualize in continuity due to their oblique path, and interference from the shoulders.
> - High resolution ultrasound has the potential to allow in depth visualization of the brachial plexus and peripheral nerves. Preliminary studies of peripheral nerves are encouraging [9,10] and suggest that in the initial period following injury, prior to haematoma transformation into scar tissue, high resolution ultrasound may permit early detection of ruptures and other injuries to the nerves.

The patient underwent detailed electrophysiological examination 10 months post-injury, and Quantitative Sensory Testing (QST) almost 12 months from injury. The results are shown in Tables 19.2 and 19.3. They are of limited use in the left upper limb, as they reflect the second, more distal injury of the ulnar nerve, with the median and radial nerves affected by the severe soft tissue damage to the left forearm. The late F wave response was detectable in the right upper limb.

> ❂ **Learning point** Electrophysiological studies
>
> Neurophysiological investigations have a role in determining conduction across a lesion from the outset. Although they are difficult to interpret in the context of nerve injury at multiple levels.
>
> - SSEPs establish the presence or absence of a lesion proximal to the sensory dorsal root ganglion.
> - Standard nerve conduction studies assess large, fast-conducting, alpha and beta nerve fibres, which mediate fine touch (velocity 40–60m/s), and deep afferent pathways.
> - Small, myelinated (velocity 3–10m/s; A delta) fibres and non-myelinated (C) fibres are involved in pain and temperature sensation, and require the specialized techniques of QST.
> - Electromyography records and analyses the spontaneous, insertional, and volitional electrical activity of the muscle.
> - Neurapraxia is demonstrated by conduction block or slowing at the level of the lesion, and normal conduction distal to the lesion.
> - Axonotmesis leads to fibrillations, compound sensory action potential (CSAP) and compound motor action potential (CMAP) reduction in proportion to the axonal loss. The latter manifest at least 7 days after injury, once Wallerian degeneration has occurred.
> - Neurotmesis is demonstrated by fibrillation potentials and absent CSAPs and CMAPs
>
> Intra-operative neurophysiological testing is invaluable. It can guide dissection, identify the region of nerve injury, protect against iatrogenic damage, and monitor function in both sensory and motor nerves [1].

Table 19.2 Neurophysiological results

Motor conduction studies	Right	Left
Median (to abductor pollicis brevis (APB))	Latency from wrist:4.1ms amplitude:0.6mV latency from elbow: variable	Absent
Ulnar (to abductor digiti minimi)	Latency from wrist: 3.2ms Amplitude: 2mV Latency below elbow: 8.1ms Amplitude: 2mV Latency above elbow: 9.7ms Amplitude: 2mV MCV (wrist to elbow): 47m/ms MCV (across elbow): 52m/ms	Absent
Sensory conduction studies		
Median (terminal phalanx of middle finger to palm and wrist)	Latency: 2.3ms Amplitude: 5μV SCV: 53m/ms	Absent
Median (index proximal phalanx to wrist)	Latency: 2.3ms Amplitude: 1.2μV SCV: 54m/ms	Absent
Ulnar (little finger to wrist)	Latency: 1.9ms Amplitude: 2μV SCV:56m/ms	Absent
Radial (first metacarpal to forearm)	Latency: 1.7ms Amplitude: 8μV SCV: 54m/ms	Absent
Lateral antebrachial	Latency: 1.6ms Amplitude: 5μV SCV: 50m/ms	absent
Medial antebrachial	Latency: 2.0ms Amplitude: 3μV SCV: 66m/ms	Absent
Electromyography (EMG)		
Deltoid	Few fibrillations and positive sharp waves; excess polyphasics, moderately reduced, 2mV	Polyphasics, moderate, 3–4mV
Infraspinatus	Polyphasics, moderate, 3–4mV	Not assessed
Biceps	Polyphasics, moderate, 3–4mV	Polyphasics, moderate/ reduced, 2–3mV
Triceps	Polyphasics, moderate, 3–4mV	Polyphasics, moderate, 2–3mV
Brachioradialis	Polyphasics, moderate, 3–4mV	Not assessed
FDS	Polyphasics, moderate, 3–4mV	Not assessed
FDP	Polyphasics, moderate, 3–4mV	Not assessed
Interossei (first dorsal)	Few units only	No units
APB	Few units only	Few units only

ms: millisecond; mV: millivolts; μV: microvolts; MCV: motor conduction velocity; SCV: sensory conduction velocity in metre/microsecond

Table 19.3 Quantitative Sensory Testing

QST	Right	Left
Thermal thresholds	Normal	Normal, but elevated in hypothenar region
Vibration thresholds	Mod. elevated right index finger and thumb	Elevated in index (marginally), ring and little fingers
Joint position sense	Preserved	Preserved aside from little finger
Pin prick	Normal	Reduced in little finger and ulnar border of forearm; hypersensitivity C5
Monofilaments	Normal	Mod. elevated in arm and hand at No.10
Sweating	Preserved in palm	Preserved in palm

mod.: moderately.

The patient continues to undergo intensive inpatient neuro-rehabilitation, currently targeting the range of movement throughout the upper limbs, together with strengthening exercises, and intermittent splinting of the left upper limb.

Discussion

This patient had many potential reasons for his sensory and motor deficits. He was initially quadraplegic, which suggested a cervical cord injury. With the episodes of hypovolaemic and subsequent septic shock, and the preferential recovery of the lower limbs, poor perfusion of the cervical cord and, hence, the possibility of a central cord syndrome was considered. Anterior cord injury was another potential diagnosis, while a partial Brown–Séquard syndrome may be postulated, as multiple brachial plexus nerve root avulsions carries the inevitably degree of CNS involvement. However, the patient's tone always remained normal. Other potential diagnoses included ITU polyneuropathy, hypoperfusion of the brachial plexus bilaterally, and blast injury to the brachial plexus bilaterally. The polyneuropathy of critical illness has been postulated to be a neurological manifestation of the systemic inflammatory response syndrome [11]. Corticosteroids and neuromuscular blocking agents, poor glycaemic control, and immobility may also be contributory factors [12,13], as may a low albumin. Critical care polyneuropathy may be induced by a diffuse compartment syndrome, with increased pressure in the endoneurial, perineurial, and epineurial compartments.

Evaluation of the left upper limb in this case was complicated by the extensive destruction of muscle and skin, the anklyosis of the left elbow, and the presence of an ulnar nerve lesion, i.e. a second level peripheral nerve lesion, which was grafted soon after injury. The neurophysiological studies, at 10 months post-injury, indicate moderate function of the proximal muscles of the left upper limb. The left median nerve and superficial radial nerve are in continuity, as shown by the preservation of sensation, and the activity of muscles supplied by the median nerve. The absence of conduction on the formal neurophysiological testing, at 10 months post-injury, is predictable, due to the forearm soft tissue destruction and ulnar nerve lesion. The Tinel's sign over the left ulnar nerve indicates axonal severance with regeneration

❝ Expert comment Preganglionic brachial plexus lesions

Root avulsion can be detected by the electrodiagnostic triad of:

- Normal CSAP and a preserved histamine response.
- Denervation of paraspinal muscles.
- Loss of the SSEP.

This triad, together with evidence of fibrillations and absence of voluntary motor unit activity in peripheral muscles supplied by the root, distinguish a proximal lesion from more distal pathology [1].

❝ Expert comment

In blast injury, the patient is exposed to a shock wave at close range, without any fracture, or signs of significant soft tissue injury. The underlying mechanism is, as yet, not fully understood. Large fibre conduction recovers, but the small fibres repair more slowly, and sometimes imperfectly [14].

❝ Expert comment

It is generally advocated that patients with traumatic peripheral nerve injuries, including closed brachial plexus traction lesions, should undergo surgery as early as possible, as this has been shown to optimize recovery. In this case, however, bilateral exploration of the brachial plexus was not advised. This was due to the patient's poor systemic state and multiple co-existing injuries. Furthermore, in the acute stage, there was no definitive evidence of brachial plexus nerve damage amenable to surgical intervention.

through the graft. Indeed, subsequent electrophysiological studies show early recovery, although the graft of the left ulnar nerve.

A diagnosis of bilateral brachial plexus conduction block at the root level was reached in this patient due to the notable absence of pain, lack of Horner's sign, intact phrenic nerves, and absence of supraclavicular or infraclavicular Tinel's sign. These features together with the neurophysiological results indicate a preganglionic conduction block, rather than an avulsion or rupture. There is evidence of physical continuity of motor axons to the small muscles of the right hand. The EMGs at 10 months post-injury showed only a few motor axons under volition, but clear evidence of continuity. These features are consistent with considerable axonopathy. On the right, the F wave indicated at least partial preservation or continuity of the large afferent and efferent myelinated pathways. To date, the right C6, C7, and C8 roots have shown better recovery than C5 and T1. However, the prognosis is favourable, especially as sympathetic function throughout the right upper limb is present. The QSTs show all modalities recovering, even the finer fibres.

✓ Evidence base Outcome following brachial plexus injury

- Kato et al. [15] studied 137 patients who underwent brachial plexus repair. Of the sixty who underwent early surgery (within 1 month), 56.7% had a good result, i.e. the patient regained at least one function. Of those in whom surgery was delayed by more than 6 months, only 13.6% showed a good result.
- Berman et al. [16] showed that repair of the plexus offers the patient the possibility of pain relief. Of 116 patients with proven root avulsions who underwent nerve transfer and/or grafting, 88% experienced severe pain pre-operatively. This was reduced to 34% at 3 years post-operatively. These findings are supported by later work [15,17]. Hence, even when repair fails to restore worthwhile function, reinnervation by some means alleviates pain. It seems that reinnervation of muscle is more important than that of the skin.

✚ Clinical tip Surgical intervention for traumatic brachial plexus lesions

- The avulsed ventral root may be repaired by:
  - Transfer to an adjacent ruptured stump.
  - Transfer to a normal nerve (for example, the spinal accessory nerve).
  - Rarely, by direct repair to a stump in the spinal canal.
  - By re-implantation.

- Preganglionic avulsion lesions of the brachial plexus may be considered for re-implantation, if within 1 month of injury. Contraindications include severe head, chest, or visceral injuries, rupture or occlusion of the subclavian or vertebral artery, cervical or upper thoracic vertebral fractures, and spinal cord injury. These exclusion criteria do eliminate approximately 25% of individuals who present with avulsion injury. The pure lateral approach, as detailed in [18], allows access to the intra- and extraspinal regions of the brachial plexus. It involves exposure of the anterior and posterior tubercles, and the transverse processes at the relevant spinal levels. The posterior tubercle and part of the lateral mass are then resected to allow direct access to the spinal cord. The dura is opened longitudinally and the grafts fed through the intervertebral canals and implanted via small slits in the pia as close to the ventral root exit zone as possible. Published results of long-term functional recovery are encouraging, although sample size is small [19, 20, 21].
- The approach to post-ganglionic lesions is dependent on the target region of the brachial plexus [1] describes a medial extension of the transverse supraclavicular approach, which he and Bonney adopted. It allows access to the first part of the subclavian and vertebral arteries and the whole of the brachial plexus. Fiolle and Delmas [22] added a vertical limb to the transverse supraclavicular wound, with the potential to display the supra-, retro-, and infraclavicular plexus, the second part of the subclavian artery to the terminal axillary artery, and the subclavian and axillary veins deep to the clavicle. The infraclavicular part of the brachial plexus can be displayed by full opening of the delto-pectoral interval, and division of the pectoralis minor tendon. Finally, the posterior subscapular route provides access to the most proximal parts of the nerves [23].

> **❝ Expert comment** Peripheral nerve surgery
>
> - External neurolysis involves dissection outside of the epineurium, i.e. freeing the nerve from a constricting or distorting agent.
> - Internal or interfascicular neurolysis requires exposure of the bundles by epineurotomy and their separation.
> - Nerve repair entails the restoration of healthy conducting elements without tension. This may be by direct suture or grafting. The nerve must be adequately prepared, that is, the ends cut back progressively, until healthy bundles are exposed. This may be 1–2mm in an urgent case, typically 5–10mm, but up to 4cm in delayed cases or where infection has occurred. Intra-operative neurophysiological assessment is used in conjunction with visualization and gentle palpation of the nerve. If the gap after resection is small and the repaired nerve lies without tension, little mobilization of the nerve is required and end-to-end suture is appropriate. This involves matching bundle (fascicle) to bundle, with additional epineurial sutures. This is rarely appropriate in supraclavicular brachial plexus injuries. Grafting is undertaken using cutaneous nerves from the damaged limb if feasible. In brachial plexus surgery, this is typically the medial cutaneous nerve of the forearm (MCNF), taken through a straight incision. The sural nerve is also often required, which is taken through a midline incision running laterally in the distal aspect of the leg, to a point mid-way between the posterior aspect of the lateral malleolus and the lateral margin of the Achilles tendon. In cases where C5 and/or C6 are ruptured or avulsed, the superficial radial nerve makes an excellent graft, and the lateral cutaneous nerve of the forearm may also prove useful. The grafts are cut to the appropriate length and sewn into place, the suture uniting the epineurium of the graft to the perineurium of the stump bundle. The repaired nerve must lie in healthy tissue, with full thickness skin overlying.
> - Nerve transfer is appropriate in cases of brachial plexus root avulsion not amenable to reimplantation. Nerve transfer has the optimum chance of success if it is transferred to a nerve and muscle of roughly equivalent size, without an interposed nerve graft [24].
> - Muscle transfers may be used once the neurological prognosis is known.

The patient continues to work with an extensive multi-disciplinary neuro-rehabilitation team. To date, his management has rested on accurate diagnosis and prognostic information, together with intensive neuro-rehabilitation. Stiffness in the shoulders continues to be addressed, as does that in the small joints of the hands. Surgery is now indicated to overcome the clawing of the right MCP joints. Although small muscle activity continues to recover, their weakness rules out useful function in his dominant hand. Extensor carpi radialis longis (ECRL) transfer via Brandt's method is planned, followed by resurfacing of the left forearm together with an assessment of the continuity of musculotendinous units. This would provide the left median and ulnar nerves with the best possible conditions for recovery.

> **✪ Learning point** Rehabilitation
>
> Neuro-rehabilitation is a mainstay of treatment for patients with peripheral nerve lesions. Active and close involvement of relevant surgical specialties is also essential. Further operative procedures may form an integral part of the rehabilitation process, to manage neuropathic pain, decompress nerves, or provide full thickness skin cover to aid pain management and enhance nerve regeneration [14]. Neuro-rehabilitation involves a MDT whose purpose is to:
>
> - Objectively assess disability and accurately measure the outcome of treatment.
> - Reduce the degree of disability by physical and other therapies.
> - Return the patient to his/her original work, a modified role, or to alternative employment.
> - Restore the patient's ability to live in his/her own home, to enjoy recreation and social interaction, and to be independently mobile.
>
> Neuro-rehabilitation often involves functional splinting, which may prevent deformity, enhance use by placing joints in a useful position, and strengthen selective muscles [1].

A final word from the expert

Peripheral nerve injuries offer many challenges, especially those that are proximal, involving the nerve plexus, and/or are complicated by other injuries. Secondary distal damage to a peripheral nerve can further confuse the clinical picture. A thorough history and examination, together with appropriate imaging and neurophysiological investigations, allow accurate diagnosis and prognosis. The management of such severe blast injury to peripheral nerves is a new phenomenon requiring further research. In this case, a diagnosis of conduction block at the root level was made using all available clinical details and investigations. Despite the patient's quadriplegic presentation, a positive prognosis was delivered. Further neuro-rehabilitation, in its broadest sense, remains the long course ahead for this patient.

References

1. Birch R. Surgical disorders of the peripheral nerves, 2nd edn. London: Springer-Verlag, 2011.
2. O'Brien M. Aids to the examination of the peripheral nervous system, 5th edn. Kidlington: Saunders/Elsevier, 2010.
3. Bonney G. Clinical Neurophysiology in Peripheral Nerve Injuries. In: R Birch, G Bonney, CB Wynn Parry (eds), Surgical disorders of the peripheral nerves (pp. 196–8). Edinburgh: Churchill Livingstone, 1998.
4. Seddon HJ. Three types of nerve injury. Brain 1943; 66: 237–88.
5. Tinel J. Nerve wounds. London: Balliere Tindall and Co., 1917. [Authorised translation by F Rotherwell, revised and edited by CA Joll.]
6. Hems TEJ, Birch R, Carlstedt T. The role of magnetic resonance imaging in the management of traction injuries to the adult brachial plexus. Journal of Hand Surgery 1999; 24b: 550–5.
7. Tavakkolizadeh A, Saifuddin A, Birch R. Imaging of adult brachial plexus traction injuries. Journal of Hand Surgery 2001; 26B: 183–91.
8. Carvalho GA, Nikkhah G, Matthies G, et al. Diagnoses of root avulsions in traumatic brachial plexus injuries: value of computerised tomography myelography and magnetic resonance imaging. Journal of Neurosurgery 1997; 86: 69–76.
9. Cokluk C, Aydin K. Ultrasound examination in the surgical treatment for upper extremity peripheral nerve injuries. Part I: Turkish Neurosurgery 2007a 17: 197–201.
10. Cokluk C, Aydin K. Ultrasound examination in the surgical treatment for upper extremity peripheral nerve injuries. Part II: Turkish Neurosurgery 2007b 17: 277–82.
11. Visser LH. (2006). Critical illness polyneuropathy and myopathy: clinical features, risk factors and prognosis. European Journal of Neurology 2006; 13: 1203–12.
12. Schweickert WD, Hall J. ICU-acquired weakness. Chest 2007; 11: 1541–9.
13. Latronico N, Bolton CF. Critical illness polyneuropathy and myopathy: a major cause of muscle weakness and paralysis. Lancet Neurology 2011; 10: 931–41.
14. Birch R, Eardley WGP, Ramasamy A, et al. Nerve injuries sustained during warfare: Part II: Outcomes. Journal of Bone and Joint Surgery (British) 2012; 94B: 529–35.
15. Kato N, Htut M, Taggart M, et al. The effects of operative delay on the relief of neuropathic pain after injury to the brachial plexus. Journal of Bone and Joint Surgery 2006; 88B: 756–9.
16. Berman J, Taggart M, Anand P, (1995) The effects of surgical repair on pain relief after brachial plexus injuries. In: Association of British Neurologists Proceedings, University of Liverpool, April 1995, JNNP; 44: 5–7.

17. Taggart M. (1998) Relief of pain with operation. In:Birch R, Bonney G, WynnParry CB. (eds) Surgical disorders of the peripheral nerves. Edinburgh: Churchill Livingstone, 373–405.

18. Camp SJ, Carlstedt T, Casey ATH. Technical note: pure lateral approach to intraspinal re-implantation of the brachial plexus. Journal of Bone and Joint Surgery (British) 2010; 92B: 975–9.

19. Carlstedt T. (2007) Central nerve plexus injury. In:T Carlstedt,(ed.), Central nerve plexus injury. London: Imperial College Press.

20. Carlstedt T, Anand P, Hallin R, et al. Spinal nerve root repair and reimplantation of avulsed ventral roots into the spinal cord after brachial plexus injury. Journal of Neurosurgery 2000; 93: 237–47.

21. Carlstedt T, Grane P, Hallin RG, et al. Return of function after spinal cord implantation of avulsed spinal nerve roots. Lancet 1995; 346: 1323–5.

22. Fiolle J.Delmas J. In: CG Cumston (transl. ed.), The surgical exposure of the deep seated blood vessels (pp. 61–7). London: Heinemann, 1921.

23. Kline DG, Kott J, Barnes G, et al. Exploration of selected brachial plexus lesions by the posterior subscapular approach. Journal of Neurosurgery 1978; 49: 872–9.

24. Addas BMJ.Midha R. Nerve transfers for severe nerve injury. Neurosurgery Clinics 20: Peripheral Nerve Injury 2009; 20(1): 27–38.

Spontaneous intracerebral haemorrhage

Peter Bodkin

Expert commentary Patrick Statham

Case history

A 68-year-old man presented to his local emergency department with a left hemiparesis of sudden onset. His background medical history included poorly-controlled hypertension, ischaemic heart disease, and previous TIAs. He was medicated on amlodipine 5mg, aspirin 75mg, dypiridamole 100mg tds, and simvastatin 20mg. Blood parameters, including clotting, were within normal range.

On admission, his conscious level was normal, but he had MRC grade 3/5 weakness of the left upper and lower limb. Cranial nerves were normal apart from a left upper motor neurone facial palsy. His blood pressure was 210/105 in the emergency department. A CT brain scan (Figure 20.1) revealed a right frontal intracerebral haematoma (41 × 53 × 39mm, approximately 42mL; see Learning point: estimation of volume of intracranial haemorrhage). Antiplatelet agents were immediately stopped.

> **⊗ Learning point** Estimation of volume of intracranial haemorrhage
>
> An ellipsoid can be described by its Cartesian coordinates of:
>
> - The largest cross-sectional diameter.
> - A second diameter drawn at right angles to the first.
> - The height of the ellipsoid [1].
>
> Volume $= (4\pi/3) \times (a/2) \times (b/2) \times (c/2)$
>
> If π is approximated to 3 the equation simplifies to:
>
> Volume $= (a \times b \times c)/2$
>
> In practice, the axial image with the largest cross-sectional area of clot should be chosen, and a and b values measured in centimetres. The c value should be worked out by counting the number of slices the intracranial haemorrhage (ICH) is visible on and multiplied by the slice thickness in centimetres. A value in millilitres will be given. There has been proven to be a very close correlation between this method of volume estimation and computer-assisted planimetric image analysis [2].

He was initially managed conservatively with careful control of his blood pressure by labetolol infusion with a target systolic blood pressure of below 180mmHg.

Between days 1 and 5 he remained neurologically stable. On day 6 he became increasingly drowsy and confused, with eye opening to speech and speech limited to occasional words (E3 V3 M6). His eyes were noted to be deviated to the right at rest. A repeat CT brain showed haematoma expansion causing increased mass effect (Figure 20.2). There were no systemic factors contributing to his deterioration.

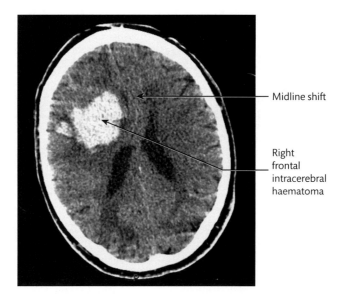

Figure 20.1 Patient's initial CT. Non-contrasted axial image showing haematoma in the right frontal lobe with effacement of the right frontal horn and 4mm of midline shift.

⭐ **Learning point** Frontal eye fields [3]

Horizontal conjugate gaze deviation towards the side of a lesion (Prévost or Vulpian sign) may be a result of damage to the frontal eye fields (FEFs). These are located in the posterior part of the middle frontal gyrus and adjacent precentral sulcus (Brodman areas 6 and 4). The FEFs are involved in complex neural pathways, modulating responses from visual and other stimuli for horizontal saccadic and pursuit movements, ultimately via the abducens nucleus. For pursuit movements, the dorsolateral pontine nucleus, cerebellum, and vestibular nucleus are intermediaries; for saccades the superior colliculus and paramedian pontine reticular formation (PPRF) play important roles. Oculocephalic manoeuvres and caloric stimulation can typically override the gaze palsy. A seizure focus in the region of the FEF will cause deviation of gaze *away* from the side of origin.

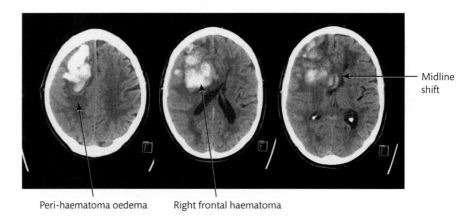

Figure 20.2 Preoperative CT. Non-contrasted axial slices demonstrating significantly larger right frontal haematoma with mid-line shift now of 1cm.

The balance of risk versus benefit at this point favoured surgical evacuation, which was discussed with his family. A right frontal burr hole was created under general anaesthesia, and a Dandy cannula was used to aspirate the clot. This was done with a freehand technique. The most appropriate entry point and target depth had been planned based on measurements in axial, sagittal, and coronal planes. 30mL of dark blood clot was aspirated. The brain was seen to relax after clot aspiration.

✚ Clinical tips Burr hole aspiration of intracerebral clot

Minimally-invasive techniques for clot aspiration are an attractive treatment option to avoid the inevitable trauma of craniotomy with corticotomy, brain retraction, etc. Aspiration may be most accurately performed with stereotactic methods using the same equipment as for tumour biopsy or shunt placement. Alternatively, modern digital imaging software usually provides measuring tools so that a target can be localized from anatomical landmarks using reconstructed 3D images. Given that the clot was large and in a relatively non-eloquent region of the brain, we felt that this method was appropriate. Adjunctive methods of dissolution of the clot may also be used (see Discussion). In this case, we were fortunate that the clot had largely liquefied, given that it was 6 days old.

Following surgery, he recovered to being mildly confused (GCS E4 V4 M6). His hemiparesis (MRC 3/5) persisted. A post-operative CT showed markedly improved appearances (Figure 20.3. He was discharged to a rehabilitation unit, where his neurological deficit improved such that he was mobile with a Zimmer frame and independent of most activities of daily living.)

Unfortunately, he presented again 3 months later with a left-sided basal ganglia bleed with intraventricular extension (Figure 20.4). This may well relate to his being recommenced on antiplatelet agents 2 weeks previously. Further surgery was not undertaken at that point.

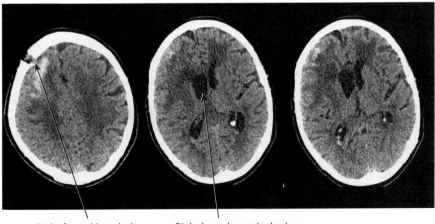

Right frontal burr hole   Right lateral ventricular horn

Figure 20.3 Post-operative CT 2 days following surgery. Non-contrasted axial slices showing minimal residual haematoma and resolution of mid-line shift.

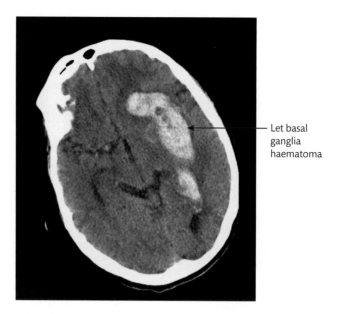

Let basal ganglia haematoma

Figure 20.4 3 months later - CT non-contrasted axial image showing extensive left basal ganglia and intraventricular haemorrhage.

> **❝ Expert comment**
>
> Primary intracerebral haematoma (PICH) represents the end stage of a longstanding disease. Removing a haematoma may reduce the immediate risk to life, but at the cost of residual disability. Careful discussion with the patient and relatives is vital to prevent misunderstandings in the weeks and months following intervention. This should start before referral for 'urgent' neurosurgery. Secondary intracerebral haematoma is a very different surgical problem, which has to be considered on the merits of the underlying disease.

Discussion

In 1888, the Glasgow surgeon Sir William Macewen described the first operation to evacuate an ICH [6]. Since then, the surgeon's role in the treatment of haemorrhagic stroke has been highly controversial. Deciding on the best management of these patients in relation to operative versus non-operative treatment, management of hypertension, choosing between different operative techniques and timing of surgery is a challenge faced by neurosurgeons on a daily basis.

Spontaneous ICH may be classified as primary or secondary. Secondary ICH includes those due to:

- Trauma.
- Structural lesions, such as aneurysms, AVMs, cavernomas, and neoplasms.
- Haemorrhage into arterial or venous infarctions.

Neoplasms that have a particular tendency to bleed include melanoma, choriocarcinoma, thyroid, and renal cell carcinoma. However, due to its high prevalence, the commonest metastasis to cause haemorrhage is from carcinoma of the lung. Primary ICH is related to hypertension, amyloid angiopathy, and coagulopathy, and accounts for 78–85% of all cases. The incidence is 24.6 per 100,000 person years, more than twice that of SAH [7]. It affects in the order of 2 million people worldwide per annum.

✪ Learning point Anticoagulation following intracranial haemorrhage

There is some evidence to suggest that deep nuclear ICH patients at high risk of thromboembolic disease, that is, those with atrial fibrillation (AF) or pulmonary embolism (PE), may benefit from treatment with anticoagulation [4]. For those with lobar haemorrhages, however, the risks of anticoagulation outweigh any benefits as their risk of recurrence is higher (4.4 versus 2.1% per patient-year) [5].

Risk factors fall into non-modifiable and modifiable categories. Race and age are important non-modifiable factors. The incidence of ICH is slightly higher in men [9] and is higher in Japanese, Chinese, and African American populations. Age plays a significant role, with risk doubling every decade after 35. Those under 45 are much more likely to have an underlying lesion. The most significant modifiable risk factor is hypertension, which is present in 75% of cases [10]. The increasingly effective management of hypertension has reduced the incidence of ICH in some populations over the last few decades [11]. Conversely, ICH may be a direct consequence of anticoagulation treatment. Long-term anticoagulation increases the risk of ICH eight- to eleven-fold, and causes haemorrhages twice the volume, on average, compared with non-anticoagulated patients. The mortality is also significantly increased (60–65%). Most bleeds occur in the first 6 months of treatment [12]. Aspirin therapy also increases the risk, but by much less (0.7% compared with 0.37% with placebo). Thrombolysis for myocardial infarction and ischaemic stroke also carries a significant risk (0.4–1.3% [13] and as much as 11%, respectively [14]). Alcohol consumption may also contribute, probably due to its adverse effect on clotting and a direct effect on blood vessel walls. Intake of more than two standard units of alcohol per day doubles the risk of ICH. Smoking has only a modest effect, if any.

Primary ICH makes up 10–20% of all strokes, but has a far higher mortality rate, up to 40–45% in the first month compared with ischaemic stroke (Figure 20.5) [17].

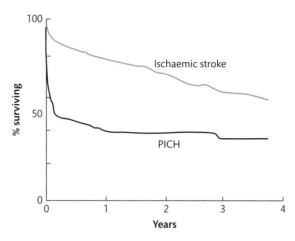

Figure 20.5 Kaplan–Meier plot showing long-term survival following first-ever stroke due to PICH or cerebral infarction.

Source: Dennis MS, Burn JPS, Sandercock PAG, BamfordJM, Wade DT, Warlow CP: Long-term survival after first-ever stroke: The Oxfordshire Community Stroke Project. Stroke 1993;24:796–800.

At 1 year, only around 25% are independent in activities of daily living with 10–15% alive, but dependent. The new-onset seizure rate is 4.6–8.2% [18].

Common sites for ICH include the deep structures of the periventricular white matter, caudate nucleus, globus pallidus, putamen, internal capsule, and thalamus (50%), in the gray matter or subcortical white matter (lobar (35%), cerebellum (10%), and brainstem (6%) [20]). On a histological level it has been shown that degenerative changes within the cerebral blood vessels, often attributable to chronic hypertension, are responsible for leakage of blood into the brain parenchyma. This is mainly seen at or near the bifurcation of small arteries, 50–700μm in diameter [21]. Charcot and Bouchard described micro-aneurysms, sites of fibrinoid necrosis of the subendothelium, which have been implicated in underlying PICH. It has been difficult to establish conclusively, however, whether these lesions are the source of hypertensive ICH.

Expert comment

A number of factors have been identified that predict outcome. The functional outcome risk stratification scale (FUNC) score brings together the most important predictors (ICH volume, age, ICH location, GCS, pre-ICH cognitive impairment) to give a likelihood of functional independence 90 days after PICH [19]. Some studies have shown absolute values for clot size predictive of death or survival, for instance, all patients in a cohort study with haematomas greater than 85cm³died with or without surgery, whereas all patients with haematoma less than 26cm³ survived without surgery [24].

Learning point Cerebral amyloid angiopathy

Lobar or subcortical haemorrhages, especially in the elderly, are often caused by amyloid angiopathy. This results from the deposition of beta-amyloid in the media and adventitia of small cerebral arteries and capillaries. There is loss of smooth muscle cells, vessel wall thickening, luminal narrowing, concentric splitting of the vessel wall, and micro-aneurysm formation. The result is cortical and subcortical micro-infarctions and microhaemorrhages, some visible on DWI and gradient echo sequence MRI. Although individually clinically silent, their gradual accumulation over some years results in significant cognitive impairment. There is also some overlap with deposition of beta-amyloid in the parenchyma (Alzheimer's disease). Both are underpinned by abnormalities in the genes responsible for apolipoprotein E production [22].

There is evidence that many haematomas expand slowly over the first few hours after the initial bleed. Some sequential imaging studies have shown up to 73% demonstrate some enlargement of haematoma in the first 24 hours, the majority of this occurring within the first 4 hours [23]. This corresponds with the typical clinical presentation with a progression of neurological deficit in the early period with a minority initially presenting with dense deficits. Haematoma expansion and the development of intraventricular haemorrhage (IVH) are independent risk factors for poor outcome [24].

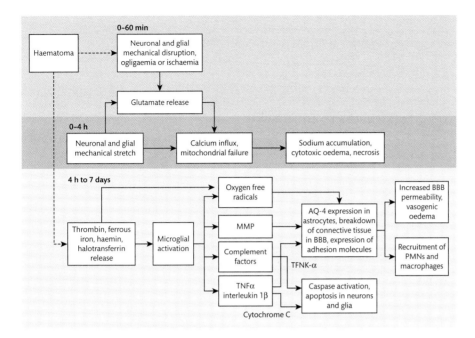

Figure 20.6 Sequence of neural damage initiated by intracerebral haemorrhage. Note that in the initial 4 hours injury is caused by the mass effect and subsequent damage by release of breakdown products.

BBB = blood–brain barrier; MMP = matrix metallopeptidase; TNF = tumour necrosis factor; PMN = polymorphonuclear cells [1]

Qureshi AI, Mendelow AD, Hanley DF. Intracerebral haemorrhage. *Lancet* 2009; 373(9675): 1632–44.

Following haemorrhage, subsequent secondary damage may occur through a cascade of pathological processes, including cytotoxicity of blood products, hypermetabolism, excitotoxicity, spreading depression, oxidative stress, and inflammation (Figure 20.6) [25]. Resulting peri-haematoma oedema peaks around 5–6 days and lasts up to 14 days.

The optimal medical management of these patients requires co-ordinated input from prehospital care practitioners, general practitioners, A&E staff, stroke physicians, neurosurgeons, and geriatricians. Specialist stroke unit care [26], as well as neurosciences intensive care unit [27,28] has been shown to improve outcome.

Blood pressure management is a controversial, but important issue to address early on in the management of these often medically complex patients (see Evidence base: blood pressure control after primary intracranial haemorrhage).

> ✷ **Evidence base** Blood pressure control after primary intracranial haemorrhage
>
> Seventy-five percent of patients admitted with ICH have systolic blood pressure over 140mmHg, and 20% present with systolic blood pressure over 180mmHg [29].
>
> Although instinctively logical, a causal link has not been firmly established between ICH and hypertension. Blood pressure may be affected by parenchymal haemorrhage itself through activation of neuroendocrine systems and by alterations in ICP. Some studies report an inconsistent
>
> (continued)

relationship between blood pressure and haematoma expansion. There are also theoretical arguments about the balance between permissive elevation of blood pressure to maintain viability of the peri-haematoma penumbra versus lowering the blood pressure to reduce the risk of haematoma expansion.

Two recent trials have sought to clarify some of these questions. The Intensive Blood Pressure Reduction in Acute Cerebral Haemorrhage Trial (INTERACT) [30] randomized 404 Chinese patients between a target systolic blood pressure of 140 and 180mmHg. There was a weak association with reduced haemorrhagic expansion, however, secondary clinical outcomes were statistically unchanged. The Antihypertensive Treatment of Acute Cerebral Haemorrhage (ATACH) [31] had three cohorts of patients with a target blood pressure of 170–200, 140–170, or 110–140. The study did not show any difference in haematoma expansion, peri-haematoma oedema, and 3-month outcome between the groups, but with only sixty patients, the study was somewhat underpowered. Follow-up studies are under way and may advance our understanding. American and European guidelines based on Class 3 (IIb) evidence are shown (Table 20.2), but have been shown to be poorly adhered to [32].

Table 20.2 Options for urgent warfarin reversal [37]

Agent	Pros	Cons	Usefulness for urgent reversal
Vitamin K1	Widely available; inexpensive; directly reverses warfarin effect; small volume infused; low infective and thrombotic risk	Slow onset of action; possible allergy	Poor
Fresh-frozen plasma	Widely available; contains all coagulation factors; low thrombotic risk	Large volumes usually needed; requires cross-matching and thawing; slow onset of action; not negligible infective risk, possible TRALI	Fair
Prothrombin complex concentrate	Rapid onset; small volume infused; low infective risk	Expensive; variable factor concentrations in different preparations; no negligible thrombotic risk	Good
Recombinant activated factor VII	Rapid onset; small volume infused; thrombin burst; low infective risk	Very expensive; acts directly on only a single factor; INR correction may be 'lab artefact'; off label use	Good

TRALI: transfusion-related acute lung injury.

The most recent ASA/AHA guidelines [33] state:

Until ongoing clinical trials of blood pressure intervention for ICH are completed, physicians must manage blood pressure on the basis of incomplete evidence.

- If SBP is >200mmHg or MAP is >150mmHg, then consider aggressive reduction of blood pressure with continuous intravenous infusion, with frequent blood pressure monitoring every 5 minutes.
- If SBP is >180mmHg or MAP is >130mmHg, and there is the possibility of elevated ICP, then consider monitoring ICP and reducing blood pressure using intermittent or continuous iv medications, while maintaining a cerebral perfusion pressure ≥60mmHg.
- If SBP is >180mmHg or MAP is >130mmHg, and there is no evidence of elevated ICP, then consider a modest reduction of blood pressure (e.g. MAP of 110mmHg or target blood pressure of 160/90mmHg), using intermittent or continuous iv medications to control blood pressure, and clinically re-examine the patient every 15 minutes.

(continued)

According to the European Guidelines [34], routine blood pressure lowering is not recommended. Treatment is recommended if blood pressure is elevated above the following levels, confirmed by repeat measurements (class IV evidence):

- **Patients with a known history of hypertension or signs (ECG, retina) of chronic hypertension:** systolic blood pressure >180mmHg and/or diastolic blood pressure >105mmHg. If treated, target blood pressure should be 179/100mmHg (or a MAP of 125mmHg).
- **Patients without known hypertension:** systolic blood pressure >160mmHg and/or diastolic blood pressure > 95mmHg. If treated, target blood pressure should be 150/90 mmHg (or a MAP of 110mmHg).
- **A reduction of MAP by > 20%** should be avoided.
- These limits and targets should be adapted to higher values in patients undergoing monitoring if increased ICP, to guarantee a sufficient CPP>70mmHg.
- **Recommended drugs for blood pressure treatment:** iv labetalol or urapidil, iv sodium nitroprusside or nitroglycerine, and captopril (per os). Avoid oral nifedipine and any drastic blood pressure decrease.

Non-contrasted brain CT is the first line imaging modality. Gradient echo MRI can be used to detect hyperacute haemorrhage and microhaemorrhages. Ancillary studies, e.g. angiography may be used when aneurysmal/AVM haemorrhage is suspected, or delayed MRI to look for underlying cavernomas or tumours.

Activated recombinant factor VII (fVIIa) has been investigated in its capacity to limit haematoma expansion. A phase II trial showed significantly reduced haematoma volume (from 29 to 11–16%) and 90-day mortality (29% compared with 18%) [35]. A phase III trial (the FAST trial) [36] had rather less encouraging results, however. Although the effect on limiting haematoma volume was confirmed, at 3 months the percentage who were dead or disabled in the placebo group was 24%, compared with 26% and 29% in the 20μg/kg and 80μg/kg groups, respectively. In patients who develop ICH on oral anticoagulation fVIIa is an option, although an expensive one. Rapid reversal of anticoagulants not only prevents ongoing bleeding, but also allows the possibility of surgical intervention. Normalization of INR within 2 hours from hospital admission is associated with low rates of haematoma enlargement and is achieved in the majority of patients (84%) treated with prothrombin complex concentrates, while fresh frozen plasma (FFP) infusions show only a partial effect in reducing haematoma enlargement (39%) and vitamin K1 has no effects [37]. Vitamin K, however, must be given to avoid a rebound in coagulopathy.

Surgical intervention

The use of surgery for ICH is highly variable across the world with reports of 50% in German and Japanese literature, whereas other countries report 2–20% [38].

The concept of ischaemic penumbra has been used as an argument for early surgical intervention. DWI, perfusion-weighted imaging (PWI), and positron emission tomography (PET) studies do not consistently demonstrate the existence of ischaemic change in the peri-haematoma region, however [40]. Nonetheless, damage may be occurring through mitochondrial dysfunctional, leading to impaired oxidative metabolism. Raised glutamate, lactate, glycerol, and lactate/pyruvate ratio point to a biochemical, rather than ischaemic crisis. These metabolic changes are seen to reverse 24–48 hours following clot evacuation [41].

❝ Expert comment

The rationale for surgical evacuation of ICH has a sound theoretical basis. It directly addresses the damaging mass effect, prevents release of inflammatory blood breakdown products, and may improve perfusion of the vulnerable penumbra. A wide variety of surgical strategies are available—open craniotomy, frameless stereotactic aspiration, or endoscopic evacuation with or without thrombolysis [39].

✪ Evidence base Medical versus surgical treatment of intracranial haemorrhage

The investigation of the relative merits of medical versus surgical treatment of ICH has a long and illustrious history. Wylie McKissock published the first prospective randomized trial in neurosurgery on the subject in 1961 [49]. After randomizing 180 patients diagnosed by catheter angiogram and air ventriculography, surgical intervention produced no obvious advantage. The conclusion of this landmark paper was: 'We have clearly made no contribution to the treatment of primary intracerebral haemorrhage by surgery.' Most subsequent studies have supported this conclusion. The largest trial to date is the International Surgical Trial in Intracerebral Haemorrhage (STICH) led by Mendelow from Newcastle, UK and published in 2005 [50] in the *Lancet*. In summary, 1033 patients from twenty-seven countries were randomized either to early surgery (within 24 hours of randomization) or medical treatment. The results showed that 26% of surgically-treated patients had a favourable outcome compared with 24% treated medically. However, this was not statistically significant and the overall conclusion was that there was 'no benefit from early surgery compared with initial conservative treatment'. Indeed, for some groups, especially those patients presenting in a coma (where risk was increased by 8%), surgery seemed to be harmful. When one examines the Forest plots of the twelve meaningful trials (including STICH) there may, however, be a suggestion of overall benefit for surgery (odds ratio of 0.85, CI 0.71, 1.03), when the unfavourable outcome was death (Figure 20.7).

Review: Surgery in intracerebral haemorrhage
Comparison: 01 surgery v control
Outcome: 02 death

Study or sub-category	Treatment n/N	Control n/N	Peto OR 95% CI	Peto OR 95% CI
McKissock (1961)	58/89	46/91		1.81 (1.01, 3.27)
Auer (1989)	21/50	35/50		0.32 (0.15, 0.71)
Juvela (1989)	12/26	10/26		1.36 (0.46, 4.05)
Batjer (1990)	4/8	11/13		0.20 (0.03, 1.33)
Chen (1992)	15/64	11/63		1.44 (0.61, 3.40)
Morgenstern (1998)	3/17	4/17		0.71 (0.14, 3.63)
Zuccarello (1999)	2/9	3/11		0.77 (0.11, 5.62)
Cheng 2001	26/266	34/234		0.64 (0.37, 1.09)
Teernstra (2001)	20/36	20/34		0.88 (0.34, 2.25)
Hosseini 2003	3/20	9/17		0.19 (0.05, 0.72)
Hattori (2004)	9/121	20/121		0.42 (0.20, 0.92)
Mendelow (2005)	173/477	189/505		0.95 (0.73, 1.23)
Total (95% CI)	**1183**	**1182**		**0.85 (0.71, 1.02)**

Total events: 346 (treatment), 392 (control)
Test for heterogeneity: $Chi^2 = 26.29$, df = 11 ($p = 0.006$), $I^2 = 58.2\%$
Test for overall effect: $z = 1.73$ ($p = 0.08$)

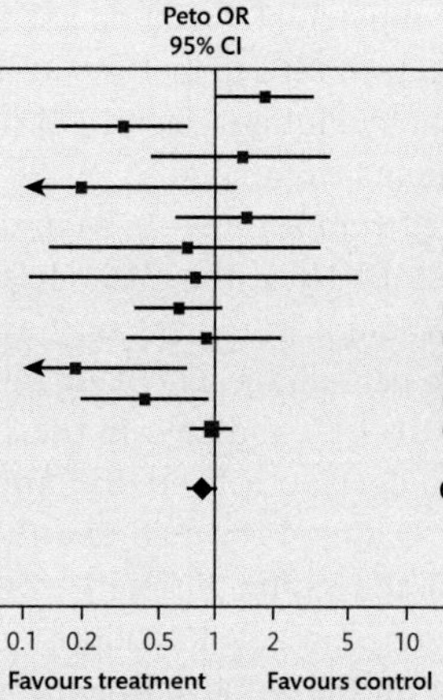

0.1 0.2 0.5 1 2 5 10
Favours treatment   Favours control

Figure 20.7 Forrest plots of twelve ICH trials [1].

Source: Mendelow AD, Gregson BA, Mitchell PM, Murray GD, Rowan EN, Gholkar AR. Surgical trial in lobar intracerebral haemorrhage (STICH II) protocol. Trials 2011:12:124. Distributed under the terms of the Creative Commons Attribution License 2.0

When subgroups are analysed, it appears that there is quite a difference in outcome in patients with IVH (42%) (favourable outcome of only 15% compared with 31% in those without IVH). A meta-analysis of purely lobar haemorrhages seems to favour surgical evacuation (Figure 20.8). Given the results of this post hoc analysis, the STICH collaborators have pointed out that the overall conclusion should be that, for certain patients with ICH, surgery can be justified. A further ongoing study (STICH II) is looking prospectively at the subgroups of patients most likely to benefit from surgery. The following lists are the criteria for this to date unpublished study (http://research.ncl.ac.uk/stich):

Inclusion criteria

- Evidence of a spontaneous lobar ICH on CT scan (1cm or less from the cortex surface of the brain).
- Patient within 48 hours of ictus.

(continued)

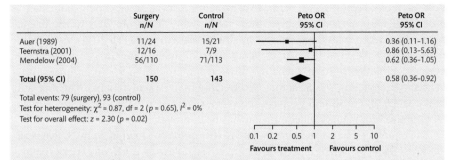

	Surgery n/N	Control n/N	Peto OR 95% CI	Peto OR 95% CI
Auer (1989)	11/24	15/21		0.36 (0.11–1.16)
Teernstra (2001)	12/16	7/9		0.86 (0.13–5.63)
Mendelow (2004)	56/110	71/113		0.62 (0.36–1.05)
Total (95% CI)	**150**	**143**		**0.58 (0.36–0.92)**

Total events: 79 (surgery), 93 (control)
Test for heterogeneity: $\chi^2 = 0.87$, df = 2 ($p = 0.65$), $I^2 = 0\%$
Test for overall effect: $z = 2.30$ ($p = 0.02$)

0.1   0.2   0.5   1   2   5   10
Favours treatment   Favours control

Figure 20.8 Forrest plot of lobar haematomas without IVH [1].

Source: Mendelow AD, Gregson BA, Mitchell PM, Murray GD, Rowan EN, Gholkar AR. Surgical trial in lobar intracerebral haemorrhage (STICH II) protocol. Trials 2011:12:124. Distributed under the terms of the Creative Commons Attribution License 2.0

- Best motor score on the GCS of 5 or 6, and best eye opening score on the GCS of 2 or more.
- Volume of haematoma between 10 and 100mL (calculated using $(a \times b \times c)/2$ method).

Exclusion criteria

- Clear evidence that the haemorrhage is due to an aneurysm or angiographically-proven arteriovenous malformation.
- IVH of any sort.
- ICH secondary to tumour or trauma.
- Basal ganglia, thalamic, cerebellar, or brainstem haemorrhage or extension of a lobar haemorrhage into any of these regions.
- Severe pre-existing physical or mental disability, or severe co-morbidity that might interfere with assessment of outcome.
- If surgery cannot be performed within 12 hours.
- If the haematological effects of any previous anticoagulants are not completely reversed.

STICH II aims to recruit 600 patients by May 2012, efforts are ongoing. There are other important trials ongoing in the subject. Clot lysis evaluating accelerated resolution on intraventricular haemorrhage (CLEAR III) is a phase III clinical trial examining how recombinant tissue plasminogen activator (rtPA), placed through EVD changes, modified Rankin score at 12 months compared with EVD alone. minimally invasive surgery plus rtPA for intracerebral haemorrhage evacuation (MISTIE) also looks at tPA, this time its effect after being placed within the clot itself. Currently (February 2012), CLEAR III is still ongoing and MISTIE has finished recruiting, but is waiting for follow-up data.

Surgical methods of intracranial haemorrhage treatment

Traditional craniotomy provides a relatively large access to the haematoma with direct visibility of the cavity wall. This allows bipolar cautery of the haematoma bed, placement of haemostatic agents, and visualization of any underlying abnormalities such as AVMs, tumours, etc. It is, of course, an invasive method with increased risk of causing damage to the cortex and white matter tracts, whilst accessing the clot. This is obviously most significant in deep-seated basal ganglia and thalamic bleeds. Neuronavigation may be usefully applied to plan the safest trajectory. Intra-operative ultrasound has also proven to be a simple and effective localization technique [42].

Less invasive methods have been applied. The simplest of these is aspiration via a burr hole, sometimes undertaken under local anaesthesia. Stereotactic aspiration in 175 patients achieved at least 50% clot removal in 75%. By contrast, 7.4 % had post-operative bleeding [43]. Fifty-two percent achieved independent outcomes at 6 months. This method may also allow the delivery of fibrinolytics to the haematoma. Catheter systems may be left in situ to allow infusion of rtPA or urokinase following aspiration of the clot. A Japanese study found only 58% of patients had evacuation of 50% of haematoma by initial aspiration, but after the urokinase infusion, the haematoma was 80% removed in more than 70% of patients. The mortality rate was 3% [44]. It should be noted, however, that no correlation between degree of clot removal and neurological outcome has been proven [45].

The endoscope has also been applied to ICH, providing a view of the haematoma cavity, so that clot can be identified and removed, allowing greater total clot removal and direct coagulation of visualized bleeding points. This is reflected in the clinical results with 96% removal in the putaminal group, 86% in the thalamic group, and 98% in the subcortical group [46].

Other mechanical devices have been described to aid haematoma evacuation, such as 'Archimedes screw' type devices, ultrasonic aspirators, and oscillating cutters.

Hemicraniectomy (without primary clot evacuation) has also been used as a treatment method. A case series of twelve patients with evacuation and hemicraniectomy had a survival rate of 92% and good functional outcome in 55% [47].

✪ **Learning box** Cerebellar haemorrhage [48]

Cerebellar haemorrhage accounts for 5–13% of spontaneous ICH and has a high mortality rate (20–75%). It can be an uncommon complication of supratentorial surgery. Kirollos [48] published one of the few prospective studies in cerebellar haemorrhage. The configuration of the fourth ventricle was used as a measure of mass effect and a guide to treatment:

- **Grade I:** fourth ventricle was not effaced or displaced from the midline.
- **Grade II:** partial effacement or shift to one side.
- **Grade III:** total effacement or brainstem distortion.

The following treatment protocol was used.

Results (good outcome)

Grade III with GCS<8 (0%), Grade III with GCS>8 (38%), Grade II with GCS<8 (57%), Grade II with GCS>8 (58%), Grade I (100%).

The importance of urgent surgical treatment of the Grade III patients before conscious level deteriorates (when outcome is universally poor) was emphasized.

A protocol for the management of infratentorial is shown in Figure 20.9 .

A final word from the expert

For most patients with PICH, surgery is not the best option, and attention to the best medical treatment is vital, with management in a dedicated stroke unit likely to confer an advantage. Where there is uncertainty, or clinical equipoise, it is most helpful to enter the patient into a prospective randomized trial, such as STICH II. This will elucidate whether the subgroup of patients who made a better recovery after surgery, such as lobar haemorrhage, did so because of surgery or from confounding factors.

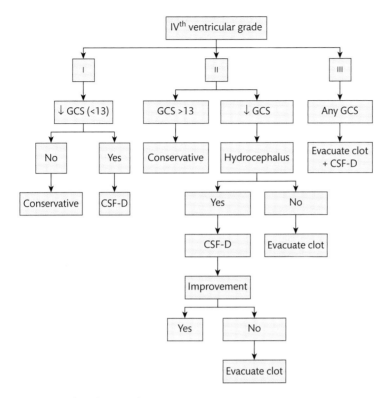

Figure 20.9 Protocol for infratentorial ICH.

Source: Ivi Kirollos RW, Tyagi AK, Ross SA, van Hille PT, Marks PV. Management of spontaneous cerebellar hematomas: a prospective treatment protocol. *Neurosurgery* 2001:49(6):1378–1387

References

1. Newman GC. Clarification of the abc/2 rule for ICH volume. Stroke 2007; 38: 862.
2. Kothari RU, Brott T, Broderick JP, et al. The ABCs of measuring intracerebral hemorrhage volume. Stroke 1996; 27: 1304–5.
3. Brazis PW, Masdeu JC, Biller J. Gaze palsy. Localization in clinical neurology. Philadelphia: Lippincott, Williams and Wilkins, 2007.
4. Eckman MH, Rosand J, Knudsen KA, et al. Can patients be anticoagulated after intracerebral hemorrhage? A decision analysis. Stroke 2003; 34: 1710–16.
5. Bailey RD, Hart RG, Benavente O, et al. Recurrent brain hemorrhage is more frequent than ischemic stroke after intracranial hemorrhage. Neurology 2001; 56: 773–77.
6. Singh RVP, Prusmack CJ, Morcos JJ. Spontaneous intra cerebral hemorrhage: non arteriovenous malformation, non aneurysm. In HR Winn (ed.), Youmans Neurological Surgery, 5th edn (pp. 1753–5). Philadelphia, PA: Saunders, 2004.
7. van Asch CJJ, Luitse MJA, Rinkel GJE, et al. Incidence, case fatality, and functional outcome of intracerebral haemorrhage over time, according to age, sex, and ethnic origin: a systematic review and meta-analysis. Lancet Neurology 2010; 9: 167–76.
8. Meretoja A, Strbian D, Putaala J,. SMASH-U: a proposal for etiologic classification of intracerebral hemorrhage. Stroke 2012 43(10): 2592–7.
9. Gupta RK, Jamjoom AAB, Nikkar-Esfahani A, et al. Spontaneous intracerebral haemorrhage: a clinical review. British Journal of Hospital Medicine 2010; 71: 499–504.
10. Butcher K, Laidlaw J. Current intracerebral hemorrhage management. Journal of Clinical Neuroscience 2003; 10(2): 158–67.

11. Lovelock CE, Molyneux AJ, Rothwell PM. Change in incidence and aetiology of intracerebral haemorrhage in Oxfordshire, UK, between 1981 and 2006: a population-based study. Lancet Neurology 2007; 6(6): 487–93.
12. Singh RVP, Prusmack CJ, Morcos JJ. Spontaneous intra cerebral hemorrhage: non arteriovenous malformation, non aneurysm. In: HR Winn (ed.), Youmans Neurological Surgery, 5th edn (pp. 1753–5). Philadelphia, PA: Saunders, 2004.
13. Camerlingo M, Casto L, Censori B, et al. Immediate anticoagulation with heparin for first—ever ischaemic stroke in the carotid artery territories observed within 5 hours of onset. Archives of Neurology 1994; 51: 462–7.
14. Pessin MS, Del Zoppo GJ, Estol CJ. Thrombolytic agents in the treatment of stroke. Clinical Neuropharmacology 1990; 13: 271–89.
15. Connolly SJ, Ezekowitz MD, Yusuf S, et al. RE-LY steering committee and investigators dabigatran versus warfarin in patients with atrial fibrillation. New England Journal of Medicine 2009; 361(12): 1139–51.
16. Rahme RJ, Bernstein R, Batjer HH, et al. Is it time to abandon warfarin and embrace oral direct thrombin inhibitors to prevent stroke in patients with atrial fibrillation? Neurosurgery 2011; 68(2): N16–17.
17. Dennis MS. Outcome after brain haemorrhage. Cerebrovascular Disease 2003; 16(Suppl. 1): 9–13.
18. Yang TM, Lin WC, Chang WN, et al. Predictors and outcomes of seizures after spontaneous intracerebral hemorrhage. Journal of Neurosurgery 2009; 111: 87–93.
19. Rost NS, Smith EE, Chang Y, et al. Prediction of functional outcome in patients with primary intracerebral hemorrhage: the FUNC score. Stroke 2008; 39(8): 2304–9.
20. Flaherty ML, Woo D, Haverbusch M, et al. Racial variations in location and risk of intracerebral hemorrhage. Stroke 2005: 36; 934–7.
21. Qureshi AI, Mendelow AD, Hanley DF. Intracerebral haemorrhage. Lancet 2009; 373(9675): 1632–44.
22. Viswanathan A, Greenberg SM. Cerebral amyloid angiopathy in the elderly. Annals of Neurology 2011; 70(6): 871–80.
23. Brott T, Broderick J, Kothari R, et al. Early hemorrhage growth in patients with intracerebral hemorrhage. Stroke 1997; 28: 1–5.
24. Davis SM, Broderick J, Hennerici M, et al. Hematoma growth is a determinant of mortality and poor outcome after intracerebral hemorrhage. Neurology 2006; 66: 1175–81.
25. Aronowski J, Zhao X. Molecular pathophysiology of cerebral hemorrhage: secondary brain injury. Stroke 2011; 42(6): 1781–6.
26. Candelise L, Gattinoni M, Bersano A. Stroke-unit care for acute stroke patients: an observational follow-up study. Lancet 2007; 369(9558): 299–305.
27. Diringer MN, Edwards DF. Admission to a neurologic/neurosurgical intensive care unit is associated with reduced mortality rate after intracerebral hemorrhage. Critical Care Medicine 2001; 29: 635–40.
28. Mirski MA, Chang CW, Cowan R. Impact of a neuroscience intensive care unit on neurosurgical patient outcome and cost of care: evidence-based support for an intensivist-directed speciality ICU model of care. Journal of Neurosurgical Anesthesiology 2001; 13: 83–92.
29. Qureshi AJ, Ezzedine MA, Nasar A, et al. Prevalence of elevated blood pressure in 563,704 adults with stroke presenting to the ED in the United States. American Journal of Emergency Medicine 2007; 25: 32–8.
30. Anderson CS, Huang Y, Wang JG, et al. Intensive blood pressure reduction in acute cerebral haemorrhage trial (INTERACT): a randomised pilot trial. Lancet Neurology 2008; 7: 391–9.
31. Antihypertensive Treatment of Acute Cerebral Haemorrhage (ATACH) investigators. Antihypertensive treatment of acute cerebral haemorrhage. Critical Care Medicine 2010; 38(2): 637–48.

32. Manawadu D, Jeerakatil T, Roy A, et al. Blood pressure management in acute intrarerebral haemorrhage. Guidelines are poorly implemented in clinical practice. Clinical Neurology and Neurosurgery 2010; 112: 858–64.

33. Morgenstern LB, Hemphill JC, Anderson C, et al. Guidelines for the management of spontaneous intracerebral hemorrhage: a guideline for healthcare professionals from the American Heart Association/American Stroke Association. Stroke 2010; 41: 2108–29.

34. Steiner T, Kaste M, Forsting M, et al. Recommendations for the management of intracranial haemorrhage. The European Stroke Initiative Writing Committee and the Writing Committee for the EUSI Executive Committee. Cerebrovascular Disease 2006; 22: 294–316.

35. Mayer SA, Brun NC, Begtrup K, et al. Recombinant activated factor VII for acute intracerebral hemorrhage. New England Journal of Medicine 2005; 352: 777–85.

36. Mayer SA, Davis SM, Begtrup K, et al. Subgroup analysis in the FAST trial: a subset of intracerebral hemorrhage patients that benefit from recombinant activated factor VII. Stroke 2008; 39: 528.

37. Masotti L, Di Napoli M, Godoy DA, et al. The practical management of intracerebral hemorrhage associated with oral anticoagulant therapy. International Journal of Stroke 2011; 6: 228–40.

38. Prasad K, Mendelowe AD, Gregson B. Surgery for primary supratentorial intracerebral haemorrhage. Cochrane Database System Review 2008; 8: C D000200.

39. Dubourg J, Messerer M. State of the art in managing nontraumatic intracerebral hemorrhage. Neurosurgery Focus 2011; 30(6): E22.

40. Kirkman MA. Debate—does an ischaemic penumbra exist in intracerebral haemorrhage. British Journal of Neurosurgery 2011; 25: 523–5.

41. Nilsson OG, Polito A, Saveland H, et al. Are primary supratentorial intracerebral hemorrhages surrounded by a biochemical penumbra? A microdialysis study. Neurosurgery 2006; 59(3): 521–8.

42. Lee J-K., Lee J-H. Ultrasound-guided evacuation of spontaneous intracerebal hematoma in the basal ganglia. Journal of Clinical Neuroscience 2005; 12: 553–6.

43. Niizuma H, Shimizu Y, Yonemitsu T, et al. Results of stereotactic aspiration in 175 cases of putaminal hemorrhage. Neurosurgery 1989; 24: 814–19.

44. Niizuma H, Otsuki T, Johkura H, et al. CT-guided stereotactic aspiration of intracerebral hematoma—result of a hematoma-lysis method using urokinase. Applied Neurophysiology 1985; 48: 427–30.

45. Choy DKS, Wu PH, Tan D, et al. Correlation of the long-term neurological outcomes with completeness of surgical evacuation in spontaneous supratentorial intracerebral hemorrhage: a retrospective study. Singapore Medical Journal 2010; 51(4): 320.

46. Kuo LT, Chen CM, Li CH, et al. Early endoscope-assisted hematoma evacuation in patients with supratentorial intracerebral hemorrhage: case selection, surgical technique, and long-term results. Neurosurgery Focus 2011; 30(4): E9.

47. Murthy JM, Chowdary GV, Murthy TV, et al. Decompressive craniectomy with clot evacuation in large hemispheric hypertensive intracerebral hemorrhage. Neurocritical Care 2005; 2: 258–62.

48. Kirollos RW, Tyagi AK, Ross SA, et al. Management of spontaneous cerebellar hematomas: a prospective treatment protocol. Neurosurgery 2001; 49(6): 1378–87.

49. Mckissock W, Richardson A, & Taylor J. Primary intracerebral haemorrhage: a controlled trial of surgical and conservative treatment in 180 unselected cases. The Lancet 1961; 278(7196): 221–226.

50. Mendelow AD, Gregson BA, Fernandes HM, et al. Early surgery versus initial conservative treatment in patients with spontaneous supratentorial intracerebral haematomas in the International Surgical Trial in Intracerebral Haemorrhage (STICH): a randomised trial. The Lancet 2005; 365(9457): 387–397.

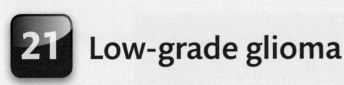

21 Low-grade glioma

Deepti Bhargava

Expert commentary Michael D. Jenkinson

Case history

A 34-year-old right-handed man presented to A&E with a single generalized tonic clonic seizure lasting 3 minutes. In the post-octal period, he recovered to a normal conscious level with no focal neurological deficits.

He was generally fit and well, a non-smoker with no significant family history. However, direct questioning revealed that he had suffered occasional headaches for the past 6 months, with exacerbation in the mornings, and he felt generally lethargic.

Routine bloods were normal. A contrasted CT head undertaken at this stage revealed a uniformly hypodense, ill-defined, non-enhancing mass lesion in the left temporoparietal region, expanding the overlying gyrus, causing a degree of midline shift (Figure 21.1). The appearances were consistent with an intrinsic primary lesion, probably a low-grade glioma. Biopsy was offered and declined by the patient. Management comprised anti-epileptic medication (phenytoin 300mg), and a 'wait and watch' policy was instituted with an initial 6-month scan followed by annual review of disease that remained stable both clinically and radiologically.

> **Expert comment**
>
> Starting anti-epileptic drugs (AEDs) after the first seizure, with consideration of surgical treatment of the epileptogenic focus early in patients with poor seizure control on medication, are two recommendations we make for low-grade glioma.
>
> **Surveillance imaging**
>
> There are no guidelines for surveillance imaging in patients being managed conservatively. MRI is the modality of choice for follow-up and should include T1 +/– gad, T2, and FLAIR. Six-monthly MRI is probably sufficient. Perfusion MRI can be useful for predicting malignant transformation. A joint or concurrent neurosurgery/neuro-oncology low-grade glioma clinic is desirable—this minimizes clinic appointments for the patient, and avoids duplication of follow-up imaging. Once all active treatment options have been exhausted, management should be transferred to the palliative care team.

After 6 years, the patient developed gradual onset expressive dysphasia over a period of 2 months. Radiologically, the tumour remained unchanged. He was seizure free on medication and did not have any adverse drug effects. After discussion, the patient consented to tissue diagnosis. The lesion being superficial, but in eloquent cortex, stereotactic biopsy from the most posterior part of the lesion was undertaken.

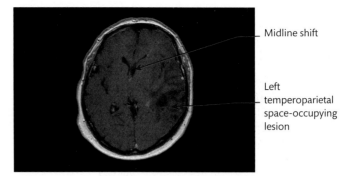

Midline shift

Left temperoparietal space-occupying lesion

Figure 21.1 T1-weighted axial MRI with gadolinium shows a non-enhancing diffuse large temporoparietal lesion with minimal surrounding oedema and midline shift.

> ⊕ **Clinical tip** Brain biopsy: techniques, limitations, and yields
>
> **Open biopsy**
>
> Under general anaesthesia via a small craniotomy. The biopsy may be:
>
> - Excisional, resecting the whole lesion.
> - Incisional, removing a tissue block without disturbing the cyto-architecture.
> - Needle aspiration, where the tissue architecture is disturbed, yielding material for cytology.
>
> Open biopsy is most suitable for superficial lesions, particularly where meningeal biopsy is also required. It may be difficult to localize the region of interest in ill-defined lesions. The diagnostic yield is variable and depends on the diagnosis.
>
> **Stereotactic biopsy**
>
> Under general or local anaesthesia, via a burr hole using 3-D co-ordinates from a contrasted CT/ MRI scan. Stereotaxy may either be frame based or frameless, using neuronavigation techniques. This technique is most suitable for deep/eloquent/small/heterogeneous lesions. It should not be undertaken if the patient has a bleeding diathesis or low platelet count. The diagnostic accuracy using stereotactic biopsy is between 82 and 99 % [1] and is better for cases with enhancing lesions.
>
> The diagnostic yield of a biopsy can be improved with the use of an intra-operative smear/ frozen section. Smearing tissue on a microscope slide reveals lesion cytology. Freezing a block of fresh tissue and cutting thin sections with a cryotome allows the tissue architecture to be preserved, and demonstrates the histological appearances. Generally, after sending fresh tissue, the surgeon waits for the results before either closing the wound or obtaining more tissue if necessary. The accuracy of frozen section or of a smear is comparable, but intra-operative smears are quicker and provide additional cytology characteristics to aid the formal pathology diagnosis [2,3].

Biopsy revealed mildly atypical neoplastic glial cells with a fibrillary and myxoid background consistent with grade 2 oligodendroglioma. The case was discussed and a decision made to offer the patient procarbazine-lomustine (CCNU)-vincristine chemotherapy. This decision took into account the location within eloquent brain and his Karnofsky score of over 90. The disease remained clinically and radiologically stable for another 8 years. However, there was then obvious growth of the tumour on contrasted MRI scan, although it remained non-enhancing (Figure 21.2) and there was recurrence of his seizures.

Functional MRI for motor and language mapping (Figure 21.3) was undertaken. This revealed close proximity of the tumour to speech pathways.

The patient subsequently underwent awake craniotomy and subtotal resection of low-grade glioma.

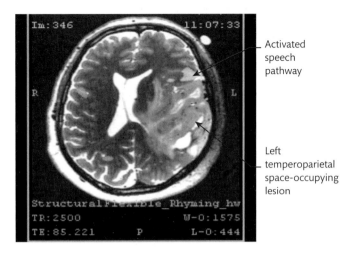

Figure 21.2 T1-weighted axial MRI with gadolinium contrast showing small irregular enhancing lesion in the resection cavity at 10 months.

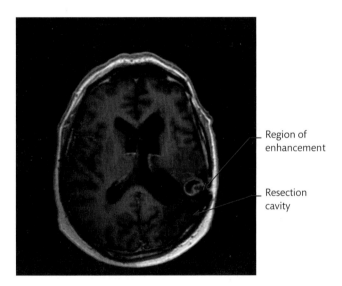

Figure 21.3 T2-weighted axial functional MRI shows close proximity of the tumour to speech pathways.

➕ **Clinical tip** Awake craniotomy with speech mapping

The operation commences with the patient intubated and under general anaesthesia. The cortical surface is exposed give a 2-cm clearance around the tumour margin. The anaesthetist then lightens the sedation and the patient is extubated. Electrical stimulation of the cortex is performed, while the patient interacts generally with tasks of naming and numbering. Each site is tested three times. Tumour resection is undertaken with the patient awake and any areas where electrical stimulation hampers speech are spared with a 1-cm margin. White matter mapping is also possible to attempt preservation of relevant tracts. Once the desired resection is achieved, the patient is re-intubated for craniotomy closure. Functional deficits, if any, after such resections are typically transient and, although they may be encountered immediately in the post-operative period in up to a third of patients, only 1.6% are left with permanent deficits after 6 months [4].

Histology revealed grade 2 oligodendroglioma without any features of malignancy. Post-operatively, he developed transient expressive dysphasia, right homonymous hemianopia, and mild paraesthesia in right upper limb.

As resection was limited due to the presence of functional tissue, a post-operative MRI scan revealed a sizable residue. Adjuvant radiotherapy was administered, after which he suffered mild cognitive and memory deficits. He was referred for neurorehabilitation, where he made good progress.

However, after initial improvement, a further increase in seizure frequency occurred and right upper limb sensory symptoms worsened over a period of the next 10 months. Repeat MRI scan at 10 months revealed an area of enhancement in the resection cavity (Figure 21.2). A change of grade was further suggested on MR spectroscopy (Figure 21.4).

The consensus view of the MDT was that he would not benefit from further surgery or radiotherapy. The patient currently has a KPS of 80 and is receiving temozolamide chemotherapy.

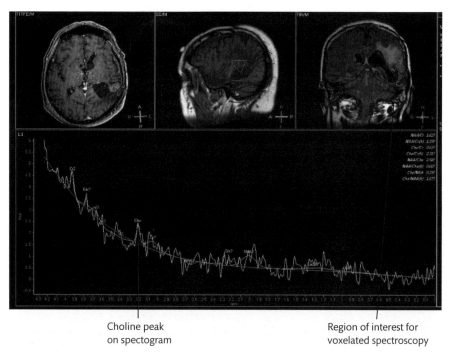

Choline peak
on spectogram

Region of interest for
voxelated spectroscopy

Figure 21.4 MR spectroscopy imaging with metabolic signature of enhancing voxels showing increased cellularity (increased choline: Cho), indicating likely change of grade.

> ✪ **Learning point** Metabolic markers in MR spectroscopy (Table 21.1)
>
> **Table 21.1 Metabolic markers in MR spectroscopy**
>
> | Metabolites | Clinical significance in brain tumours |
> |---|---|
> | NAA (N-acetyl-aspartate) | Neuronal marker, lower in primary brain (glial) tumours. NAA/Cr ratio has inverse relation to grade of glioma |
> | Cho (choline) | Marker of cellular proliferation, increases with tumour grade in glioma. Cho/Cr ratio direct relation to grade of glioma |
> | Cr (creatinine) | Stable brain metabolite in grey and white matter, used as internal reference for determining metabolite ratios |
> | Lipid | Marker of necrosis or proliferation in absence of necrosis |
> | Lactate | Marker of anaerobic glycolysis. Lipid and lactate increase with grade of glioma, combined lipid–lactate peak: reliable marker to distinguish Grade II, III, and IV glioma |

Discussion

Low-grade gliomas are diffusely infiltrating brain tumours, comprising WHO grade II astrocytomas, grade II oligodendrogliomas, and oligoastrocytomas. Despite the name, low-grade gliomas are not benign lesions. These tumours have growth potential and can undergo malignant transformation to high grade tumours. Death is usually due to malignant change. With recent advances in neurobiology, diagnostic imaging, surgical technology, and adjuvant therapies, the management of these tumours has undergone a paradigm shift [5].

Low-grade gliomas comprise 15% of all primary brain tumours. They are more common in Caucasian men, the most common age at onset being the fourth decade. Primarily supratentorial in adults, these lesions have a predilection for the insula and the supplementary motor area [6]. Exposure to ionizing radiation is the only definitive causative factor [7]. They are more commonly seen in patients with neurofibromatosis-1 and Li–Fraumeni syndrome, but no familial tendencies have been noted. IgE levels have been found to have an inverse relation to glioma risk and survival [6].

Histological characteristics determine the classification of these lesions and have a direct bearing on prognosis. Astrocytomas are thought to be the more aggressive with a median survival of 6–9 years; oligodendrogliomas have a relatively better prognosis with a median survival of 9–12 years. The mixed oligoastrocytomas fare somewhere in between [1]. Recent studies show that oligoastrocytomas are monoclonal indicating a common lineage for these tumour subtypes. Amongst astrocytomas, there are three further histological subtypes—fibrillary, protoplasmic, and gemistocytic. The fibrillary variety is most common. A high number of gemistocytes indicates less time to progression and a higher risk of upgrading to higher WHO grades.

★ **Learning point** Histological sub-typing of diffuse low-grade glioma (Table 21.2)

Table 21.2 Histological sub-typing of diffuse low-grade glioma

	Astrocytoma	Oligodendroglioma	Oligoastrocytoma
Image			
Morphology	Low to moderate cellularity, and minimum cellular and nuclear atypia	Uniform cells with round nuclei and scant cytoplasm—fried egg appearance. Loose fibrillary matrix traversed by delicate branching vessels, dividing the tumour into pseudolobules—chicken wire pattern	Mixed areas of astrocytic and oligodendroglial differentiation
Biomarkers	GFAP, vimentin, S-100 protein	No specific markers, identified by absence of typical astrocytic markers	No specific markers
Genetics	Heterozygosity on 17p and heterozygosity of TP53	1p19q co-deletion is most common, seen in 40–70% oligos	30–70% have 1p19q c0-deletion, 30% have TP53 and 17p mutation. All cells in a given tumour are monoclonal

❝ Expert comment

The three most relevant favourable genetic markers include 1p/19q loss, MGMT promoter hypermethylation, and *IDH1* mutation. Testing for these is increasingly being made available in the NHS. While 1p19q simply suggests better outcome, *IDH* and *MGMT* mutations are important in predicting the response to temozolamide chemotherapy.

★ Learning point

Lack of enhancement on MR is not necessarily predictive of low-grade as there is a 50% error rate in diagnosis on imaging grounds alone. The risk of anaplasia in non-enhancing lesions increases with age. Pre-operative metabolic imaging to guide stereotactic biopsy improves diagnostic accuracy up to 100% [6].

Genetic profiling has further advanced our knowledge of these subtypes and their clinical behaviour. Of clinical relevance, *P53* and *PDGF* mutations are associated with astrocytomas and with upgrading. 1p19q loss of heterozygosity is associated with oligodendroglial lineage. Tumours with this mutation have better response rates to temozolamide chemotherapy. *IDH* mutations are associated with better prognosis; *IDH1* is more common in astrocytomas and *IDH2* in oligodendrogliomas. Methylation of MGMT can be found in all histological subtypes and is again associated with a better response to temozolamide [6].

Seizures, often simple partial, complex partial, or generalized tonic clonic, are the most common presentation in 80–90% of patients with low grade glioma (LGG), followed by headaches and focal deficits. Close proximity to the cortex is likely to be responsible for this picture.

Typical radiological findings are of a diffuse, hypodense lesion on CT. Structural MRI, which has been traditionally used for diagnosing LGG's, shows a hypo-intense lesion on T1, and hyperintense on T2 and FLAIR sequences, but patchy enhancement is seen in 15–39% [7]. Cystic degeneration and calcification are common in oligodendroglial tumours.

Advanced imaging techniques have helped to further define tumour characteristics. Low-grade gliomas are hypometabolic on PET. MR spectroscopy shows high choline (increased membrane synthesis), low N-acetyl aspartate (neuronal marker), and no lactate or lipid (no necrosis).

Voxels with choline peaks offer targets for biopsy. MR spectroscopy can also be used in follow-up to distinguish recurrence or change of grade from radiation necrosis, both of which present with enhancement on MRI. Phosphocoline increases with cell density, while glycerophosphocholine increases with Ki-67 proliferation index [8].

The prognosis of LGGs is variable. Based on a meta-analysis, the following factors have been shown to decrease survival:

- Age over 40.
- Tumour size ≥6cm.
- Tumour crossing the midline.
- Neurologic deficits.
- KPS ≤70.
- Enhancement on imaging.
- Residual tumour volume greater than 1cm.

Rate of tumour growth on serial imaging is the most reliable indicator of time to progression and likelihood of malignant change [9]. Class I evidence supports age over 40 years and presence of pre-operative neurological deficits as adverse prognostic factors. Evidence for neuro-imaging findings is Class II [10].

While wait and watch was an accepted policy in management of these tumours, recent evidence has challenged this approach. Modern protocols start with anticonvulsants for symptom control and steroids if there are features of raised ICP [9].

Further management is guided by both patient and tumour characteristics. If the lesion is diffuse and in highly eloquent cortex MRI-guided stereotactic biopsy is offered. Molecular profiling of the tumour accompanies this. Biopsy may be followed by procarbazine carvincrisitine vincrisitine (PCV) or temozolamide chemotherapy, especially if the tumour is 1p19q or *MGMT* mutant, if the tumour demonstrates 'high risk' features or if radiotherapy is not appropriate.

If the tumour has relatively discrete margins in brain tissue, where a macroscopic resection will be possible without compromising function, maximum safe surgical resection of all hyperintense tissue on FLAIR sequences should be attempted. This will improve overall and progression-free survival and gives improved seizure control, as well as providing better tumour sampling for histology. Total/near total resection decreases the incidence of recurrence, the risk of malignant transformation, and improves progression-free survival (PFS) and overall survival (OS) (Class III) [11]. Complex partial and generalized tonic clonic seizures, as well as seizures of short duration responsive to AEDs are best controlled with surgery. Extent of resection of the tumour also has important impact on seizure control with gross total resection achieving much better control than partial/subtotal resection [12]. Use of fMRI, awake craniotomy, intra-operative imaging, and cortical and sub-cortical mapping are all useful adjuncts in achieving the surgical goal.

⊕ Clinical tip

Anticonvulsants may increase or decrease the metabolism of chemotherapeutic agents (cytochrome p 450). In patients with a single seizure, immediate treatment with AEDs reduces seizure frequency. There is no role for prophylactic AEDs.

❝ Expert comment

Surgical adjuncts in the macroscopic resection of low grade gliomas (LGGs)

- Intra-operative cortical stimulation mapping is typically used for speech and motor mapping. The technique is detailed in the description of awake craniotomy. Risks of permanent damage are substantially reduced.
- Intra-operative tractography/subcortical electrical mapping is performed in a similar manner to cortical mapping. The technique is most useful for tumours involving the optic radiation, speech tracts, and descending motor fibres in that order.
- Intra-operative ultrasound correlates poorly with MRI and generally results in larger post-operative residual tumour volumes when compared with MRI directed resections. It may have a role in centres, where intra-operative MRI is not available or the patient has a contraindication for MRI scanning.
- Intra-operative MRI is the most useful for LGG, as it may be difficult to differentiate glioma intra-operatively from normal brain tissue. Sequential intra-operative MR is ideal. Operative time is substantially increased, but the need for early second surgery is curtailed and better tumour resection is possible. In the ideal setting, one would use intra-operative MR with direct cortical stimulation mapping to achieve maximal functional resection.

✚ Clinical tip

Identification and resection of the epileptogenic focus through electrocorticography is likely to enhance seizure control after resection. Long duration (multifocality) and hippocampal atrophy suggest poor seizure control post-operatively. Seizure control is an index for quality of life in these patients, but surgery is not targeted at epileptogenic foci for those with minimal seizure frequency or well-controlled disease on medication. In patients with good seizure control post-operatively, seizure recurrence usually indicates tumour progression.

The timing and role for adjuvant/neo-adjuvant therapy in these patients is being extensively researched. According to current evidence early (primary adjuvant) versus delayed (upon recurrence) radiotherapy does not bestow any overall survival advantage. Although improved PFS was demonstrated for patients treated with immediate RT, this did not translate into improved OS (Class I)- EORTC 22845 (reference here).

The benefit of progression-free survival gained from early radiotherapy is offset by the resultant neurotoxicity. As such radiotherapy is mainly reserved for high risk cases or upon tumour progression. Optimal dosage is considered to be 50–54Gray since studies show no difference when compared with a higher dose [*EORTC 22844* and *NCCTG* investigated higher v/s lower dose of RT showed no advantage for higher doses (Class I)] and the benefit is reduced neurotoxicity [9].

Traditionally, chemotherapy was not thought to be very effective in this setting. As detailed above, genetic profiling of these tumours has changed this perspective. Temozolamide and PCV regimens are both being extensively investigated in multicentre trials. *RTOG 9802* investigated RT plus early chemotherapy versus chemotherapy at progression. PFS, but not OS were improved (Class I). However, beyond 2 years, the addition of PCV to RT conferred a significant OS and PFS advantage, reducing the risk of death by 48% and progression by 55%, suggesting a delayed benefit for chemotherapy. Grade 3–4 toxicity was higher amongst patients receiving RT + PCV (67 versus 9%; Class I).

Patient wishes and aspirations are always important, and need to be considered in all decision making, as is the discussion of all cases in the neuro-oncology multidisciplinary meeting.

A final word from the expert

The optimal management of low-grade glioma remains to be defined. The majority of tumours are located within eloquent brain and affect young people. Management aims to stabilize tumour, whilst preserving quality of life. Four points summarize the future direction of LGG management:

- There is a paradigm shift towards early aggressive resection to functional limits defined by intra-operative brain mapping to encompass the FLAIR signal abnormality.

- Functional remodelling of eloquent brain regions allows further tumour resection.

- Neo-adjuvant chemotherapy can reduce tumour size to enable complete resection of the FLAIR signal.

- Supra-complete tumour resection with a 2-cm margin beyond the FLAIR signal abnormality may potentially 'cure' low-grade glioma, but long-term outcome data are awaited.

References

1. Greenberg M, Duckworth EA, Arredondo N (6the edn). Handbook of Neurosurgery. Thieme Medical Publishers, Incorporated, November 2005.
2. Woodworth GF, McGirt MJ, Samdani A, et al. Frameless image-guided stereotactic brain biopsy procedure: diagnostic yield, surgical morbidity, and comparison with the frame-based technique. Journal of Neurosurgery 2006; 104 (2): 233–7.
3. Hayden R, Cajulis RS, Frias-Hidvegi D, et al. Intraoperative diagnostic techniques for stereotactic brain biopsy: cytology versus frozen-section histopathology. Stereotactic Functional Neurosurgery 1995; 65 (1–4): 187–93.
4. Sanai N, Berger MS. Operative techniques for gliomas and the value of extent of resection. Neurotherapeutics 2009; 6 (3): 478–86.
5. Potts MB, Smith JS, Molinaro AM, et al. Natural history and surgical management of incidentally discovered low-grade gliomas. Journal of Neurosurgery 2012; 116 (2): 365–72.
6. Sanai N, Chang S, Berger MS. Low-grade gliomas in adults (Review). Journal of Neurosurgery 2011; 115 (5): 948–65.
7. Cavaliere R, Lopes MB, Schiff D. Low-grade gliomas: an update on pathology and therapy. Lancet Neurology 2005; 4: 760–70.
8. McKnight TR, Smith KJ, Chu PW, et al. Choline metabolism, proliferation, and angiogenesis in nonenhancing grades 2 and 3 astrocytoma. Journal of Magnetic Resonance Imaging 2011; 33 (4): 808–16.
9. Gilbert MR, Lang FF. Management of patients with low-grade gliomas. Neurology Clinic 2007; 25: 1073–88.
10. Pignatti F, van den Bent MJ, Curran D, et al. Prognostic factors for survival in adult patients with cerebral low grade glioma. Journal of Clinical Oncology 2002; 20: 2076–84.
11. Smith JS, Chang EF, Lamborn KR, et al. Role of extent of resection in the long-term outcome of low-grade hemispheric gliomas. Journal of Clinical Oncology 2008; 26: 1338–45.
12. Englot DJ, Berger MS, Barbaro NM, et al. Predictors of seizure freedom after resection of supratentorial low-grade gliomas. A review. Journal of Neurosurgery 2011; 115 (2): 240–4.

22 Intracranial arteriovenous malformation

Jinendra Ekanayake

⊕ Expert commentary Neil Kitchen

Case history

A 54-year-old right-handed man was admitted with a 2-week history of left-sided headaches, visual disturbance, and difficulties with short-term memory. Examination revealed a right-sided temporal hemianopia.

Nine years previously, following a brief loss of consciousness at home, investigations had revealed a left-sided occipital arteriovenous malformation (AVM) with a 3.5-cm nidus, and associated deep venous drainage (Spetzler–Martin Grade 4). He remained entirely asymptomatic following this event, which was diagnosed as an unrelated vasovagal episode. It was initially decided that the management should be conservative, given the incidental discovery of the AVM.

> **✪ Learning point** Surgical operability and the Spetzler–Martin grade
>
> The Spetzler–Martin classification (1986) was proposed as a means of defining surgical operability [1]. It is based on three components—nidus size, venous drainage, and proximity to eloquent brain regions. Eloquent brain is given a somewhat broad description, including primary motor, sensory, visual and language cortices, as well as the thalamus, hypothalamus, brainstem, and cerebellar peduncles.
>
> Table 22.1: The percentage of patients with a major neurological deficit (defined as hemiparesis aphasia, and/or hemianopia) increases as the Spetzler–Martin grade rises.
>
> **Table 22.1 Correlation of AVM grade with surgical results***
>
> | Grade | No. cases | No deficit | | Minor deficit | | Major deficit | | Death (%) |
> |---|---|---|---|---|---|---|---|---|
> | | | No. | % | No. | % | No. | % | |
> | I | 23 | 23 | 100 | 0 | 0 | 0 | 0 | 0 |
> | II | 21 | 20 | 95 | 1 | 5 | 0 | 0 | 0 |
> | III | 25 | 21 | 84 | 3 | 12 | 1 | 4 | 0 |
> | IV | 15 | 11 | 73 | 3 | 20 | 1 | 7 | 0 |
> | V | 16 | 11 | 69 | 3 | 19 | 2 | 12 | 0 |
> | Total | 100 | 86 | 86 | 10 | 10 | 4 | 4 | 0 |
>
> *Exceptions to this include if the patient has repeated haemorrhages, or progressive neurological deficit, the presence of flow-related aneurysms (amenable to surgery or endovascular treatment) and steal-related deficits (amenable to endovascular treatment) [2].
>
> The grade is the sum of the three individual components scoring AVMs from I to V (Table 22.2). A further grade has been proposed, VI, to define 'inoperable'. Despite criticisms related to nidus heterogeneity, eloquence, and infratentorial AVMs, the system has been prospectively validated and remains in common usage.
>
> (continued)

Table 22.2 Spetzler–Martin grading scale for AVMs

Feature	Score
<3 cm	1
3–6 cm	2
>6 cm	3
Location	
Non-eloquent cortex	0
In/ adjacent to eloquent cortex	1
Venous drainage	
Superficial only	0
Deep	1

Spetzler and Ponce have proposed a recent revision (2011) to this classification to reflect treatment strategies (Table 22.3) [2]. The grouping of the grades into a three-tier system was based on a pooled analysis of outcome in 1476 patients taken from seven surgical series. Predictive accuracies for surgical outcomes were found to similar when comparing surgical outcomes between the five-tier and three-tier system [2,3].

Table 22.3 Spetzler- Martin grading scale for AVMs

Class	Spetzler-Martin Grade	Treatment
A	I &II	Microsurgery
B	III	Multimodality
C	IV & V	No treatment*

❝ Expert comment Unruptured AVMs—to treat or not to treat?

Current best evidence in relation to treatment is from the ARUBA trial (A Randomised Trial in Unruptured Brain Aneurysms) reported by Mohr et al (2013) [4]. It was a prospective, parallel-design randomized controlled trial (NHS class A) which was stopped early, with a follow-up of 33 months. Eligibility was age 18 years or over, no previous haemorrhage or intervention, in patients with brain AVMs (bAVMs) considered suitable for obliteration. 226 patients were recruited between 2007–2013; 114 patients were randomised to intervention, 109 patients to best medical management (7 patients crossed to the intervention arm, without suffering a bleed). 5 were treated with surgery, 30 with embolisation, 31 with radiotherapy, 28 with a multimodality approach. The primary outcome measured were symptomatic stroke or death; secondary outcome measures were clinical impairment, defined as 2 or higher on the modified Rankin Scale.35/114(30.7%) patients in the treatment arm vs 11/109 (10.1%) patients in the medical arm reached the primary endpoint. 17/109 (38.6%) treated patients, and 6/109 (14%) of the patients managed medically reached the secondary endpoint. The authors concluded that medical management was therefore superior to intervention for unruptured bAVM patients at 33 months.

Russin and Spetzler (2014) provided a critique of the study and its findings, citing design flaws, lack of standardisation of the treatment arm , and inadequate study detail (i.e. 726 patients were eligible, 226 patients were enrolled- 177 patients were managed outside of the randomisation process) [5]. Nonetheless, the findings of the ARUBA trial provide important evidence on the management of unruptured aneuryms, and is supported by the Scottish Intracranial Vascular Malformation Study (SIVMS) which was carried out between 1999–2003. This was a smaller prospective observational study, with a 3 year outcome, which found an increased risk of a poor outcome in patients receiving treatment, and those with large AVMs [6].

On his most recent admission, CT imaging once again confirmed the presence of the AVM. There was no evidence of an intracranial bleed or brain swelling associated with the AVM.

CT angiography and digital subtraction angiography (DSA) revealed that the AVM was principally supplied from the left posterior cerebral artery, with pial supply from the left anterior and middle cerebral arteries. Drainage was through a single arterialized vein into the straight sinus (Figure 22.1a–d).

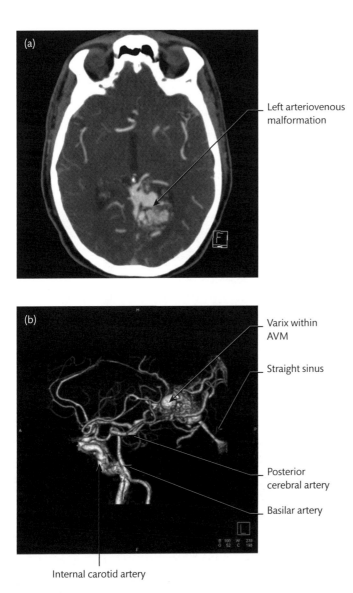

Figure 22.1 (a) CT angiogram axial section. There is a serpiginously-enhancing lesion in the left occipital lobe. The appearances are those of an AVM with no evidence of acute haemorrhage. (b) CT angiogram sagittal 3D reconstruction. The nidus is fed mainly by the left PCA with venous drainage into the vein of Galen. (c,d) DSA: left vertebral artery injection, anteroposterior and lateral views, respectively.

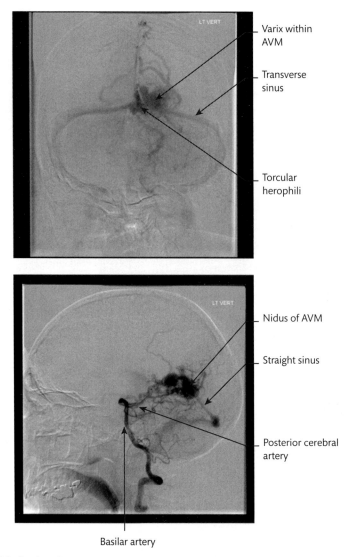

Figure 22.1 Continued

In view of the size and location of the AVM, the recommendation of the neuro-vascular multidisciplinary meeting was staged endovascular embolization. At the time of his first embolization, performed via internal carotid and vertebral artery catheterization, 50% of the nidus was obliterated (Figures 22.2a,b).

> ✪ **Learning point** Staged embolization and stereotactic radiosurgery
>
> In large lesions, which are considered to be unfavourable for surgery, staged embolization followed by SRS has been used. Embolization has two goals:
>
> • Targeted eradication of AVM-related aneurysms and fistulae.
> • Volumetric reduction.
>
> By reducing the size of the nidus, a larger dose of stereotactic radiation can be prescribed in order to increase the probability of nidus obliteration without increasing the risk of complications. Many
>
> (continued)

radiosurgery centres now avoid embolization before treatment for large AVMs, preferring instead to stage the radiosurgery either by volume (with different components of the nidus being treated on each occasion) or by dose, with suboptimal doses being used on two or more occasions.

Gobin and colleagues treated 125 inoperable AVM patients with embolization prior to definitive treatment with SRS. Embolization resulted in total occlusion in 11.2% of AVMs and, in 76%, was reduced enough to allow SRS. Subsequent SRS produced total occlusion in 65% of these cases.

No complications were associated with SRS. There was morbidity of 12.8% and a mortality of 1% following embolization. The haemorrhage rate for the partially embolized AVMs was 3% per annum [7].

The patient subsequently underwent three further embolization procedures with a progressive reduction in the size and flow rate of the AVM (Figure 22.3).

Following a further multidisciplinary assessment, gamma knife radiosurgery was advised and subsequently delivered. Normally, follow-up after radiosurgery would

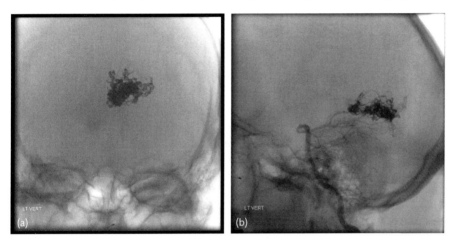

Figure 22.2 (a,b) Post-embolization DSA/left vertebral injection anteroposterior and lateral views.

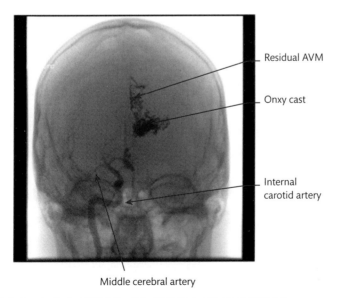

Residual AVM

Onyx cast

Internal carotid artery

Middle cerebral artery

Figure 22.3 Post-embolization DSA/left vertebral injection, anteroposterior view.

involve annual MRI scans as a preliminary indication of nidus obliteration. This will often require 2–3 years, but may occur up to 4 years after treatment. If there are no obvious flow voids in the area of treatment, digital subtraction angiography is indicated to confirm obliteration. Retreatment with radiosurgery is possible and would normally be recommended if obliteration has not occurred within 4 years.

✪ Learning point Stereotactic radiosurgery

This is typically reserved for compact lesions, usually less than 3cm in size. It is currently the preferred treatment strategy for the majority of patients, unless there are very good clinical reasons to prefer surgery (e.g. treatment of the AVM during removal of an ICH, patient preference after careful counselling).

After treatment, which may take up to 48 months to obliterate the nidus, there is a risk of haemorrhage. Annual haemorrhage rates have been estimated at 4.8–7.9% per year for the first 2 years*, then 2.2–5% in the third, fourth, and fifth years. Notably, if the nidus is obliterated, the risk of haemorrhage is near zero. In the optimal case, i.e. small nidus, uncomplicated location, complete obliteration can be achieved in at least 90% of cases, although this decreases significantly for larger AVMs (i.e. treatment volumes of 20cm^3) [4].

The technique allows a high dose of radiation to be delivered to a focal brain region, while minimizing radiation to surrounding normal brain. It is therefore ideal for centrally-located lesions, such as the brainstem, thalamus, and basal ganglia. Lim and colleagues have also demonstrated its successful use in patients with medically intractable seizures. Furthermore, it may be used in those with multiple lesions [8], such as in familial syndromes [9,10].

*The risk of haemorrhage in the first 2 years following SRS is higher than the annual risk of haemorrhage in an untreated unruptured AVM, i.e. 2.4%.

❝ Expert comment Surgery for arteriovenous malformations

With the advent of endovascular obliteration and gamma knife radiotherapy, neurosurgical intervention is no longer the commonest modality of treatment for intracranial AVMs in most centres. The main benefit of surgery is of an immediate cure. Following dural opening, surgical technique involves delineation of the malformation, elimination of superficial feeding vessels, circumferential dissection of the nidus with control of the deep arterial pedicles and transection of the venous system. A haemosiderin or gliotic rim, or acutely haemorrhagic clot itself may provide a plane of dissection around the nidus, see figure 22.5.

It is critically important to identify arterialized veins before resection. If there is any doubt a temporary clip maybe used, as premature coagulation of a draining vein may result in catastrophic haemorrhage.

Sylvian fissure lesions are prone to *en passage* vessels, which must be skeletonized and preserved, with resection only of the small side branches feeding the nidus.

It is of vital importance to plan the surgical approach well in advance of surgery, using pre-operative MRI and angiogram imaging to establish the position of probable feeding and draining vessels

---

✪ Learning point Arteriovenous malformations and driving

In the UK, there are very specific guidelines regarding AVMs and driving, with the diagnosis of an AVM potentially having a significant impact on the livelihood of professional drivers. Decisions are made on the background of the history and examination, e.g. incidental AVMs versus ruptured AVMs, supratentorial versus infratentorial location (Tables 22.4 and 22.5), and related seizures.

Please see the DVLA website for more information: http://www.dft.gov.uk/dvla

(continued)

Table 22.4 Supratentorial AVMs cars/ bikes (Group 1) lorries/ large goods vehicle (LGV) (Group 2)

Pathology	Group 1 recommendation	Group 2 recommendation
Incidental		
No treatment	Retain licence	Permanent refusal
Treatment	As for ICH presentation	Refusal unless cured and 10 years seizure free
ICH presentation		
Craniotomy	6/12 off driving	Refusal unless cured and 10 years seizure free
Embolization/SRS	1/12 off driving	Refusal unless cured and 10 years seizure free
No treatment	As above	Permanent refusal

Table 22.5 Infratentorial AVMS

Pathology	Group 1 recommendation	Group 2 recommendation
Incidental		
No treatment	Retain	Individual assessment
Treatment	Can drive once no disability	Refusal unless cured/no disability
ICH presentation		
Craniotomy	Retain unless disability affecting driving	Refusal unless cured
Embolization/ SRS	As above	As above
No treatment	As above	Permanent refusal

> ✚ **Clinical tip** Risk of arteriovenous malformation rebleeding
>
> Several morphological and angio-architectural factors have been examined with regards to the risk of rebleeding, with a considerable degree of variability in the results [11].
>
> • Previous rupture.
> • Annual rupture rate of 6% (first 5 years)/cumulative 5-year risk 26%.
> • Associated aneurysms.
> • Deep venous drainage.

Discussion

AVMs were first described by Virchow in 1851, although clinical descriptions of extracranial vascular abnormalities date back to the Ebers Papyrus (*c.* 1500 BC). The first complete neurosurgical excision of an intracranial AVM is credited to Emile Pean in 1889 who removed a right-sided 'central' tumour in a 15-year-old boy with left-sided seizures.

> ✪ **Learning point** Arteriovenous malformations—an embryological versus developmental abnormality
>
> AVMs may develop during embryonic development- the two main hypotheses regarding their pathogenesis include:
>
> • Embryonic agenesis of the capillary system.
> • Retention of the primordial connection between arteries and veins [12].
>
> (continued)

Despite this, they are believed to be dynamic biological entities, rather than static congenital vascular lesions.

Although certain genes are associated with the development of AVMs (e.g. ALK-1 in hereditary haemorrhagic telangiectasia, (HHT)) and their rupture (e.g. ApoE e2), there is clear evidence of de novo formation and active growth post-natally. This would suggest a more complex mechanism, including environmental contributions to the expression of genes involved in angiogenesis and vascular repair. It is of note that, in certain cases, AVMs have been observed to regress and disappear completely [13].

AVMs are associated with several rare hereditary conditions including: HHT, von Hippel–Lindau disease, Sturge–Weber disease, and Wyburn–Mason syndrome. They are rarely familial, having been described in only twenty families (forty-four cases) [14]. See Figure 22.4

Arteriovenous malformations of the brain are complex vascular lesions with a number of associated neuroparenchymal, haemodynamic and angio-architectural changes. The fundamental abnormality is one or more direct fistulous communications between afferent feeding arteries and efferent draining veins, without the presence of an intervening capillary bed. The increased blood flow through these arteriovenous shunts causes the characteristic changes of vascular dilatation, tortuosity, and the formation of the 'nidus', an intervening network of vessels.

They may be found in either the brain or the dura. Note arteriovenous fistulae (AVFs) differ only in the absence of an intervening nidus.

> ✪ **Learning point** Arterial contributions to the nidus
>
> Identifying the arterial supply to the AVM is particularly important within the context of surgical disconnection prior to excision of the AVM. Valavanis (1996) described three types of supply [15].
>
> - Direct or terminal feeders.
> - Dedicated vessels terminating in the nidus, arising from main arteries.
> - Indirect feeders.
> - 'Satellite' branches from an artery in close proximity to the nidus.
> - 'En passant' vessels.
> - These are functional vessels and, in addition to supplying the nidus, pass through to supply normal brain tissue beyond.

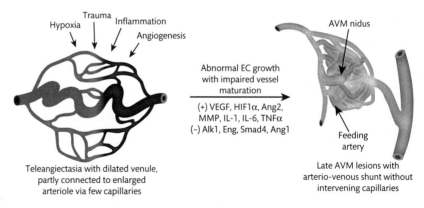

Figure 22.4 AVMs are fast-flow lesions wherein feeder arterioles shunt directly to veins without intervening capillaries. Candidate disease-associated molecules that are upregulated (+) or downregulated (−) are shown. EC, endothelial cell

(Taken from Storkebaum et al., 2011 [15])

Clinical presentation

These are rare lesions (0.14% incidence, 0.001–0.52% prevalence), but are important as they tend to affect young patients who are frequently otherwise healthy [24].

They typically present as ICHs accounting for 2% of all strokes and 4% of intracranial haematomas overall, but up to 38% in 15–45-year-olds. Haemorrhage is associated with a 5–10% risk of death, and 30–50% chance of permanent or disabling neurological deficits [25].

Other presentations include seizures, which are the second most common presentation (20% of patients, with higher risk in large AVMs i.e. >6cm [28]), Less commonly, ipsilateral headaches, and focal neurological deficits (temporary, fixed, or progressive) in 3–10% of patients due to mass effect and haemodynamic disturbances. At least 15% of patients with AVMs at the time of detection are asymptomatic, and this figure will increase with greater access to MRI scanning [29].

CT imaging is routinely used in the acute setting of haemorrhage/ICH presentation, allowing identification of the bleed and/or infarct. Unruptured AVMs may be identified by prominent calcification (20–30%). CT angiography provides good delineation of vascular anatomy, particularly with 3D vascular reconstruction. However, digital subtraction catheter angiography remains the gold standard allowing for

In addition to the above, which were found to be independent risk factors on multivariate analysis, other authors [6,27] identified the importance of intra-nidal pressure and included the following:

- Single draining vein.
- Venous stenosis.

*Other important studies include Ondra et al. (1990) [26], and Stapf et al. (2006) [25].

evaluation of venous outflow obstruction, associated aneurysms, feeding artery/arteries, and venous drainage. MRI/MRA enables the best assessment of the anatomical relationships to neighbouring brain structures (i.e. 'eloquence'). Functional MRI and diffusion tensor imaging can further help to identify eloquent areas (i.e. language, motor, etc.) and associated white matter tracts, respectively.

AVMs and Epilepsy

The cause of epileptogenesis is still unclear. Focal cerebral ischaemia as a result of arteriovenous shunting has been suggested, as has ischaemia in the surrounding brain regions, as a result of steal phenomena. Gliotic brain tissue within the nidus, and in the surrounding brain regions may also contribute to secondary epileptogenesis

Nonetheless Yeh et al. operated on twenty-seven patients with epilepsy with seizure-elimination in twenty-one patients. They concluded that excision of an AVM must also include removal of the epileptogenic focus [19].

More recent studies of seizure outcomes after radiosurgery have demonstrated very promising results and deserved particular consideration (62% [20] and 80% [21]). It has been suggested that beneficial effects on seizure control occur even before complete obliteration, although this provides the best seizure-free results However, new-onset seizures can be a complication of radiosurgery [22].

There are fewer reports of seizure control after embolization, although this likely to reflect that it primarily used as an adjunctive procedure in multimodality treatment [23].

Treatment

The treatment of AVMs uses three modalities, alone or in combination. They are microsurgery, embolization, and radiosurgery. The manner in which these are applied take into account patient factors (i.e. age, co-morbidities, mode of presentation), AVM factors (size, location, Spetzler–Martin grade), and available expertise.

Microsurgical approaches afford direct visualization of anatomy with control of feeding vessels, but are offset by the attendant risks of open surgery, together with the technical expertise required for correct vessel delineation. It potentially offers immediate and complete cure and, for some surgeons, is the preferred first line treatment for SM grade I and II AVMs, see figure 22.5. Complications following surgery have been variously classified as major and minor neurological deficits. They are related to the location of the lesion, with size, deep venous drainage, and the presence of associated aneurysms increasing the surgical risk. Complications include aphasia, hemianopia, hemiparesis, and death. A recent meta-analysis reported a morbidity of 8.6% and mortality of 3.3%, after mostly surgical treatment, in a series of 2452 patients [31]. The surgical risk for morbidity and mortality for Spetzler–Martin grade of less or equal to 3 has been reported to be 2–6.3% and 0–2%, respectively. The surgical risk for morbidity and mortality for Spetzler–Martin grade IV and V has been reported to be 9–39% and 0–9%, respectively.

Stereotactic radiotherapy provides the least invasive treatment option. The most important factor for nidus obliteration is the dose of radiation delivered. The safe dose correlates inversely with volume, in that the larger the lesion, the smaller

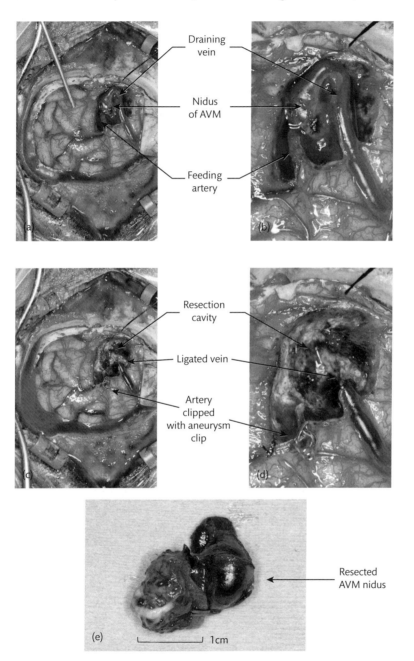

Figure 22.5 Intraoperative images of an occipital AVM showing cardinal anatomy (a,b) i.e. feeding artery, draining vein, and the AVM nidus. Postoperative images showing the resected AVM nidus and the residual postoperative cavity(c,d,e).

the dose that can be given without a high risk of radionecrosis of surrounding brain. Other factors include the size of the nidus (e.g. ideally <3cm), the nidus angio-architecture (e.g. compact versus diffuse nidus), intranidal aneurysms, venous drainage, eloquent location, and previous haemorrhage. A compact nidus is a better target compared with plexiform or diffuse lesions, as they have no neural tissue inside the target volume, enabling larger does to be prescribed. It may take up to 4 years for complete obliteration of the nidus, during which time the patient continues to be at risk of haemorrhage (5% per year: see Learning point: stereotactic radiosurgery). Multiple series have been published regarding the different techniques used for radiosurgery, including proton beam, gamma knife, linear accelerator (LINAC) and CyberKnife. A recent meta-analysis of sixty-nine cohorts (twenty-two gamma knife, thirty-six LINAC) by Beijnum et al. (2011) found a 40% 2-year obliteration rate [28]. The probability of obliteration depends on the administered dose, which is influenced by the location of the AVM. Obliteration is produced by radiation-induced damage to the endothelium of the arterial wall, resulting in smooth muscle proliferation with subsequent luminal occlusion. Complications of radiosurgery include white matter oedema, seizures, radiation necrosis, and haemorrhage.

Embolization can be used as a pre-operative adjunct to surgery, leading to decreased operating times, transfusion requirements, morbidity, and mortality. As a primary modality, it offers relatively low cure rates (5–20%) with a risk of subsequent recanalization, although the use of new embolic agents, such as onyx, holds promise (15–50%). It may be offered as a primary treatment option in selected patients, i.e. for small deep-seated thalamic or basal ganglia AVMs, with one or two feeding arteries providing immediate protection against recurrent and immediate haemorrhage. Complications may be permanent or temporary, and are usually neurological deficits related to inadvertent embolization of arteries supplying healthy brain or obliteration of the venous outflow, leading to ICH. They include haemorrhage (2–5%), permanent neurological deficits (2–5%), and death (1%).

> **Learning point** Guidelines for treatment
>
> **SM I, II**
> - SRS.
> - Microsurgery (patient preference, surgery for haematoma).
>
> **SM III**
> - Microsurgery/radiosurgery +/– endovascular therapy.
>
> **SM IV, V**
> - Observation.
> - Consider tailored treatment if risk of haemorrhage/repeat.
> - Bleeds.
>
> In practice, SM grade III are the most challenging malformations to treat, representing a heterogeneous mix of pathology. This group has been subdivided into IIIA (>6cm) that are best treated with embolization and surgery, and IIIB (small, i.e. deep venous drainage and in eloquent cortex [32]) that are best treated with radiosurgery

⊗ **Learning point** Aneurysms and AVMs

Aneurysms occur in approximately 20–25% of patients with AVMs. They may be incidental, in a separate vascular territory, or they may be 'flow related' on feeding vessels. These latter aneurysms are thought to arise secondary to the hyperdynamic circulatory state induced by the AVM. Intranidal aneurysms may also occur.

It is not clear if there is an increased risk of haemorrhage in AVMs with aneurysms. In a small study of ninety-one patients with unruptured AVMs Brown et al. demonstrated an increased risk of ICH at 1 year in patients with an AVM and an aneurysm (7% cf. 3% with only an AVM) [33].

In the presence of haemorrhage, a number of studies have suggested that the AVM is more likely to be the cause of the haemorrhage except in the posterior fossa. Intranidal aneurysms have been suggested to be associated with an increased risk of haemorrhage, as have those associated with a pedicle or feeding artery [31].

In the setting of a non-haemorrhagic presentation, aneurysms that are distal or flow-related are likely to regress with treatment of the AVM, whereas this is unlikely in those arising on the circle of Willis.

❝ Expert comment Multimodality treatment

A staged multimodality approach is often recommended for complex AVMs, or after treatment failure, on a case-by-case basis. It combines the advantages of the individual treatments, and may be the safest approach for some AVMs. However, it does result in an additive risk; Beijnum et al (2011) on meta-analysis found that embolization after SRS was associated with increased risk of haemorrhage and other complications [28].

⊗ **Learning point** Occlusive hyperaemia versus normal perfusion pressure breakthrough

Following AVM resection, haemorrhage and cerebral oedema is occasionally seen in the cortex surrounding the resection cavity. Two prevailing hypotheses attempt to explain this phenomenon, although it is likely that they are not mutually exclusive, potentially forming a spectrum of complex haemodynamic changes seen in and around AVMs.

The **'normal perfusion pressure breakthrough'** hypothesis, put forward in 1978 suggests that the surrounding parenchyma of an AVM is chronically hyperperfused, with impaired autoregulation. As such, it becomes vulnerable to uncontrolled hyperaemia, oedema, and potential 'breakthrough' bleeding upon the restoration of normal perfusion pressures, following removal of the AVM [29].

The 'occlusive hyperaemia' hypothesis (1993) suggests stagnant arterial flow to the AVM, and obstruction to venous outflow of the surrounding parenchyma results in a hypoperfused and ischaemic state, which is worsened following resection [6].

A final word from the expert

The future management of these lesions will lie in better defining the natural history versus interventions in unruptured AVMs (ARUBA results), in clarifying the use of radiation in large AVMs (dose reduction/fractionation/partial volume treatments), and in the continuing evolution and assessment of endovascular technologies against the background of what is emerging as an increasingly benign disease.

The emergency or urgent treatment of ruptured AVMs requires experience and skill in determining the correct treatment sequence, and should be restricted to those centres capable of providing the full range of expertise required.

References

1. Spetzler RF, Martin NA. A proposed grading system for arteriovenous malformations. Journal of Neurosurgery 1986; 65 (4): 476–83.
2. Spetzler R, Ponce F. A 3-tier classification of cerebral arteriovenous malformations. Clinical article. Journal of Neurosurgery 2011; 114 (3): 842–9.
3. Houdart E, Gobin YP, Casasco A, et al. A proposed angiographic classification of intracranial arteriovenous fistulae and malformations. Neuroradiology 1993; 35: 381–5.

4. Mohr JP, Parides MK, Stapf C, et al. Medical management with or without interventional therapy for unruptured brain arteriovenous malformations (ARUBA): a multicentre, non-blinded, randomised trial. Lancet. 2013;383 (9917):614–621.

5. Russin J, Spetzler R, Neurosurgery. Commentary: the ARUBA trial. Neurosurgery. 2014. 75 (1): E96–E97

6. al Rodhan NR, Sundt TM, Piepgras DG, et al. Occlusive hyperaemia: a theory for the hemodynamic complications following resection of intracerebral arteriovenous malformations. Journal of Neurosurgery 1993; 78 (2): 167–75.

7. Gobin YP, Laurent A, Merienne L, et al. Treatment of brain arteriovenous malformations by embolization and radiosurgery. Journal of Neurosurgery 1996; 85 (1): 19–28.

8. Lim YJ, Lee CY, Koh JS, et al. Seizure control of gamma knife radiosurgery for non-hemorrhagic arteriovenous malformations. Acta Neurochirurgica 2006; 99: 97–101.

9. Kikuchi K, Kowada M, Sasajima H. Vascular malformations of the brain in hereditary hemorrhagic telangiectasia (Rendu-Osler-Weber disease). Surgical Neurology 1994; 41: 374–80.

10. Yahara K, Inagawa T, Tokuda Y, et al. [A case of multiple cerebral arteriovenous malformations treated by gamma knife radiosurgery]. No Shinkei Geka—Neurological Surgery 1995; 23: 1121–5.

11. Choi JH, Mohr JP. Brain arteriovenous malformations in adults. Lancet Neurology 2005; 4: 299–308.

12. Hashimoto N, Nozaki K, Takagi Y, et al. Surgery of cerebral arteriovenous malformations. Neurosurgery 2007; 61: 375–87; discussion 387–9.

13. Nehls DG, Pittman HW. Spontaneous regression of arteriovenous malformations. Neurosurgery 1982; 11: 776–80.

14. Herzig R, Burval S, Vladyka V, et al. Familial occurrence of cerebral arteriovenous malformation in sisters: case report and review of the literature. European Journal of Neurology 2000; 7 (1): 95–100.

15. Storkebaum E, Quaegebeur A, Vikkula M, Carmeliet P. Cerebrovascular disorders: molecular insights and therapeutic opportunities. Nature Neuroscience. 2011;14 (11): 1390–1397

16. Valavanis A. The role of angiography in the evaluation of cerebral vascular malformations. Neuroimaging Clinics of North America 1996; 6 (3): 679–704.

17. Hofmeister C, Stapf C, Hartmann A, et al. Demographic, morphological, and clinical characteristics of 1289 patients with brain arteriovenous malformation. Stroke 2000; 31: 1307–10.

18. Hoh BL, Chapman PH, Loeffler JS, et al. Results of multimodality treatment for 141 patients with brain arteriovenous malformations and seizures: factors associated with seizure incidence and seizure outcomes. Neurosurgery 2002; 51: 303–9; discussion 309–11.

19. Yeh HS, Kashiwagi S, Tew JM, Jr, et al. Surgical management of epilepsy associated with cerebral arteriovenous malformations. Journal of Neurosurgery 1990; 72: 216–23.

20. Trussart V, Berry I, Manelfe C, et al. Epileptogenic cerebral vascular malformations and MRI. Journal of neuroradiology.\ Journal de Neuroradiologie 1989; 16: 273–84.

21. Yeh HS, Privitera MD. Secondary epileptogenesis in cerebral arteriovenous malformations. Archives of Neurology 1991; 48: 1122–4.

22. Heikkinen ER, Konnov B, Melnikov L, et al. Relief of epilepsy by radiosurgery of cerebral arteriovenous malformations. Stereotactic & Functional Neurosurgery 1989; 53 (3): 157–66.

23. Lv X, Li Y, Jiang C, et al. Brain arteriovenous malformations and endovascular treatment: effect on seizures. Interventional Neuroradiology 2010; 16: 39–45.

24. Hernesniemi JA, Dashti R, Juvela S, et al. Natural history of brain arteriovenous malformations: a long-term follow-up study of risk of hemorrhage in 238 patients. Neurosurgery 2008; 63: 823–9; discussion 829–31.

25. Stapf C, Mast H, Sciacca RR, et al. Predictors of hemorrhage in patients with untreated brain arteriovenous malformation. Neurology 2006; 66: 1350–5.
26. Ondra SL, Troupp H, George ED, et al. The natural history of symptomatic arteriovenous malformations of the brain: a 24-year follow-up assessment. Journal of Neurosurgery 1990; 73 (3): 387–91.
27. Pollock BE, Flickinger JC, Lunsford LD, et al. Factors that predict the bleeding risk of cerebral arteriovenous malformations. Stroke 1996; 27: 1–6.
28. van Beijnum J, van der Worp HB, Buis D, et al. Treatment of brain arteriovenous malformations: a systematic review and meta-analysis. Journal of the American Medical Association 2011; 306 (18): 2011–19.
29. Spetzler RF, Wilson CB, Weinstein P, et al. Normal perfusion pressure breakthrough theory. Clinical Neurosurgery 1978; 25: 651–72.
30. Spetzler RF, Hargraves RW, McCormick PW, et al. Relationship of perfusion pressure and size to risk of hemorrhage from arteriovenous malformations. Journal of Neurosurgery 1992; 76 (6): 918–23.
31. Turjman F, Massoud TF, Vinuela F, et al. Correlation of the angioarchitectural features of cerebral arteriovenous malformations with clinical presentation of hemorrhage. Neurosurgery 1995; 37: 856–60; discussion 860–2.
32. de Oliveira E, Tedeschi H, Raso J. Comprehensive management of arteriovenous malformations. Neurological Research 1998; 20 (8): 673–83.
33. Menghini VV, Brown RD, Jr, Sicks JD, et al. Clinical manifestations and survival rates among patients with saccular intracranial aneurysms: population-based study in Olmsted County, Minnesota, 1965 to 1995. Neurosurgery 2001; 49: 251–6; discussion 256–8.

INDEX

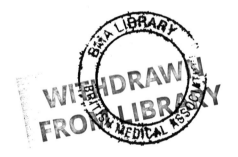